British Women Surgeons and their Patients, 1860–1918

When women agitated to join the medical profession in Britain during the 1860s, the practice of surgery proved both a help (women were neat, patient and used to needlework) and a hindrance (surgery was brutal, bloody and distinctly unfeminine). In this major new study, Claire Brock examines the cultural, social and self-representation of the woman surgeon from the second half of the nineteenth century until the end of the Great War. Drawing on a rich archive of British hospital records, she investigates precisely what surgery women performed and how these procedures affected their personal and professional reputation, as well as the reactions of their patients to these new phenomena. Also published as open access, this is essential reading for those interested in the history of medicine. *British Women Surgeons and their Patients, 1860–1918* provides wide-ranging new perspectives on patient narratives and women's participation in surgery between 1860 and 1918. This title is also available as Open Access.

CLAIRE BROCK is Associate Professor in the School of Arts at the University of Leicester. She is the author of two monographs, *The Feminization of Fame, 1750–1830* (2006) and *The Comet Sweeper* (2007), and the editor of *New Audiences for Science: Women, Children, and Labourers* (2013). Brock won the British Society for the History of Science's international Singer Prize for young scholars (2005) and received a Wellcome Trust Research Leave Award (2012–2014) for *British Women Surgeons and their Patients, 1860–1918*.

British Women Surgeons and their Patients, 1860–1918

Claire Brock

University of Leicester

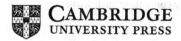

CAMBRIDGE
UNIVERSITY PRESS

CAMBRIDGE
UNIVERSITY PRESS

University Printing House, Cambridge CB2 8BS, United Kingdom

One Liberty Plaza, 20th Floor, New York, NY 10006, USA

477 Williamstown Road, Port Melbourne, VIC 3207, Australia

314-321, 3rd Floor, Plot 3, Splendor Forum, Jasola District Centre, New Delhi - 110025, India

79 Anson Road, #06-04/06, Singapore 079906

Cambridge University Press is part of the University of Cambridge.

It furthers the University's mission by disseminating knowledge in the pursuit of education, learning and research at the highest international levels of excellence.

www.cambridge.org
Information on this title: www.cambridge.org/9781316637494

First published 2017
First paperback edition 2019

A catalogue record for this publication is available from the British Library

ISBN 978-1-107-18693-4 Hardback
ISBN 978-1-316-63749-4 Paperback

Cambridge University Press has no responsibility for the persistence or accuracy of URLs for external or third-party internet websites referred to in this publication, and does not guarantee that any content on such websites is, or will remain, accurate or appropriate.

Contents

Figures and Table

Figures

Table

Illustrations

Acknowledgements

The research for this project was immeasurably assisted by a Wellcome Trust Research Leave Award (WT096499AIA), held between 2012 and 2014, which allowed me to concentrate exclusively upon it. I would like to thank the Trust for their ongoing faith in the value of the history of medicine, the medical humanities and work which doesn't fit into neat categories.

I would like especially to thank the following, who, hopefully, know why they're here: Julie Coleman; Gowan Dawson; Jennian Geddes; Elizabeth Hurren; Steve King; Bernie Lightman; Hilary Marland; and Peter Stanley. Audiences, over the past five years, at Bart's Pathology Museum, the Royal College of Surgeons, and the Universities of Portsmouth and Warwick have been particularly helpful to me. At Cambridge University Press, Lucy Rhymer has been a fantastic editor. The two anonymous reviewers were the best an author could wish for in many ways: thank you very much.

Some parts of chapter 1 have appeared as 'Risk, Responsibility and Surgery in the 1890s and Early 1900s', *Medical History*, 57.3 (July 2013), 317–37, reprinted with permission of Cambridge University Press and 'Surgical Controversy at the New Hospital for Women, 1872–1892', *Social History of Medicine*, 24.3 (December 2011), 608–23, reproduced by permission of Oxford University Press.

I have been to archives across the length and breadth of the country for this project and would like to thank all those who have assisted me. Victoria Rea has to come first, because I spent most of my time, in freezing cold and boiling hot weather, at Belsize Park, when the Royal Free Hospital Archives were located there. As anyone who ever went there will know, there was something special about this place and I'm sorry it's no longer there. Thank you also to the staff at Birmingham City Archives, Brotherton Library, Leeds, Edinburgh University Library, Ipswich Record Office, London Metropolitan Archives, Mitchell Library, Glasgow, and the Women's Library, London.

To my family, in old and New South Wales, there are very few words to express my gratitude. My parents, Siân and Paul Brock, my sister, Helen Giddings, and my grandparents, Vera and Francis Connolly, have been with me every step of the way. My other grandparents, the late Ann and Fred Brock, are no longer here to be thanked in person, but cannot be left out. Ben Dew has learned far more about women's health in this period than anyone should ever have to know. He has, however, never grumbled when I have enthused at length about surgery nor groaned (too much) when I have told him horrifying tales from the archives. I don't know what I would do without him, nor without his love and understanding. This book (gory bits and all) is for him.

Introduction: Disapproval, Curiosity, Amusement, Obstinate Hostility?
Women and Surgery, 1860–1918

In the second half of the nineteenth century, significant changes in surgical practice coincided with the entrance of women into the medical profession. The links between the two, however, have never been explored. From the very early days of women's attempts to become doctors, it was the possibility of them performing surgery which most haunted critics and friends alike, as well as potential patients. In April 1859 the *British Medical Journal* presented a disturbing vision for its readers. Imagine a female surgeon:

the Semiramis of surgery, a Fergusson in woman's outward guise, amputating a thigh, or removing a diseased jaw or elbow-joint, aided by assistants of like sex and mind, and surrounded by a host of fair damsels, who regard the proceedings of the operator with that appreciation of the cool head and the ready hand which medical students so well know how to feel! Imagine some fair and amiable damsel, a female Rokitansky, poring with inquisitive eye over a collection of ulcerated Peyer's patches or a piece of softened cerebral substance, or assiduously endeavouring to ascertain, by the aid of the microscope, the presence or absence of fatty degeneration in a piece of heart-tissue, or to determine the nature of a tumour which her associate Semiramis has just removed! Call to mind all things that are done in the ordinary course of hospital duties, or even of general practice in town or country; and imagine, good reader, if you can, a British lady performing them.

Women who would practise medicine and surgery must do so wholly; there is no shirking the obligation. If they attempt to do less, they will fail in the duty they undertake; and the male sex will have an unfair advantage over the female, in being able to command a higher exercise of professional skill and knowledge.[1]

Although represented as unthinkable when considered in the same breath as British ladies, the female surgeon was to become a more real addition to the medical profession in the next half-century than the author of this article could have ever envisaged. Without the requisite attainments, women would be unable to prove their medical and surgical capabilities;

---

[1] 'Room for the Ladies!', *British Medical Journal* (*BMJ*) 1.119 (9 April 1859), 292–4; 293.

with them, they would succeed in carrying out all the professional duties expected, regardless of their status as 'British ladies'. This was something the scoffing writer recognised, even if he did not believe in women ever attaining such qualities.

The professional expectations placed upon women medical practitioners were exacerbated by the lack of opportunities to advance clinical skills. This was especially evident in surgery, where women were doubly hampered by social proprieties, as well as professional prejudice against lancet-wielding females. Attain the requisite 'qualities', however, they did. By September 1914, Louisa Garrett Anderson could provide a view of an operating theatre staffed by women which would have startled the author of 'Room for the Ladies!' in its similarity to his nightmarish vision:

> We have a lot of surgery: sometimes I am in the theatre from 2 to 9 or 10 at night, and have eight or more operations. The cases come to us very septic and the wounds are terrible. Today we are having an amputation of thigh, two head cases perhaps trephine and five smaller ones. We have fitted up a satisfactory small operating theatre in the 'Ladies Lavatory' which has tiled floor and walls, good water supply and lighting. I bought a simple operating table in Paris and we have arranged gas rings and fish kettles for sterilisation.[2]

A woman surgeon, surrounded by others of her sex, carrying out complex procedures on men and without male assistance would have been enough of a surprise. The location of the theatre, in an unmentionable all-female space, made aseptic with domestic and culinary accoutrements would surely have been the final straw. More familiar, however, would have been the reaction, as detailed by Garrett Anderson's colleague, Flora Murray, to the female surgeon's desire to do something to help as the Great War began. 'The feeling of the Army Medical Department towards women doctors could be gauged by the atmosphere in the various offices with which business had to be done', sighed Murray: 'In one there was disapproval; in another curiosity and amusement; in a third obstinate hostility.'[3] While concessions had been made towards the female surgeon by 1918, reactions all too similar to those encountered nearly sixty years before were still to be seen and heard.

British Women Surgeons explores the crucial period between 1860 and 1918. These years witnessed a number of key developments in the history of medicine and surgery, alongside women's official entry into the

---

[2] Louisa Garrett Anderson to Elizabeth Garrett Anderson, Hôpital Auxiliaire, Hôtel Claridge, Paris, 27 September 1914, 7LGA/2/1/09, The Women's Library, London School of Economics.

[3] Flora Murray, *Women as Army Surgeons* (London: Hodder and Stoughton, n.d. [1920]), p. 126.

medical profession and increased campaigning for social and political rights. In *Making a Medical Living* (1994), Anne Digby has identified this period as vital to the development of the medical marketplace.[4] The second half of the nineteenth and early twentieth century saw the growth in the medical and social importance of the hospital and work on the history of surgery locates, at this juncture, both changing (lay and medical) perceptions of the surgeon and alterations in surgical practice. These adjustments were stimulated by, amongst others, anaesthetics and asepsis, the development of surgical instruments, changes in anatomical and physiological understanding, and the advent of the X-ray. It is my intention in this book to assess the position of the woman surgeon at this exciting moment in history. I will argue that she is a pivotal figure who intersects with such social, medical and surgical developments and whose place in the history of medicine has been long neglected. With the exception of research into women's participation in the medical and surgical mobilisation of the Great War, the qualified female surgeon has not been the focus of historical analysis.[5] While women's entry into the medical profession in the mid-nineteenth century has proved a popular area of research, what resulted from this experiment has barely been considered.[6] Therefore, I will not re-examine the much-told narrative of women's battle to join the professional ranks. Rather, I want to explore

---

[4] Anne Digby, *Making a Medical Living* (Oxford: Oxford University Press, 1994).

[5] The recent work of Jennian Geddes has transformed this field. See, for example, 'Deeds *and* Words in the Suffrage Military Hospital in Endell Street', *Medical History* (*MH*), 51.1 (January 2007), 79–98; 'The Women's Hospital Corps: forgotten surgeons of the First World War', *Journal of Medical Biography*, 14.2 (May 2006), 109–17.
   Women's role in surgery before 1800 has also been investigated. See, for example, Celeste Chamberland, 'Partners and Practitioners: Women and the Management of Surgical Households in London, 1570–1640', *Social History of Medicine* (*SHM*), 24.3 (December 2011), 554–69 and A.L. Wyman, 'The Surgeoness: The Female Practitioner of Surgery 1400–1800', *MH*, 28.1 (January 1984), 22–41.

[6] With the notable exception of two still unpublished theses: Mary Ann C. Elston, 'Women Doctors in the British Health Services: A Sociological Study of their Careers and Opportunities', PhD thesis, University of Leeds, 1986, and Elaine Thomson, 'Women in Medicine in Late Nineteenth and Early Twentieth-Century Edinburgh: A Case Study', PhD thesis, University of Edinburgh, 1998. For the Scottish context, see also Wendy Alexander, *First Ladies of Medicine* (Glasgow: University of Glasgow Wellcome Unit for the History of Medicine, 1987) and M. Anne Crowther and Marguerite Dupree, *Medical Lives in the Age of Surgical Revolution* (Cambridge: Cambridge University Press, 2007). More recently, for the Irish context, Laura Kelly, *Irish Women in Medicine, c.1880s–1920s* (Manchester: Manchester University Press, 2013). For examinations of individual medical women in America, see Carla Bittel, *Mary Putnam Jacobi and the Politics of Medicine in Nineteenth-Century America* (Chapel Hill, NC: University of North Carolina Press, 2009), Ellen S. More, *Restoring the Balance: Women Physicians and the Profession of Medicine, 1850–1995* (Cambridge, MA and London: Harvard University Press, 1999), and, more specifically focused on surgery, Regina Morantz-Sanchez, *Conduct Unbecoming a Woman* (New York: Oxford University Press, 1999).

what happened once that initial fight was won. Given the assumption that it would be impossible for women to perform surgery for mental, physical and moral reasons, their reaction to this discipline needs to be measured. Why was surgery considered particularly inappropriate, or appropriate, for women? What surgical procedures did women carry out and where did they operate? Did they attempt controversial surgery and what was their attitude to the increasing fears about malignant disease, frequently encountered in gynaecological cases at the turn of the twentieth century? What role did women surgeons play in the Great War at the front, but also at home, where unprecedented opportunities came their way? What was the experience of those who were operated upon by female surgeons and who were they? These questions will allow an exploration, through printed sources, private letters and case notes, of the ways in which the woman surgeon participated in the developments, controversies and changing public perception of surgery and the surgeon between 1860 and 1918.

For medical and lay alike, surgery in this period exemplified both the progressive nature of science and technology and the corresponding fear that surgeons had too much power over their patients. No longer had the operator to utilise brute strength to hack off limbs as quickly as possible before the patient bled to death; with anaesthesia and asepsis, time and care could be taken to ensure a successful procedure was performed while the patient was insensible. Areas of the body could be treated surgically in ways they could never have been before without a prone patient and an aseptic operating theatre and surgeon. In 1890, Sir Thomas Spencer Wells looked back upon half-a-century of surgical progress and concluded with a reassuring glimpse into the next century:

And for our younger Fellows and Members – for the surgeons of the future – may we not be confident that with the energetic spirit of inquiry now awakened, with an enlightened determination to apply all the resources of modern scientific discovery to the perfecting of our art with a conscientious aim at making it as truly conservative as is compatible with usefulness and progress and with honourable feeling and highly cultivated judgment, directing hands delicately and expressly trained, we may augur for the surgeons of the coming time an influence supremely beneficent for mankind, and promise to its devotees the dignity and distinction justly earned by their life-giving and health-preserving work.[7]

For Spencer Wells, surgeons were conscientious and restrained, preserving health rather than wilfully encouraging illness for personal profit. The professional body was refined, diligent and possessed a delicacy of

---

[7] Sir T. Spencer Wells, 'The Bradshaw Lecture on Modern Abdominal Surgery', Part II, *BMJ*, 2.1565 (21 December 1890), 1465–8; 1468.

touch. Fundamental to Spencer Wells' assessment was his careful mention of the need to make surgery 'truly conservative' in order to advance the profession. This was a deliberate attempt to deflect attention away from the sort of surgery – knife-wielding, radical, heroic – which characterised earlier periods, and towards procedures which conserved and protected. Spencer Wells' account of surgical progress, with its fastidious and benevolent tone, aimed to counter past horrors with a record of innovation, development and perfection, coupled with the 'honourable feeling and highly cultivated judgment' of the thoughtful surgeon. This spirited defence sought to challenge those who doubted the wisdom of risky procedures.

For some, however, very little had changed. Surgery was still unnecessary butchery. It was harder to shake off the trade associations than Spencer Wells believed: surgeons were still viewed as aspiring, not actual gentlemen. The development of antiseptic and aseptic procedures may have made surgery less painful both for patient and operator, but theoretical advance was not always followed by practical adoption.[8] Spencer Wells' field – abdominal surgery – was visceral, bloody and brutal, and, by implication, so was the abdominal surgeon. Accusations of wilful carelessness dogged the surgical profession in the late nineteenth and early twentieth centuries. What surgeons viewed as perfecting their craft through experimentation could be seen by others as reckless concern for reputation rather than for the patient's needs.[9] Surgical independence – both from other surgeons and from the team who assisted an operation – meant that the surgeon stood aloof, distant from any regulation. The *British Journal of Surgery* (*BJS*) was established in 1913, and a year later it led with a telling editorial about surgical practices in early twentieth-century Britain. Currently, 'workers' were 'isolated from one another', which slowed progress and ensured irregular outcomes. '[W]hereas', the 'Introductory' continued, 'if they could act together, not only would individual surgeons gain in breadth of view and soundness of conclusion, but there would certainly result a general advance in knowledge which only comes with co-operative effort.' The journal had been set up to counter the 'individualistic, competitive and secretive' bent of surgery, by

---

[8] On the varying degrees of procedural adoption, see Michael Worboys, *Spreading Germs* (Cambridge: Cambridge University Press, 2000).

[9] Sally Wilde's work has been the most recent and illuminating exploration of risk and experimentation in surgery. See *The History of Surgery*, at www.thehistoryofsurgery.com; 'Truth, Trust, and Confidence in Surgery, 1890–1910: Patient Autonomy, Communication, and Consent', *BHM*, 83.2 (Summer 2009), 302–30; and with Geoffrey Hurst, 'Learning from Mistakes: Early Twentieth-Century Surgical Practice', *Journal of the History of Medicine and Allied Sciences* (*JHMAS*), 64.1 (January 2009), 38–77.

providing a 'common meeting place [...] to which all contribute', and 'the gatherings of an association which all [could] attend'.[10] Although 'the business' of surgery took place behind closed doors, the *BJS* reassured its readers that surgical 'science' was 'altruistic, public, and above all, co-operative'. That it took until the second decade of the twentieth century to establish a general surgical publication implies professional unity had not yet been achieved. Co-operation in surgical enterprise was necessary, not already apparent.

Indeed, the history of surgery in general has suffered from critical neglect, akin to the closed world of the operating theatre described above. What had once resembled a public performance had largely retreated into a private, sterile space by the start of the twentieth century.[11] More than thirty years ago, Christopher Lawrence expressed surprise at the scant attention paid to surgery in the history of medicine.[12] Recently, Thomas Schlich has reiterated the call for more analysis of surgical knowledge and practice, which has 'attracted little serious historical interest'.[13] Both mention women's history as an exception to the silence, but Lawrence remarks that work in this area renders surgery marginal to the primary focus on gender. Indeed, women's history has a curious attitude to surgical procedure. Too often, in this discipline, women are the victims of brutal male operators who seek to mutilate the weak and defenceless.[14] Ludmilla Jordanova has gone so far as to claim that '[c]learly, surgery is a male act'.[15] Lawrence relates this attitude to the thrustingly 'masculine' language surrounding surgical procedures; actions characterised by 'power, penetration and pleasure; of nature being unveiled, revealed, known and conquered'.[16] Consequently, research on women's place in

---

[10] 'Introductory: The Need of Co-operation in Surgical Enterprise', *British Journal of Surgery*, 2.5 (1914), 1–3; 1.

For more on professionalization in general from the late nineteenth century onwards, see Harold Perkin, *The Rise of Professional Society*, second edition (London and New York: Routledge, 2002) and Anne Witz, *Professions and Patriarchy* (London and New York: Routledge, 1992).

[11] Thomas Schlich, 'Surgery, Science and Modernity: Operating Rooms and Laboratories as Spaces of Control', *History of Science*, 45.3 (September 2007), 231–56.

[12] Christopher Lawrence, 'Democratic, divine and heroic: the history and historiography of surgery', in Lawrence, ed., *Medical Theory, Surgical Practice* (London and New York: Routledge, 1992), pp. 1–47; p. 10.

[13] Thomas Schlich, *The Origins of Organ Transplantation* (Rochester, NY: University of Rochester Press, 2010), p. 8.

[14] For the classic example of female patient as victim, see Mary Poovey, '"Scenes of an Indelicate Character": The Medical "Treatment" of Victorian Women', *Representations*, 14 (Spring 1986), 137–78. For a response to Poovey, see Morantz-Sanchez, *Conduct Unbecoming*.

[15] Ludmilla Jordanova, *Sexual Visions* (Madison, WI: University of Wisconsin Press, 1989), p. 153.

[16] Lawrence, 'Democratic, divine and heroic', p. 31.

the history of surgery has always placed them 'under the knife', as patients rather than surgeons.[17] The history of surgery itself might have benefited from research into women's position within it, but women have correspondingly suffered by being reduced to passive objects, operated upon rather than operating.

Certainly, the linguistic frisson embedded in the surgical act affected discourse surrounding the rights and wrongs of the woman surgeon from the outset. As a 1908 article by Theodore Dahle in the *Sunday Chronicle* put it, with scarcely disguised excitement: 'Women like men must school themselves to see glittering, keen-edged knives parting live human flesh.'[18] The sharp and sparkling instruments dazzle in this image; the sense that the operation is illicit, but enthralling, is compounded by the sharp cuts made and the living, breathing nature of the body which is being 'parted'. Dahle rightly considered the performance of surgery as something which would affect any operator, regardless of sex. To carry out a surgical procedure requires nerve, courage, strength and the confidence to take responsibility for the action performed. It is important not to forget, however, that surgery needs enthusiasm for carving through flesh and bone. As the ongoing debate about women's suitability for diplomas of the Royal College of Surgeons revealed only too evidently, when medical women had been assimilated into other parts of the profession, they were far from accepted in the operating theatre as late as the 1890s. While some members were in favour of women's entry simply because they would never attain the masculine strength to compete on level terms with men, the views of others were exemplified by a Dr Barnes, who noted that:

surgery, of all other things, was the highest grade of the profession, demanding, as it did, the highest talent, skill and mental and physical powers, and those, he thought, did not belong to women. [...] Surgery belonged to men and strength, and where strength was there the great amount of gentleness lay. It was simply a horrible thing for him to see women operate. They might be gentle in their minds, but they certainly had not the power which was necessary to perform serious surgical operations. He thought it was a degrading thing to admit women to the study of medicine in any branch, and it applied most strongly to surgery.[19]

[17] Ann Dally, *Women Under the Knife* (London: Hutchinson Radius, 1991).
[18] Theodore Dahle, 'A Great Medical School for Women and its Work', *Sunday Chronicle* (undated, but from internal evidence, 1908), in *London School of Medicine for Women and Royal Free Hospital Press Cuttings, Volume IV: January 1904–August 1915*, H72/SM/Y/02/004, London Metropolitan Archives (hereafter LMA).
[19] 'Royal College of Surgeons of England. Annual Meeting', *BMJ*, 2.1819 (9 November 1895), 1176–1178; 1178. Barnes can be one of two men of this name who were Fellows at the time, both of whom were general surgeons: John Wickham Barnes (1830–1899); or Robert Barnes (1817–1907). See *Plarr's Lives of the Fellows* at livesonline.rcseng.ac.uk.

Such paradoxical, and clearly deliberate, grounding of gentleness in strength showed both the desperate attempt of some members of the RCS to exclude the weaker sex on physical and moral grounds, and also the Victorian surgeon's insecurity about his own place within the profession and within society. Specialty, Barnes concluded, was far beyond the capability of the average female; confine women, by all means to operating upon their own in 'the inferior grades of obstetrics and gynaecology', but do not allow them even then to perform complex procedures, for which they are unfit.

'Fitness' to operate was a constant refrain when surgeons of both sexes were discussed. Of course, this meant fitness in the sense of aptitude, but also the ability to maintain composure and health throughout any surgical procedure. I have chosen to date this book from 1860 because this was when Elizabeth Garrett Anderson first decided to make medicine her profession.[20] It was also the first time a woman with such an ambition in Britain experienced an operation, not as a patient, but as a future practitioner. In a letter to her friend Emily Davies, Garrett Anderson described the experience, witnessed while ostensibly nursing at Middlesex Hospital. Given the assumption that women would not be able to stand the strain of surgery as onlookers, let alone operators, Garrett Anderson's reaction was intriguing:

It was a stiffish one, and I did not feel at all bad, the excitement was very great but happily it took the form of quickening all my vitality, instead of depressing it. I was excessively tired after it was all over, but this effect will soon cease I should think. I stood with all the pupils in the theatre, and they gave me the best place for seeing and then took no more notice of me, which was exactly the right style.[21]

Neither displaying weakness nor feeling faint, Garrett Anderson actually tired herself out with the physical thrill of the situation. Indeed, four days later, she noted that '[i]t is rather provoking that people will think so much of the difficulties, in spite of my assurances that far from their being appalling I am enjoying the work more than I have ever done any other study or pursuit'.[22] It is also noticeable that the male medical students chivalrously allowed Garrett Anderson the best viewpoint during the operation. We can only conjecture why this happened, but when she enquired about pursuing her chosen career, Garrett Anderson was

---

[20] I will refer to women doctors by their best-known names throughout, to avoid confusion.
[21] Elizabeth Garrett Anderson to Emily Davies, Bayswater, Wednesday 5 September 1860, HA436/1/1/1: Letters from Elizabeth Garrett Anderson to Emily Davies: June–December 1860, Ipswich Record Office, Suffolk.
[22] Elizabeth Garrett Anderson to Emily Davies, 9 September 1860, 9/10/015, ALC/2905, The Women's Library.

repeatedly put off by those who suggested that any business involving cutting open bodies, dead or alive, would be 'too much for any woman to stand with enough composure of mind to study'.[23] That her only exhaustion was from excitement meant that Garrett Anderson held up mentally and physically to the challenge.

Surgery required both a strong stomach and a steady hand. As satirical periodical *Punch* put it in one of its many skits on women doctors, entitled 'Chloe, M.D.', in July 1876: 'the Surgeon, who needs, that his work may be done, / Lion's heart, Eagle's eye, Lady's hand – must have Manhood and Genius in one'. Underneath its mockery, *Punch* revealed the complexity of the surgeon's task, as well as the multifaceted nature of surgery itself. In spite of the link implied between feminine touch and surgical procedures, 'Chloe, M.D.' denied women the facility to cope with the demands of the operating theatre: 'She that once at blood's flowing had swooned, / With the deftness of feminine fingers might tenderly bandage a wound'.[24] Here, 'feminine fingers' could swiftly perform the simplest of remedies, but, overcome with fear at a more severe injury, lacked the steadiness, pluck and nerve needed by a surgeon. Swooning at the sight of a cadaver was (and still is) a regular part of medical education. Although it was not a part which the profession desired to acknowledge, it was an attribute which was expected of, and indeed foisted onto, disruptive, ineffective women when faced with the unpleasant results of a dissection or an operation. It was precisely this presumed inability to cope with the unruly body, however, that medical women used again and again to their advantage. When she later came to contribute a chapter for women medical students to an 1878 textbook, Garrett Anderson countered any suggestion that alleged female delicacy would lead to collapse in the face of dissection or surgery. This was contrasted, in the same publication, with hints for male counterparts at potential distress. Charles Bell Keetley's *The Student's Guide to the Medical Profession*, although occasionally reading like a boys' adventure story, opened its discussion of dissection with the information that it will be 'repulsive at first' and recommended '[k]eeping your knives sharp'.[25] Garrett Anderson's advice firmly denied any feeling as strong as repulsion and suggested, in a professional manner, that the experience was more intriguing than troubling: 'I know of nothing in the medical education especially distasteful to female students. Everyone expects to dislike dissecting, but as a matter of fact no

23 Elizabeth Garrett Anderson to Emily Davies, Aldeburgh, January 1861, HA436/1/1/2, Ipswich Record Office.
24 'Chloe, M.D., On Mr Cowper-Temple's Bill', *Punch*, Saturday 15 July 1876, 24.
25 Charles Bell Keetley, *The Student's Guide to the Medical Profession* (London: Macmillan, 1878), p. 25.

one does – it is found to be extremely interesting'. As an extension of this argument, '[i]t is very natural', remarked Garrett Anderson, that surgery should 'attract [ladies] more than medicine', because, in common with their male contemporaries, it was 'much more interesting'.[26] According to Garrett Anderson, confident behaviour was only to be expected of the female medical student, who was 'naturally' led towards the physical and intellectual challenges posed by surgery.

This ability to remain calm and upright was insisted upon repeatedly by women doctors in spheres as diverse as periodical articles and Select Committees. The interview format beloved of New Journalists in the 1890s allowed curious outsiders glimpses into the world of the female medical student. And, of course, the first thing most wanted to know was how women coped with the more squeamish aspects of their education. An article entitled 'How the Medicine Woman is Trained', published in the *Sketch* in June 1898, showed a fascination with whether or not girls have 'nerve, pluck, and endurance sufficient to carry them through the long course of work'. The secretary of the London School of Medicine for Women (LSMW), Miss Douie, retorted: 'I have never seen a girl faint in the operating theatre, though male students often do in their early days. I do not know of any girl who has given up the work after beginning it.' Amusingly enough, the male journalist, although stressing that he did not 'shrink from [exploring] the dissecting-room', was forced to conclude that 'it was not a pretty sight from the layman's point of view, although the room is pretty, very light, and very airy'.[27] The stylistic repetition, focusing attention on the spaciousness of the room, actually has the effect of stressing the claustrophobia felt by this 'layman', as he was forced to look away from the unattractive sights.

Male queasiness was evident in a completely different form when reading Garrett Anderson's evidence to the 1891 House of Lords Select Committee on Metropolitan Hospitals.[28] Their Lordships displayed a distinctly unworldly attitude when quizzing their witness, becoming perplexed at her achievements. Lord Zouche asked Garrett Anderson whether she 'performs operations'; Garrett Anderson replied: 'Yes, we perform ovariotomy, and similar operations'. Earl Cathcart then enquired, a little incredulously, 'Do you think that women have strength enough of wrist to do those things?', to which his witness replied simply:

---

[26] 'A Special Chapter for Ladies Who Propose to Study Medicine', in ibid., pp. 42–8; p. 47.

[27] S.L.B., 'How the Medicine Woman is Trained', *Sketch*, 15 June 1898, in *Royal Free Hospital Press Cuttings, Volume 3: May 1878–January 1904*, H72/SM/Y/02/003, LMA.

[28] Evidence of Mrs Elizabeth Garrett Anderson, M.D., 5 March 1891, *Select Committee of House of Lords on Metropolitan Hospitals* (1890–1891), 16452–531.

'Yes'. Having carried out countless surgical procedures herself, Garrett Anderson must have found the disbelief at female physical prowess amusing. Indeed, there is a real sense in Garrett Anderson's evidence that she enjoyed teasing her naïve interlocutors, but, as the last question makes clear, she also desired to stress female commitment to their education and, later, to their career. Indeed, Garrett Anderson had 'heard of men fainting occasionally', but did 'not know that I have ever heard of any of our women fainting' at what the Earl of Arran claimed were 'the terrible sights and scenes in the operating theatre'. Women, assured Garrett Anderson, had far more than strong wrists; constitutionally they were thoroughly sound, unlike some of their more precious male colleagues. But she was careful not to alienate her audience and added, craftily, 'but I daresay it takes both of them a little time to get used to it'. This balanced response, of course, although not removing the previous comment, tempered it, without losing her implication.

Time and again, excitement, rather than the potential 'terrors' posed by surgery, dominated nineteenth- and early twentieth-century accounts by and about the woman surgeon. Mary Scharlieb, who became one of the foremost early women surgeons, looked back with fondness in her 1924 *Reminiscences* upon the rough and ready surgical procedures in India, where she began her career: her sister as anaesthetist, her maid as assistant surgeon and her 'Mahommedan ayah' in charge of the carbolic spray for antiseptics.[29] Similarly, Isabel Hutton, whose *Memories* (1960) explored her studies at the University of Edinburgh in the early 1900s, offered one of the most detailed and fascinating accounts of women's medical education. Hutton's 'hankering' after the surgical wards distracted her from medicine; but it was also the difference between the patients which convinced her of the attraction of surgery.[30] In spite of contemporary assumptions about institutional oppression, surgical patients were not at all coerced into their operations; neither were they hopeless and despairing: the victims of a butcher's knife.[31] For Hutton, the 'excitement, stimulation and drama of the surgical side' was matched by 'the cheerful, hopeful patients; there was always some gaiety and a joy shared by all when an anxious case came through its ordeal and joined

---

[29] Mary Scharlieb, *Reminiscences* (London: Williams and Norgate, 1924), pp. 111–12.
[30] Isabel Hutton, *Memories of a Doctor in War and Peace* (London: Heinemann, 1960), p. 203.
[31] See, for example, the work of medical man Edward Berdoe, who, as 'Aesculapius Scalpel', wrote damning indictments of surgical heartlessness in the fictional *St Bernard's* (London: Swan Sonnenschein & Co., 1887), and *Dying Scientifically* (London: Swan Sonnenschein & Co., 1888).

the ranks of the gay and gossipy convalescents'.[32] By contrast, on the medical side: 'the whole tempo was very slow'. Although Hutton put surgery to the back of her mind as she progressed through her degree, the 'hankering' only left her when she joined the Scottish Women's Hospitals to serve in Serbia during the Great War, as we shall see in chapter 4. Then, despite 'little experience', she performed, like other women, and, of course, men, in her situation, specialist operations for which she had never been trained. Although Hutton had finally followed her desires, she also could not resist noting that her wartime experience was 'possibly [the most worthwhile] of my life. It was a time of strain and of anxiety, but it was a period of achievement and happiness for us all.'[33] Hutton and her fellow wartime female surgeons throve upon the excitement of the unknown, and had a thrilling taste of what might have been.

As the previous examples imply, once women began to practise surgery, those reporting on the development sought to mesh two previously unthinkable categories together. By masculinising female operators or feminising surgery polar opposites began to merge into something more palatable. Intrigue about the budding female surgical practitioner sent journalists to investigate these hybrid creatures. In *Photographing Medicine*, Daniel M. Fox and Christopher Lawrence have remarked that published images of medical students taught in laboratories were not as popular in Britain as in America.[34] British women medical students, however, were perpetually photographed in laboratory situations, and described again and again in dissecting rooms.[35] The *Sketch* reporter was joined by a number of other brave souls who ventured into the LSMW in the 1890s and early 1900s. Whereas the former choked on the atmosphere, a *Daily Mail* correspondent simply could not come to terms with what he witnessed in 1898. He was put in his place before he had even been taken on a tour of the building by the formidable Miss Douie. 'Never suggest', he warned, 'that constant contact with suffering and the attendant horrors of the surgical table tend to harden a woman or deaden her susceptibilities.' Taken – noticeably – to the 'door' of the dissecting room, a merry scene was witnessed across the threshold:

---

[32] Ibid., p. 50.   [33] Ibid., p. 203.

[34] Daniel M. Fox and Christopher Lawrence, *Photographing Medicine* (New York and London: Greenwood Press, 1988), p. 46.

[35] For an opposite view, which focuses on female practitioners being represented in comfortable spaces such as the common room at the LSMW in order to 'cosmeticise or render more palatable the essentially shocking impact of knowing women had worked on anatomy in the dissecting room', see Carol Dyhouse, 'Driving Ambitions: Women in Pursuit of a Medical Education, 1890–1939', *Women's History Review*, 7.3 (1998), 321–43; 323.

I could see in a long well-lighted room three tables, at each of which attractive girls were seated, their heads bent upon their work of dissection, and their hands busy. At the centre table two gladsome students, delving with nimble hands, passed at intervals to lean forward upon their work, and exchange the merry quiplet. So happy were they that they might have been snipping out patterns for summer frocks or dissecting merely a tender duckling at the supper table.[36]

As 'the sweet girls carved on in silence', the reporter's attention was only briefly drawn to the 'indescribable things on the table', which he imagined would 'probably have smiled' at the profound interest taken by the 'bright-eyed girls' in their 'muscular organisation'. In order to cope with what he saw on his tour around the school, the reporter was compelled to feminise the actions of the would-be practitioners. By likening their cutting action to that of a dress pattern or the dissection of a small, weak animal, it became both acceptably feminine and harmless. Neither were the students scarred by their studies; they remained jolly, content and dedicated to their work.

Female reporters were equally confused about how to represent a woman surgeon. Prize-winning former student of the LSMW, Adela Knight, the first Australian woman to qualify in medicine, caught the eye of a *Lady's Pictorial* representative at the New Hospital for Women in 1898. 'Very sweet and gentle' was the verdict of the paper, which admired her 'soothing such of the patients who were tired and fretful'.[37] Such a portrait, more suitable to a nursemaid than a talented house surgeon, belied the skill which had earned Knight her academic distinction. However, the admiration did not stop at Knight's sweet nature. Attention turned swiftly to her attire: 'this lady did not show that contempt for awkward appearance with which some lady medical students, even those present on the occasion may be charged'. While her 'tasteful and well-fitting' ensemble removed Knight from any accusations of masculinity or blue-stockingness, it also proved that the woman surgeon could carry out her work while dressing in a becomingly feminine manner. Nothing was shocking or odd about Adela Knight. Indeed, '[s]he gives the impression of being the right woman in the right place'. When Knight died unexpectedly less than a year later, at the age of 25, obituaries lauded her qualities and lamented the ending of a career which had promised so much.[38]

---

[36] 'Lady Doctors', *Daily Mail*, 3 June 1898, in *RFH Press Cuttings, Volume III*.

[37] 'Opening of the New Hospital for Women', *Lady's Pictorial*, 26 July 1890, in *Newspaper Cuttings: New Hospital for Women, 1871–1968*, H13/EGA/144, LMA.

[38] See, for example, 'Miss Adela McCulloch Knight, M.B. Lond.', *Queen*, 30 May 1891 and 'The Late Miss Knight', *Lady's Pictorial*, 23 May 1891, 44, in *RFH Press Cuttings, Volume III*.

Adela Knight was neither anomalous nor ill-suited to her role. Instead, her 'right[ness]' meant that she fitted her position perfectly.

Knight's death reminded the press of the untimely demise of a previous distinguished student of the LSMW six years before: Helen Prideaux. In an unfortunate coincidence, Knight had been the recent recipient of the prize named in Prideaux's honour. This funding had allowed Knight to travel to Vienna, where she contracted her fatal illness.[39] Prideaux's death, at the age of 27, had been hastened by diphtheria, caught while working as a house surgeon at Paddington Children's Hospital. As Elston has remarked, she was the first woman to obtain a post in open competition in a London voluntary hospital.[40] Surprisingly, the reaction of the medical press to her death brought this young woman squarely into the profession for which she had given her life. Prideaux's *BMJ* obituary labelled her 'one of the most brilliant and widely known' of LSMW graduates. At Paddington, she obtained 'long desired' 'intimate clinical study', but her happiness lasted only for a month. The obituary detailed at great length her decline, along with the 'terrible sufferings' she experienced after a tracheotomy and a laryngotomy, as she fought for breath. Although she was 'acutely conscious' of her likely fate, 'she felt no alarm': 'but, with a self-control, courage, and determination which were wonderful, she assisted in carrying out all the treatment, no matter how painful'. 'No complaint of her great sufferings escaped her'; 'entire self-sacrificing power' was hers to the last. The loss of this 'above all womanly' person, whose 'unusual moral and physical courage' and 'fine intellect' was devastating for her friends, for the medical profession, but also for society itself.[41] While this eulogy was certainly written by a fellow medical woman, the press coverage of Helen Prideaux's death was fascinating. Indeed, she was later utilised as an example of professional dedication, regardless of sex.

For Sir William Gull, who led the meeting held to establish a fund in her memory, Prideaux 'had vindicated the right of woman to take the highest position in a difficult and intellectual profession'. By 'leading the honours list' and obtaining the University of London's Gold Medal in Anatomy, she had 'swept away' prejudice 'from the path of all who might follow her'. As a former opponent of women's entry into the medical profession, Gull's change of heart was remarkable. Now that women had established their rights to a medical education, he could no longer object.

---

[39] Mrs Fenwick Miller, 'The Ladies' Column', *Illustrated London News*, 2719 (30 May 1891), 715.

[40] Elston, 'Women Doctors in the British Health Services', pp. 157–8.

[41] 'Obituary: Frances Helen Prideaux', *BMJ*, 2.1301 (5 December 1885), 1089.

'The spirit of medicine' was, after all, Gull proclaimed, 'one of intellectual freedom'; to rise above prejudice and objection was the highest possible objective in establishing an award. Women's work, such as that performed by Helen Prideaux, reflected well upon the whole profession, not simply the female part of it.[42] Similarly, the initial announcement of her death had caused the *BMJ* to reflect on the wider consequences of medical and surgical work for all practitioners. In an article entitled 'The Perils of Medicine', the death of one 'of the most distinguished and most promising of the lady-graduates of medicine' was described as 'so painful'. 'Cut down at the commencement of her career', Prideaux had shared in the lot befalling those who took 'fatal risks' in the practise of their craft. Alongside the death from scarlet fever of an equally qualified male contemporary, St Thomas' house surgeon, Robert Lawson, the year had ended sadly with the 'cut[ting] off' of two young hopefuls. The periodical did not choose to separate the events; instead the focus turned to every victim of professional duty. Lawson and Prideaux were but two examples of those who had been struck down by their very dedication to patient and profession. Both were designated, alongside fallen comrades, as 'soldier[s] of medicine'.[43] Rather than isolating Helen Prideaux as an example of a woman unable to cope with her circumstances, the profession rallied around its own, simultaneously lamenting and championing the sacrifice.

Whereas we have seen the move towards a qualified acceptance of the woman surgeon both by press and profession alike in the last two decades of the nineteenth century, some felt that a change in surgery itself had made this possible. When it looked back upon anaesthesia's golden jubilee in 1896, the *Hospital* remarked that the past fifty years had seen a dramatic change in the ways in which surgery was performed, but also in the composition of operating theatre personnel. In the past, before anaesthesia, surgical procedures were carried out solely to conserve life or limb and were few in number. Now, patients could elect to undergo surgery, with the knowledge that they could be cured by the operation. Genuine 'surgical usefulness' had, therefore, been a result of recent developments. So far, so familiar. However, the periodical then turned towards another consideration; one which it felt is 'of hardly inferior weight to' the benefits afforded to the patient. Indeed, in an extension of the argument put forward by Thomas Spencer Wells,

---

[42] 'Sir William Gull on the Admission of Women to the Medical Profession', *BMJ*, 1.1313 (27 February 1886), 414–15; 414.
[43] 'The Perils of Medicine', *BMJ*, 2.1301 (5 December 1885), 1076.

with anaesthetics in use, a class of men have espoused the surgical art, and continue to adopt it in ever-increasing numbers, who, under the older conditions of surgical practice, would not have been willing – would not, indeed, have been able – to practise surgery at all. The pre-anaesthetic surgeon was often spoken of as a 'butcher'; and the term was in those days hardly one of disparagement. If the surgeon was a cultured man, with the skill of the competent butcher thrown in, so much the better both for himself and the patient. But the days of 'swift' operations are over, never, we may hope, to return. Now, thanks entirely to anaesthetics, the surgeon is not a 'butcher', but an 'artist'; a skilled user of the finest tools – of tools which can be manipulated without any distracting thought, and employed with the calm deliberateness needed to secure the highest possible result which the scientific conservation of life and structure and function can possibly attain.[44]

In other words, surgery had become more acceptable, more palatable: sensitive, one might add. Surgical art was now skilful, requiring gentleness and artistry. The instruments of the trade had been honed into superlative aids. No longer brutal tools to butcher flesh, they were not wielded, but utilised delicately as an extension of knowledgeable, refined fingers. By the turn of the nineteenth century, those who would not have been considered suitable to carry out surgical procedures had been drawn into the profession, attracted by its increasingly sophisticated outlook.

Although this is, of course, an idealised depiction of impossibly painless, bloodless surgery, by 1900, the sense that an operation was no longer traumatic, for surgeon or for patient alike, was a very real one. If, as *Punch*'s 'Chloe, M.D.' had argued in the 1870s, surgeons needed a 'Lady's Hand', then women were seen as perfect operators. Far from having an unsuitable physique for surgery, female hands, smaller and more dexterous, were ideal for the fiddly, complex procedures being developed thanks to an unconscious patient. In his free time, famed surgeon Frederick Treves liked to observe Mary Scharlieb operate because 'her movements, her sureness, her delicacy, were invaluable to watch'.[45] Louisa Garrett Anderson too wrote of Scharlieb's 'slender hands seeming to go everywhere with marvellous speed'.[46] Nimble, swift and, most importantly, sure of her direction, it was the sheer choreography of Scharlieb's surgical prowess which entranced. Anaesthesia encouraged skilfulness – a very different sort from that of the days of 'butchery'. Some,

---

[44] 'The Jubilee of Anaesthesia', quoted verbatim from the *Hospital*, in *Times*, 35023 (Friday 16 October 1896), 7.

[45] P.H., 'Women in Medicine', *Lady's Pictorial*, 20 August 1910, in *RFH Press Cuttings, Volume IV*.

[46] Louisa Garrett Anderson, *Elizabeth Garrett Anderson 1836–1917* (London: Faber and Faber, 1939), p. 242.

according to Elizabeth Garrett Anderson, even preferred the female hand to conduct an operation. In an undated speech, from the late 1890s or early 1900s, Garrett Anderson remarked, ironically, that 'the demand for medical aid from women is much more pronounced on the surgical than on the medical side. It is precisely what I think was <u>not</u> expected in the early days'. Surgery now took 'the place of honour' at women's hospitals. 'Even husbands, the most critical of judges', Garrett Anderson continued, 'say not rarely how glad they are to trust their wives into women's hands.' Once, indeed, a patient's husband said to a member of the NHW's staff that '"for medical treatment they had a very good man where they lived but that when it came to a cutting business he preferred a woman"'.[47] For one, unidentified female doctor, however, women had become 'magnificent surgeons' in order to abolish surgical procedures, save in case of accidents.[48] By perfecting operative techniques and by practising methods which 'tend to prevention', women surgeons were dedicated to becoming the best in order to put an end precisely to unnecessary surgical interference. Thanks to ancillary, but fundamental, changes in the ways in which surgeons operated, a feminised, sanitised surgery had resulted by the first decades of the twentieth century.

This 'new' surgery was one in which women could and did participate. Indeed, despite predictions to the contrary, women's initial achievements in the medical profession were primarily surgical. By the end of the period covered by this book, Christine Murrell was able to claim that surgical success was greater than medical in financial terms because of the high fees women could command: ultimately £1,000 to £2,000 a year for her services.[49] In the early years, beyond the greater press coverage given to Garrett Anderson's solo attempts to gain her education piecemeal or the heavily publicised battles at the University of Edinburgh, where Sophia Jex-Blake and others were fighting the authorities, solid success was being achieved more quietly. The Birmingham and Midland Hospital for Women (BMHW) was the first institution in the country to appoint a female house surgeon in 1872. Even though the relevant examining bodies in Britain had yet to open their courses to women and the other

[47] Elizabeth Garrett Anderson, 'Notes from an Address', Miscellaneous Documents, HA436/6/2, Ipswich Record Office. Dated to the late 1890s or early 1900s from internal evidence of a 'forty or fifty year' period since women began to demand entry to the medical profession.

[48] P.H., 'Women in Medicine'.

[49] Christine M. Murrell, 'The Medical Profession Including Dentistry', in Edith J. Morley, ed., *Women Workers in Seven Professions* (London: George Routledge & Sons, 1914), pp. 137–67; p. 158.

two candidates were registered men, Louisa Atkins' Zurich qualification was accepted by the board of the hospital.[50] A year later, Joseph Chamberlain could report that this bold, original and pioneering experiment was an enormous success. 'A fair field and no favour should be given to a competent lady candidate', he remarked, adding that 'the accession of that lady to the number of practitioners of surgery would be welcomed'. Atkins' 'zeal and ability' had been recognised by colleagues and patients alike; the former, indeed, had regarded her as 'he could not say confrère, but as a consoeur'.[51] She was the same as them, but different, yet this did not affect the way in which she was treated. Her appointment was not a one-off experiment by the BMHW either. During the 1870s alone, signalling their commitment to supporting women's progress in vital junior posts, the institution employed two further women house surgeons: Edith Pechey and Annie Reay Barker.[52]

Female medical students looked with pride upon those whom they placed in the vanguard of their profession. The 'Topical Song' at the 1895 LSMW Christmas entertainment singled out surgical achievements to be celebrated:

> One step we have made which alone brings renown,
> Five London BS's are gems in our crown;
> We have passed cent. per cent., and whatever may be,
> Our successors in this can't do better than we.
> And we do not stop short of the highest degree,
> For we've got an MS who was trained at the Free![53]

For these students, each step forward, each examination success should be celebrated, no matter how small; every increment was a move towards acceptance. What is also noticeable here was camaraderie. If the wider world chose to dismiss achievements, then they were recognised and promoted within the small community of current and ex-students. Despite

---

50   See entry for 16 July 1872, Minute Book of the Medical Committee, June 1871 to March 1892, HC/WH/1/5/1 and 'Special Meeting', 23 July 1872, Board of Governors Meetings Minutes: 29 May 1872–29 March 1892, HC/WH/1/1, Birmingham City Archives, Library of Birmingham. On the hospital itself, see Judith Lockhart, 'Women, Health and Hospitals in Birmingham: The Birmingham and Midland Hospital for Women', PhD thesis, University of Warwick, 2008.

51   Joseph Chamberlain speaking at the Annual Meeting, reported in *The Third Annual Report of the Birmingham and Midland Hospital for Women* (Birmingham, 1874), pp. 5–8; p. 5.

52   See Minute Book of the Medical Committee, 31 July 1875 for Pechey's appointment; 13 June 1876 for Barker's, HC/WH/1/51, Birmingham City Archives.

53   'Topical Song. Sung at the Christmas Entertainment, 1895', *London (Royal Free Hospital) School of Medicine for Women Magazine*, 3 (January 1896), 117. Future references to this periodical will be shortened to *L(RFH)SMWM*. The 'MS' is Louisa Aldrich-Blake.

ongoing antagonism towards medical women, the song reserved, surprisingly, a cheer for the RCS:

> There is still one advance we should much like to see
> In a body inclined too conservatively;
> So deficient in morals they thought that we were,
> They feared we might rise to their President's chair.
> Though physicians were snuffy, the surgeons were kind –
> Operations compel a more radical mind:
> But if FRCS and MRCP
> Are denied us, we'll flourish the London MD.[54]

While it was not until 1908 that the vote to allow women to join the RCS was finally won, and the first Fellow, Eleanor Davies-Colley, was admitted in 1911, pressure had been mounting in the 1890s.[55] The *Daily Graphic* reported in November 1895 that 'women must see very little to discourage them' in having lost the vote only by a 'very small majority'.[56] Indeed, the RCS' Council as a body had been largely in favour of the admission of women to its examination; it was the Royal College of Physicians who denied, in the necessary conjoint assessment, overall victory. It is hardly a wonder that the students saw a cause to laud the 'kind' RCS in their 'Topical Song'.

Surgical recognition was important because it was the final hurdle in women's professional acceptance. Membership of the Royal Colleges was the ultimate public attainment, but it is vital to acknowledge that, behind the scenes, in operating theatres of varying sizes across the country, numerous women were carrying out surgery, however slight those procedures might have been. As Christopher Lawrence remarks, 'surgical practise of the simplest sort must have been one of the commonest encounters in the history of medicine'.[57] So, even if those designated 'surgeons' were fewer in number than other practitioners, as was the case too with male colleagues, it does not follow that most medical women did not encounter any surgery at all after completing their degrees. While acknowledging the prevalence of minor surgical procedures in the lives of patients and practitioners alike, *British Women Surgeons* will focus primarily upon institutional contexts, because this was where most surgery

---

[54] Ibid.
[55] For Davies-Colley's achievement in November 1911, see 'Hospital and School News' and 'Examination Results', *L(RFH)SMWM*, 8.51 (March 1912), 36; 43; 44.
[56] 'Royal College of Surgeons. The Council and the Admission of Women', *Daily Graphic*, 16 November 1895, in *RFH Press Cuttings, Volume 3*. The vote was narrowly lost by 48 votes in favour of women's admission to 58 against. See 'The Royal College of Surgeons', *BMJ* (9 November 1895).
[57] Lawrence, 'Democratic, Divine, and Heroic', p. 10.

took place between 1860 and 1918.[58] I have also chosen to focus primarily upon metropolitan institutions, as many medical women practised in London, alert to the surgical opportunities to be gained by remaining in the capital.[59] However, this does not mean that women did not practise elsewhere, as the country-wide backgrounds of those who served during the Great War will illustrate in the final two chapters of this book. Additionally, there has been a corresponding dearth of studies on hospitals in which women worked. While some supported women's surgical ambitions, others did not. It is vital to remember, however, that even if many hospital boards were antagonistic to women surgeons across the period covered by this book, those who wanted to specialise in surgery found ways of so doing. There was little point lamenting a sorry lot when initiative, and, very importantly, sound financial backing, meant that jobs could be created for women surgeons. If the British mind, as Christine Murrell put in in 1914, was naturally slow to admit women to positions of responsibility, then 'heavily handicapped' women had retaliated by 'taking matters into their own hands' and establishing their own institutions.[60] From Elizabeth Garrett Anderson's St Mary's Dispensary, opened in 1866, to Maud Chadburn and Eleanor Davies-Colley's South London Hospital for Women and Children, which was completed half a century later, this book explores the work actually carried out by women surgeons, rather than the more usual focus on the missed opportunities. Without denying that those who chose surgery as a career were few, for whatever reason, the woman surgeon was a reality through this period. Women encountered more obstacles than their male colleagues, of course, but the ways in which they operated between 1860 and 1918 present a more fascinating, varied picture than one which removes surgical agency from them altogether.

Indeed, the majority of surgery in institutional contexts performed by women was of a serious kind and it is upon this field that *British Women Surgeons* will concentrate. Far from working towards the abolition of surgical practice, women contributed actively to the operative itch which characterised the end of the Victorian period and the first two decades of the twentieth century. As More's analysis of American gynaecological cases suggested, 'women initially were more willing to

---

[58] Joel D. Howell, *Technology in the Hospital* (Baltimore, MD: Johns Hopkins University Press, 1995).

[59] Digby notes that '[h]onorary hospital appointments were of even greater importance to the career of a surgeon than to a physician' *Making a Medical Living*, p. 33; for the concentration of medical women in London, see ibid., p. 167.

[60] Murrell, 'The Medical Profession', p. 154.

operate than men'.[61] Every surgeon, regardless of sex, discovered that confidence was gained through operating, even if every patient suffering from the same condition presented different problems. In *Seven Lamps of Medicine* (1888), Scharlieb claimed succinctly that surgical 'knowledge is power, and the feeling of power contributes greatly to the calmness and dexterity from which it is performed'.[62] This book charts the growth of women's surgical experience from the faltering first days of male assistance to the positions of responsibility attained during the Great War on the home and the battle fronts. In so doing, it will provide the 'much-needed case studies of specific institutions', which Elston called for in 2001.[63] Women may have worked primarily in female-run institutions, but they did not designate them 'special' hospitals and were insistent on their general status.[64] The treatment of particular groups – namely, women and children, until the Great War – must not be equated with narrow and limited expertise.[65] Indeed, smaller, women-run hospitals such as the New Hospital for Women (NHW) and the South London Hospital for Women (SLHW) treated a far wider range of conditions than the RFH, where women were in charge of the Gynaecological Department from 1902, precisely because of their claim to generalism. The smallest institutions where theatre facilities were not as developed, such as the initially six-bed Edinburgh Hospital for Women and Children, saw an increase in surgical procedures in the early twentieth century. Only minor surgery had been performed in the first decade and a half of the hospital's existence, but, coinciding with Elsie Inglis' appointment as junior surgeon and gynaecologist, 'operations [became] more important than has been the case in recent years'. The patients seen that year suffered from complaints which were 'more of an acute character'.[66]

---

[61] More, *Restoring*, p. 53.

[62] Mary Scharlieb, *Seven Lamps of Medicine* (Oxford: Horace Hart, 1888). See also Owen H. Wangensteen and Sarah D. Wangensteen, *The Rise of Surgery* (Folkestone: Dawson, 1978) about the acquisition of surgical technique through experience (p. 236).

[63] Mary Ann Elston, '"Run by Women, (mainly) for Women": Medical Women's Hospitals in Britain, 1866–1948', in Anne Hardy and Lawrence Conrad, eds., *Women and Modern Medicine* (Amsterdam: Rodopi, 2001), pp. 73–107; p. 74.

[64] This was, of course, in opposition to the way in which special hospitals were emerging at the time. See George Weisz, *Divide and Conquer* (New York: Oxford University Press, 2006).

[65] For example, Geddes remarks that women's surgical practise was 'almost exclusively gynaecological' before 1914. See 'Deeds *and* Words', 85, and 'The Doctors' Dilemma: Medical Women and the British Suffrage Movement', *Women's History Review*, 18.2 (April 2009), 203–18; 205.

[66] 'Medical Officer's Report', *Twenty-Seventh Annual Report of the Edinburgh Hospital and Dispensary for Women and Children, 1905–1906* (Edinburgh, 1905), p. 5, LHB8/7/26, Bruntsfield Hospital and Elsie Inglis Memorial Maternity Hospital Archives, Lothian Health Services Archive, Edinburgh University Library, Edinburgh.

It was medical women's realisation that their patients both wanted and needed surgery, in combination with their own desire to provide such services, that saw many female-run institutions becoming increasingly surgical centres by 1918.

British Women Surgeons begins with an exploration of the ways in which the New Hospital for Women, established initially as a dispensary, rapidly became an institution which promoted the surgical skills of medical women. Behind the propaganda, however, things were not progressing as smoothly as the management of the NHW would have liked. Internal schisms over the ways in which Garrett Anderson operated threatened the hospital with controversy. In many ways, the New played out all the early concerns which the profession and the public had about the ability of women surgeons to carry out complex procedures, exacerbated because of insufficient specialist training. It was also a victim of its own publicity. Annual reports and newspaper columns praised the low death rates resulting from women surgeons unafraid to take a risk, but inside the hospital procedures were not going to plan. Too frequently, the male honorary consultants were performing operations, while the much-lauded female staff watched or assisted at best. With Garrett Anderson's retirement in 1892, the New's confidence was bolstered by the elevation of Mary Scharlieb to Senior Surgeon. Much more assured than her predecessor, Scharlieb instigated a new era in the hospital's surgical procedures. Ever mindful of what she owed to her team, Scharlieb placed the individual surgeon squarely within the wider network of personnel, both within and outside the operating theatre. The way in which the NHW operated in the late nineteenth century changed for the better.

In 1902, Mary Scharlieb departed for the Royal Free Hospital, in another landmark for the woman surgeon, to run the Gynaecological Department, where she was assisted by Ethel Vaughan-Sawyer. The next chapter follows her to consider the patient base at the RFH. Whom did Scharlieb and Vaughan-Sawyer treat? What surgical solutions did they offer and how did the patients react to their surgeon, the procedures they underwent and their experience of hospital life? The relationship between the working-class female patient and her practitioner has been strangely neglected, with, as Thomson laments, a focus on motherhood dominating historical analysis.[67] In order to redress this balance, my second chapter will examine the rich vein of RFH gynaecological case notes between

See also Thomson, 'Women in Medicine', p. 143 for the list of procedures; and, for Inglis, Margot Lawrence, *Shadow of Swords* (London: Michael Joseph, 1971).

[67]   Thomson, 'Women in Medicine', p. 167.

1903 and 1913 to explore the nearly 1,500 woman patients who experienced surgical treatment under Scharlieb and Vaughan-Sawyer during these years. Increasingly, as the third chapter will show, women surgeons were carrying out procedures for one of the most feared diseases of the late nineteenth and early twentieth centuries: cancer. Previous analyses of women practitioners have suggested that they were abandoning surgery in the 1910s to make way for other, less invasive procedures such as radium treatment.[68] However, in hospitals such as the NHW, the RFH and the SLHW, surgery was still the primary recourse when cancer was discovered; radiotherapy was employed only for lost causes. The first two decades of the twentieth century were an exciting time for the surgical treatment of malignant disease, when operations, such as Wertheim's for cancer of the cervix, were devised and developed in an attempt to combat this most feared killer of women in the prime of life. For female surgeons in these three metropolitan hospitals, unafraid to try new procedures, surgery was the best way to save their patients' lives. Working-class women were often blamed in the medical and lay press for their slow response to the troubling symptoms of cancer. Case notes from the RFH will be utilised to consider how such women reacted to their condition and to the resulting treatment. With such a breadth of coverage in the records of the RFH, from 1903 to 1919, the historian can follow through on those who underwent surgery for the 'cure' period of five years and more.

By the beginning of the twentieth century, women surgeons were unafraid to attempt the most complex of operations for malignant disease. Yet they would face entirely new challenges from 1914, which would try their new-found confidence. The final two chapters examine the ways in which the Great War provided exciting professional opportunities both near to the battlefield and on the home front. When offers of assistance were brushed aside in no uncertain terms by the War Office, the response was unsurprising, given over half a century of similar reactions. Firstly, the advice was ignored. And, secondly, women simply established their own hospitals in various European countries, as they had done in Britain. In so doing, they gained not only their first real experience of operating on the opposite sex, but increased professional confidence in their surgical abilities. In a conflict where injuries did not resemble anything seen before, even by the most seasoned military surgeon, women took up the challenge and learned, along with their male colleagues, how to operate

[68] See, for example, Ornella Moscucci, 'The "Ineffable Freemasonry of Sex": Feminist Surgeons and the Establishment of Radiotherapy in Early Twentieth-Century Britain', *BHM*, 81.1 (Spring 2007), 139–63.

in the theatre of war. At home, with male members of the profession, at all levels from student to consultant, leaving their posts to serve abroad, women remained to plug the gaps. An enormous growth in the number of female students of medicine was coupled with the opening of medical schools and of many general hospital appointments, both previously shut to women applicants. While some took advantage of the situation and plunged into new worlds, others remained devoted to single-sex education and, as the wartime inauguration of the SLHW revealed, female-run institutions. As locum tenens for the length of the conflict only, as they were repeatedly reminded, women took up places fully aware that the measures were temporary. In the long run, what mattered, both at home and abroad, was that newly-promised opportunities were grasped tightly because too soon they would end and the status quo would be re-established.

During the Great War, in May 1916, the *Daily Sketch* offered its readers an assessment of a once *rara avis*:

The public, as a whole, knew nothing of her, although it imagined a great deal. It imagined, for instance, that it never could bring itself to trust a woman doctor; that she would inevitably lose her nerve at the critical moment; and that she must in any case be a curious, unsexed, morbid creature to be willing to study anything so repellent and terrible as medicine. There are still individuals who think and talk thus, but the public generally knows better than this. To-day the medical woman may be found practising in quiet little south coast watering places. She is treating the wounded in great hospitals close to the firing-line in France. She is caring for the women and children of the hill-tribes in frontier towns in India. She is waiting with calm patience and unceasing labour to be taken prisoner by the enemy rather than leave her wounded patients in Serbia. She is seeing patients every morning in her house in Harley St. She is resident medical officer in hospitals all over the country, tending the sick among the civil population and the soldiers in the wards needed for the army. She is running a big practice in a provincial town and driving her car herself because the chauffeur had joined the army. She is at remote stations of the Empire upholding the honour, the goodwill, the power and the stability of the British rule.[69]

In 1860, there were no medical women. Half a century later, there were nearly a thousand living women on the Medical Register.[70] By the start of the academic year of 1918–1919, there were 665 new entrants alone to medical schools across Britain and Ireland, nearly a third of the total

---

69 'Women and the Medical Profession', *Daily Sketch*, 13 May 1916, in Letters from Elizabeth Garrett Anderson and Louisa Garrett Anderson to Miss Brooks and Miss Sage, 1910–1943, HA436/1/4/6, Ipswich Record Office.

70 Louie M. Brooks refutes that the numbers are 'small': 930 in only 34 years, 'Women as Doctors', *Pall Mall Gazette*, 20 January 1912, in *RFH Press Cuttings, Volume IV*.

number.[71] As the *Daily Sketch* piece made clear, there were still those who could not countenance a woman competently examining the bodies of others without breaking down. What is most telling about this article, though, is the sheer range of possibilities for surgical practice especially to be found by the second decade of the twentieth century, across the country and abroad. It is those potential avenues which *British Women Surgeons* will explore further, following practitioners through the closed doors of operating theatres to see what precisely went on inside. Those who chose surgery were undoubtedly few, as was the case with male colleagues, but every single medical student, of either sex, had some knowledge of surgical procedures. Indeed, whether carrying out minor procedures in general practice, assisting as house surgeons in hospitals across Britain, or operating on wounded soldiers all over Europe, women's surgical skills had never been more needed nor praised. Ultimately, this book is a history of the 'quiet perseverance' with which women surgeons operated.[72] So quietly, indeed, that their contribution to women's professional achievements, as well as their willingness to take risks, has been forgotten. That persistence can be rightly reconsidered through the wealth of archival resources available. *British Women Surgeons* will move away from previous assessments, which focus on what medical women did not achieve in this period. Instead, I will chart, unashamedly, the growth of female surgical confidence, and do so precisely through documenting the operations they performed.

[71] 'Annotations: The Supply of Medical Students', *Lancet*, 192.4952 (27 July 1918), 113.
[72] 'Women Doctors. How They Have Won Through By Quiet Perseverance', *Pall Mall Gazette*, 20 June 1913, in *RFH Press Cuttings, Volume IV*.

1 From Controversy to Consolidation: Surgery at the New Hospital for Women, 1872–1902

When Elizabeth Garrett Anderson reflected upon the next step for medical women in the 1860s, she remarked that 'it seemed to me that we <u>must</u> <u>imperatively</u> have a hospital entirely worked by qualified medical women before women would be trusted on a large scale by the outside public'.[1] This chapter considers the vagaries of surgical practice at the New Hospital for Women (NHW), the first female-only run institution in Britain, which grew out of the foundation of St Mary's Dispensary in 1866. From the outset, the Dispensary had a dual purpose, combining philanthropy with solid practical support for women doctors, who were exclusively to form the working medical staff. It would 'meet a want in a large and poor district of London, and at the same time [. . .] assist the movement in favour of admitting women into the medical profession'.[2] Between its foundation in 1866 and its transformation into the New in early 1872, the Dispensary was flooded with women both from the metropolis and from elsewhere in the country seeking the medical assistance of their own sex. The sheer demand for the services of the Dispensary, coupled with the desperate state of many of the patients, who were too ill to attend in person, and their homes too poor and dirty to permit surgical attendance, encouraged the Dispensary Committee to provide proper hospital accommodation for a new and expanded facility. While the influx of potential patients contributed to the conversion from Dispensary to hospital, the Committee noted that it was increasingly necessary, '[i]n very many cases', to offer treatment that was 'almost purely surgical'.[3] The performance of surgical procedures and the foundation of the NHW were inextricably linked in the eyes of the hospital's management and staff. As Mary Ann Elston has noted, in the second half of the nineteenth

---

[1] Elizabeth Garrett Anderson, Notes from an Address [late 1890s/early 1900s?], Elizabeth Garrett Anderson Letters and Papers, HA436/6/2, Ipswich Record Office, Suffolk; emphasis in original.

[2] Advertisement placed in *First Annual Report of the New Hospital for Women* (London: Beveridge and Fraser, 1873).

[3] Ibid.

century hospitals were founded through 'a mixture of philanthropic, professional and entrepreneurial motives', and the New was an institution 'where women could develop professional skills and achieve positions of responsibility from which they were otherwise excluded, both by overt opposition and by the limited mandate under which nineteenth-century women entered medicine'.[4] In a list of desirable 'professional skills' and in opposition to the contemporary expectations of the medical profession, surgical expertise was considered vital for the promotion of women doctors. As the first *Annual Report* of the hospital was so keen to publicise, successful surgery performed by skilful surgeons was a key aim of the New from its inception.

The *Annual Reports* listed an all-female staff, who were assisted by male consultants.[5] While the assumption was that women would carry out operations, in fact it appears that they, at least in the first decade or so of the New's existence, actually acted as assistants to the more experienced consulting surgeons. In her 1924 *Reminiscences*, Mary Scharlieb, who joined the New as a Clinical Assistant in 1888, made reference to the peculiarities of this situation. Discussing the operations at the hospital, Scharlieb recalled that Garrett Anderson was the

one member of the staff who undertook major surgery, it was she only who was competent, and indeed she was the only one who was willing to encounter the difficulties and responsibilities inseparable from such work. Sometimes she felt that in the interests of the patient a surgeon of greater experience ought to operate. When this occurred no self-love nor false shame prevented Mrs Anderson from inviting some outside surgeon to do what was necessary. On such occasions she played the part of assistant, and I have seen her meekly and carefully following the instructions of Sir Spencer Wells, Mr Knowsley Thornton, Mr Meredith and other consultants.[6]

Scharlieb's comment is fascinating in the light of Garrett Anderson's own correspondence, which suggests that she did not consider herself a surgeon. While leaving France in 1870, Garrett Anderson remarked that she had been to the Anglo-American Hospital in Sedan, where she was 'begged' by the chief surgeons 'to stay': '[They] offered me as many patients I could manage entirely to myself. I was heartily sorry I could not. Tho' surgery is not my line I should have been thoroughly glad to stay and help in that kindly stimulating atmosphere.'[7] Although she was not inclined towards surgery, the stimulation provided by the operating

[4] Elston, '"Run by Women"', p. 85.
[5] Information given in *Annual Reports*.   [6] Scharlieb, *Reminiscences*, p. 133.
[7] Elizabeth Garrett Anderson to Jane Crowe, 'On board the steamer from Antwerp to London', 16 September 1870, Elizabeth Garrett Anderson Letters and Papers, HA436/1/4/5, Ipswich.

theatre evidently persuaded Garrett Anderson to think otherwise. With an increase in the numbers of complex surgical procedures performed in the last two decades of the nineteenth century and the growth of experimentation on the operating table, Garrett Anderson was determined to push the NHW and the cause of the woman surgeon into the forefront of developments in surgery. However, in reality, the female medical staff acknowledged their own limitations, stepping back to observe procedures rather than wielding the knife themselves.

Resignations

While the female staff remained assistants rather than operators, there was a chasm between the mission statement of the NHW and the actual practice which occurred within its walls. Although she 'knew the limits of her training', Garrett Anderson sought to change procedures, insisting that medical women should do the professional work of the hospital.[8] Both Louisa Garrett Anderson and Mary Scharlieb noted that Elizabeth Garrett Anderson was the only member of staff willing to undertake major surgery, and her desire to promote the cause of the female surgeon encountered numerous difficulties from her fellow medical women. Both women expressed her dedication to education through practise, but they also revealed Garrett Anderson's fear of her own surgical inadequacies; hence her willingness 'meekly' to assist or observe. According to her daughter, each operation caused Garrett Anderson 'intense anxiety', ensuring that she 'never enjoyed operating'.[9] Too often, the reaction of the surgeon to surgical procedures is forgotten in the history of medicine; the fear and distress surgery provoked was not only that of the patients.[10] For early women surgeons, who were compelled to learn by experience, a lack of specialised training rendered every operation a risky and potentially frightening process. In a manuscript draft for a speech, Garrett Anderson remarked feelingly upon and, evidently, with personal understanding of, the effect surgery had upon the operator:

> To see a skilled surgeon do his work is a very different thing from doing it oneself. [...] In surgery the nerve has to be trained and that only is done by actual work of your own. I believe it is impossible for any but those who have gone through it to realise what a tremendous tax upon one's nerve it is to attempt a great operation, especially of the kind where exact previous knowledge of the difficulties cannot possibly be had. I speak of this with feeling because I know what it is.[11]

[8] Louisa Garrett Anderson, *Elizabeth Garrett Anderson*, pp. 242–3.   [9] Ibid., p. 242.
[10] See Peter Stanley, *For Fear of Pain* (Amsterdam: Rodopi, 2003), especially pp. 203–4.
[11] Jo Manton, *Elizabeth Garrett Anderson* (London: Methuen, 1965), p. 230.

From a generalised opening, Garrett Anderson's constant repetition of the personal pronoun, especially prominent in the last sentence, implied that holding 'one's nerve' was far from a given attribute for the surgeon. Training was essential, but when this was limited by circumstances, risks had to be taken. Behind celebration of the calm, skilful female surgeon in the New's publicity lay a more nervy reality, where ability was questioned and doubted.

If self-doubt was evident at the NHW, then resignations over the period between 1877 and 1888 revealed that concern at women performing surgical procedures was pervasive. Much has been made in previous accounts of Frances Hoggan's resignation in 1877, but other cases have been entirely passed over. Indeed, the date and circumstances of Hoggan's leaving have been confused and conflated to the extent that she appears to have resigned over operations which were not carried out until a year after she left the New.[12] Although there is indecision over when Hoggan actually left the New, there is none when it comes to why: she resigned because of controversial surgical procedures being performed by women on women.

The Minute Books of the Managing Committee, however, confirm that Frances Hoggan tendered her resignation in March 1877, giving no reason other than that she 'had quite made up her mind to take this step', and was emphatically 'Resolved' in her decision to leave. Forced, reluctantly, to accept, the Committee noted that Hoggan's 'kind and skilful labours have done much to the raise the Hospital to its present position', and that they felt 'sure that the termination of Mrs Hoggan's connexion with the Hospital will be regarded both by its supporters and by the patients with general regret'.[13] The next meeting, exactly a month later, recorded Hoggan's gratitude at the Committee's praise for her support over the past five years, but also her willingness to continue working at the New on her usual Tuesdays and Fridays until they had found a replacement.[14] Examining the cases listed in the *Annual Report* for 1877 does not elicit any evidence of an ovariotomy, successful or otherwise, having been performed that year. In 1876, however, two operations are noted specifically, neither ovariotomies: one the repair of a

[12] Louisa Garrett Anderson in *Elizabeth Garrett Anderson*, p. 243, names 1876. Mary Ann Elston in 'Anderson, Elizabeth Garrett (1836–1917)', www.oxforddnb.com/view/article30406 (accessed 21 May 2016) and 'Hoggan, Frances Elizabeth (1843–1927)', www.oxforddnb.com/view/article/46422 (accessed 21 May 2016) suggest 1872 and 1878 respectively.

[13] Minute Books of the Managing Committee of the New Hospital for Women I: November 1871–May 1882, entry for 28 April 1877, H13/EGA/19, LMA.

[14] Ibid., entry for 28 May 1877.

recto-vaginal fistula; the other a ruptured perineum. The former failed, and the latter was postponed. One of the three deaths that year arose from complications following an operation to remove a cancerous breast. This appears to have been a tricky case, involving several operations, and resultant gangrene, which in turn led to the hospital succumbing to 'erysipelas and some of the allied diseases'.[15] As a key member of the anti-vivisectionist Victoria Street Society and someone who appeared to ally herself with the ideas of Elizabeth Blackwell, the first woman doctor to be registered in Britain, Hoggan may have objected to certain surgery involving what Blackwell labelled the 'serious ethical danger connected with unrestrained experiment on the lower animals [which leads to] the enormous increase of audacious human surgery, which tends to over-power the slower but more natural methods of medical art'.[16] Maybe, given her political stance, Hoggan did resign over the prospect of female surgeons cutting up their own sex, or because surgical procedures, as they were carried out at the hospital, could be far too risky, as the events of 1876 revealed. But, she did not leave in 1877 because Garrett Anderson was performing ovariotomies, either on her own or with support from the consulting staff.

In fact, the first time this controversial procedure was carried out was a year after Hoggan's departure in 1878. As the *Annual Report* for that year trumpeted:

During the year the operation of ovariotomy has been twice performed by a member of the Hospital staff, once in private, and once in the Hospital, and in each case the patient has recovered perfectly. The Committee are not aware of this formidable operation having been ever before, in Europe at least, performed successfully by a woman.[17]

If they had objected to the procedure previously, the response was not recorded, and here the only tone was triumph and pride in Garrett Anderson's achievement.[18] Even though she was not named directly, the anonymity employed served to reflect the glory back upon the New as an institution which nurtured female surgical expertise. However, in

---

[15] *Fifth (1876) Annual Report* (1877), p. 3.

[16] Elizabeth Blackwell, *Essays in Medical Sociology* (London: Bell, 1902), p. 119. For general background information on Hoggan and her commitment to various social reforms, see Onfel Thomas, *Frances Elizabeth Hoggan* (Newport: n.p., 1971). For more on Hoggan's anti-vivisectionist activities, see Mary Ann Elston, 'Women and Anti-Vivisection in Victorian England, 1870–1900', in Nicolaas A. Rupke, ed., *Vivisection in Historical Perspective* (London and New York: Croom Helm, 1987), pp. 259–94.

[17] *Seventh (1878) Annual Report* (1879), p. 3.

[18] Manton notes that 'the management committee refused to allow the operation to take place in the hospital [but after the success of this first operation] the next case remained in the hospital', *Elizabeth Garrett Anderson*, p. 229.

this report, the Managing Committee were also compelled to report to subscribers that, along with the departure of Hoggan, the New had lost another member of staff: John Erichsen, one of the consulting surgeons. Erichsen had been a surgical advisor to the female staff from the outset, when the hospital had been St Mary's Dispensary. After 12 years of service, Erichsen left in April 1878, according to the Minutes, but continued to 'entertain the most friendly feelings towards the Institution'.[19] As the renowned author of *The Science and Art of Surgery* (first published in 1853), a well-respected and widely-used textbook, Erichsen's loss must have been a great disappointment to the New, which still needed assistance from those established members of the profession who supported medical women and the vital clinical experience they could receive at the hospital.

Erichsen had been made surgeon-extraordinary to Queen Victoria in 1876, and was Vice-President of the Royal College of Surgeons between 1878 and 1879, becoming President in 1880. Lister had been one of his house surgeons, and, as his *BMJ* obituary noted in 1896, he should be counted 'among the makers of modern surgery', with 'his sound judgment, ripened by a vast experience, which gave him an almost unrivalled clinical insight. There was no man in the profession whose opinion in a difficult case was justly held to be of greater weight.'[20] Only three years after his resignation from the New, Erichsen publicly expressed doubts over the supposed progress of abdominal surgery. *The Science and Art of Surgery* raised, but did not support, objections to operations such as ovariotomy, concluding that the discomfort was worse without action and patient death rates were not so high as other procedures to warrant surgeons abstaining from the process.[21] And yet, by August 1881, in a lecture given as President of the Surgery Section at the BMA Annual Meeting Erichsen acknowledged the 'brilliant advance' made in abdominal surgery, but felt troubled by the increasingly alarming experimental nature of his craft:

[19] Minute Books of the Managing Committee I, entry for meeting held on 4 April 1878, H13/EGA/19, LMA. While the *Annual Report* for the year 1877 is dated March 1878, and Erichsen is noted in this edition as having resigned, in fact the report was still being edited in April 1878, so this is why Erichsen's resignation appears in the earlier report rather than the one for the next year which covered 1878.

[20] For further biographical information on Erichsen, see his obituary in the *BMJ*, 2.1865 (26 September 1896), 885–887; 886, and the entry for Erichsen at: http://livesonline.rcseng.ac.uk/biogs/E000206b.htm.
      Curiously, in none of these entries is there any mention of his long involvement with St Mary's Dispensary or the NHW.

[21] John Eric Erichsen, *The Science and Art of Surgery*, fourth edition (London: Walton and Maberley, 1864), pp. 1234–5.

The uterus and the spleen, the stomach, the pylorus and the colon, have each and all been subjected to the scalpel of the surgeon; with what success has yet to be determined; and it is for you to decide whether some, at least, of these operations constitute real and solid advances in our art, or whether they are rather to be regarded as bold and skilful experiments on the endurance and reparative power of the human frame – whether, in fact, they are surgical triumphs or operative audacities. There must, indeed, be a limit to the progress of operative surgery in this direction. Are we at present in a position to define it? There cannot always be new fields for conquest by the knife; there must be portions of the human frame that will ever remain sacred from its intrusion, at least, in the hands of the surgeon. May there not be some reason to fear lest the very perfection to which ovariotomy has been carried may lead to an over-sanguine expectation of the value and the safety of the abdominal section, and exploration when applied to the diagnosis or cure of diseases of other and very dissimilar organs, in which but little of ultimate advantage, and certainly much of immediate peril, may be expected from operative interference?[22]

Was it concern at 'operative audacity', or at least the potential for an overly sanguine acceptance of mortality through experimentation, which encouraged Erichsen to resign his consulting post at the NHW? If he anticipated the growth of such procedures at the New then he was to be proved correct. From 1888, the hospital and its female surgeons made a break with the past, and, controversially, took the lead in their own operations, which provoked a storm of controversy within the New itself.

Divisions

Despite Garrett Anderson's desire for the female staff to perform surgical procedures themselves, they were still not always doing so by the mid-1880s. In March 1884, when a patient's death under anaesthetic was reported in the *Paddington Times*, it was evident that Garrett Anderson was only 'present' at the operation, while a member of the consulting staff was to perform the surgery.[23] The patient, 32-year-old spinster Sarah Brighton, had been suffering from bladder and kidney problems and had been in declining health for months. She entered the NHW after being encouraged to do so by her (male) general practitioner on 4 February. Within three weeks she was dead. A week before her death,

---

22   Erichsen, 'An Address Delivered at the Opening of the Section of Surgery', *BMJ*, 2.1075 (6 August 1881), 212–14.

23   It was W.A. Meredith who was due to operate here. See 'Correspondence: Melancholy Death in the Hospital for Women, 222, Marylebone-Road', *Paddington Times*, Saturday 15 March 1884, and an undated article from the same paper recording the inquest, *Album of Newspaper Cuttings Relating to the New Hospital for Women*, H13/EGA/144, LMA. Further references will be to *ANC*.

an operation had been decided upon in order to prolong her life. Miss Brighton readily consented to the procedure, although her condition was deteriorating rapidly; both her pulse and heartbeat were faint, she was unable to eat much and her temperature had risen to 105. The operation was considered necessary; Miss Brighton's weakness both of pulse and heartbeat would have made the induction of anaesthesia a more risky business. However, the benefits were seen to outweigh the disadvantages of application and Miss Brighton was put under 'quietly and comfortably' by Mrs Marshall, assistant physician, while Meredith prepared to operate. The completeness of Mrs Marshall's professional credentials were reiterated by Garrett Anderson; the mixture of alcohol, chloroform and ether (A.C.E.) used to anaesthetise Miss Brighton was considered, as a textbook noted two decades later, still 'nearly twice as safe as chloroform alone'.[24] Nothing unusual was noted, until Miss Brighton simply ceased to breathe. Resuscitation was continued for an hour and twenty minutes, but Sarah Brighton was dead. While her death was attributed to misadventure by the coroner, who noted that she had received every attention, Miss Brighton's brothers accused the hospital of overzealousness. One, James, wrote to the *Paddington Times* for 'the benefit of young women who contemplate going to the Hospital for Women in Marylebone-road', warning the vulnerable patient about what had happened to his sister.[25] As he claimed, she was neither taken into the hospital for an operation, nor had profited from any procedure carried out there. The first 'extreme instrument operation' caused Sarah Brighton 'great agony', while the 'last and fatal' surgery led to her death. James Brighton had requested that no operation be performed on his sister before he had consulted a medical man of his choice. Rebuffed in his attempt to do so by a recommendation to speak only with those connected to the hospital, Brighton felt he had been conspired against. The 'most encouraging and hopeful assurances of the women of the hospital' had effectively hoodwinked his weakened sister into consenting to surgery he was convinced she did not need. While the inquest into her death concluded that the hospital was not to blame for Sarah Brighton's death, such adverse publicity would not have encouraged potential patients to trust the judgement of the woman surgeon, even if it was not she who was carrying out the operation. Worse, James Brighton remarked, was the very female persuasiveness brought to bear upon a seriously ill member of the same sex. The woman

---

[24] H. Bellamy Gardener, *Surgical Anaesthesia* (New York: William Wood and Co., 1909), p. 179.

[25] Letter from James Brighton to the Editor of the *Paddington Times*, dated 6 March 1884, *Paddington Times*, Saturday, 15 March 1884, *ANC*.

surgeon could be deadly even by proxy. Such a taint of hasty recklessness would come back to haunt the hospital in the 1890s, as we shall see, when another accusation of poorly-administered anaesthesia, in addition to ongoing concerns about operative excess, forced the New on the defensive once more about its surgical practices.

If Garrett Anderson had not operated in this instance, there were other occasions when she was in charge of the procedure. While she had apparently operated alone successfully for the two ovariotomies in 1878, subsequent results were not so pleasing. When a patient died from an ovarian tumour and consequent peritonitis, the *Annual Report* for 1879 was keen to stress that no operation had been performed in this case.[26] The Managing Committee was evidently conscious of the ongoing sensitivity of the subject and wanted to protect the New from accusations of improper conduct. In 1880, though, it was noted that there had been an in-patient death from a suppurated ovarian cyst, where ovariotomy was placed in brackets after the cause of death. The patient died after the operation, but bracketing the procedure ensured that the cause of death was recorded as the suppurated cyst.[27] A similar case took place in 1881, whereby the patient had succumbed to bronchitis after an ovariotomy for an ovarian cyst. It was added that this patient was 69.[28] As the Minutes noted every year, it was Garrett Anderson herself who prepared the *Annual Report*, so a careful public presentation of controversial procedures was in the interest of the staff and, of course, the hospital, in the eyes of its subscribers and those who followed the careers of medical women.

While it is not clear precisely who was assisting whom in surgery, the impression given by the hospital was that the women were performing their own procedures at this point. However, cross-referencing the hospital records with statistics presented in print by members of the consulting staff offers a fascinating glimpse into how involved the supposed consultants to the New really were in day-to-day surgery. In May 1882, Garrett Anderson proposed that W.A. Meredith be appointed Consulting Surgeon to the hospital.[29] Meredith had assisted both Erichsen and Spencer Wells, and was clearly an impressive addition to the list of consultants.[30] In 1889, Meredith published 'Remarks on some parts affecting the

26 *Eighth (1879) Annual Report* (1880), p. 15.
27 *Ninth (1880) Annual Report* (1881), p. 15.
28 *Tenth (1881) Annual Report* (1882), p. 11; p. 3.
29 Minute Books of the Managing Committee of the New Hospital for Women, II: June 1882–March 1895; Wednesday 4 May 1882, H13/EGA/20, LMA.
30 'Obituary: William Appleton Meredith', *BMJ*, 2.2911 (14 October 1916), 542.

Mortality of Abdominal Section', which was illustrated with 'Tables of Cases'. Table I was a list of 'One Hundred and Four Completed Ovariotomies' and Table II listed 12 'Operations for the Removal of Diseased Uterine Appendages'. Of these cases, seven were from operations undertaken at the New between 1882 and 1887: five ovariotomies and two removals of appendages. Indeed, as the *Annual Report* for the hospital remarked, the increase in surgical cases was evident from 1882, when the very fabric of the NHW began to alter because of the focus on surgery. The average number of in-patients declined due to 'the presence in the Hospital of a larger number of serious surgical cases, each one of which has frequently occupied an entire ward for several weeks'.[31] In 1882, there was one operation noted for an ovarian tumour, which tallied with Meredith's list concerning his procedure at the New this year.[32] Garrett Anderson was clearly not the surgeon taking the lead here. During 1882, indeed, there was only one death over the entire year, out of the 205 patients admitted into the NHW. The previous year had witnessed five deaths out of 221 patients.

With Garrett Anderson in Australia from January to autumn 1885, the two operations noted as 'ovarian cyst' in the *Annual Report* for this year were performed by Meredith.[33] Two years later, in 1887, the patient with a dermoid ovarian cyst was also Meredith's.[34] The majority of ovariotomies occurred in 1886, when there were three operations for ovarian cyst, with one death; Meredith's patient survived, according to his statistics.[35] It is therefore likely that the patient who died was operated upon by Garrett Anderson, whose success rate that year was 50 per cent. She had written enthusiastically to her husband, who was in America, about the 'excellent' recovery of her patient and the removal

[31] *Eleventh (1882) Annual Report* (1883), p. 3.
[32] Case 29, ibid., p. 10; W.A. Meredith, 'Remarks on Some Points Affecting the Mortality of Abdominal Section. With Tables of Cases', *Medico-Chirurgical Transactions*, 72 (1889), 31–56; 45.
[33] For information about Garrett Anderson's absence, see Scharlieb, *Reminiscences*, p. 133 and Minute Books of the Managing Committee II, entry dated Wednesday 7 January 1885, H13/EGA/20, LMA: 'Mrs Anderson informed the Committee that owing to illness in her family she was about to take a voyage to Australia and should consequently be absent several months'. Her next appearance was Wednesday 4 November that year.
      The operations performed at the New are listed in Meredith, 'Remarks on Some Points', case 66 and case 74, 48–49; and number 21, *Fourteenth (1885) Annual Report* (1886), p. 12.
[34] Meredith, 'Remarks', case 98, 51; number 27, *Sixteenth (1887) Annual Report* (1888), p. 12.
[35] Meredith, 'Remarks', case 87, 50; number 17, *Fifteenth (1886) Annual Report* (1887), p. 12.

of a tumour, which had been 'a very uncommon case' and which had, consequently, been offered 'to the Museum of the College of Surgeons as [Sir Spencer] Wells says they have only one like it'.[36] This was not the last time Garrett Anderson felt misplaced confidence about her patients' futures after surgical intervention. It was this discrepancy between surgical ambition and operative success which led to resignations from the New in 1888; a year of staff losses which were instigated by Meredith himself, alarmed at what he had witnessed in the operating theatre.

Three departures from the NHW in 1888 not only revealed uncertainty over the question of female surgical aptitude, but also placed a question mark over what Elston has called 'the nucleus of a professional and a friendship network that sustained pioneering generations' in the earliest women's hospitals.[37] Meredith was the first to leave, but he was followed in swift succession by Louisa Atkins and Mary E. Dowson. Both women were renowned in different, but equally important, ways in the battle for female entry into the medical profession, as well as, more specifically, in the history of women in surgery. As we saw in the introduction, Louisa Atkins secured a controversial post as a house surgeon in 1872 at the Birmingham and Midland Hospital for Women, when she was pitted against, and beat, two men in the final stages. When Atkins left in 1874, the philanthropic physician Thomas Heslop, co-initiator of the hospital, stated feelingly that: 'the accession of that lady to the number of practitioners of surgery would be welcomed, and upon leaving that hospital, she would leave behind her a reputation, which he trusted would serve her most essentially in her whole future life'.[38] Atkins had proved that women doctors could work alongside men, and gain their respect and trust, even in surgical cases. Mary Dowson's achievements were more recent, but equally vital in advancing the cause of medical women and, most importantly, that of female surgeons. Dowson had the 'honour', as the *BMJ* put it in the summer of 1886, of becoming 'the first woman admitted as a surgeon on the roll of the Royal College of Surgeons in Ireland', thus becoming the first *qualified* female surgeon.[39] She had been working officially as the pathologist and unofficially as a 'chloroformist' at the New since 1886, but had secured surgical qualifications when the RCSI took the unprecedented step in opening

---

[36] Louisa Garrett Anderson, *Elizabeth Garrett Anderson*, pp. 243–4.
[37] Elston, 'Women and Anti-Vivisection', p. 85.
[38] *Women and Work*, 13 (Saturday 29 August 1874), 4.
[39] 'MRS. MARY E. DOWSON, L.R.C.S.I.', *BMJ*, 1.1328 (12 June 1886), 1124.

their doors to women in 1885. To lose both women, known, within the medical profession and widely amongst the newspaper and periodical-reading lay public, as surgical pioneers, was a double blow for the New.

The departures began at the start of 1888, but the impact of Meredith's resignation was such that the copy of the *Annual Report* for the previous year, held at the London Metropolitan Archives, shows his name already crossed out, and that of his successor, Knowsley Thornton, another distinguished abdominal surgeon of the Samaritan Free Hospital, added firmly in ink.[40] The Managing Committee Minutes of 1 February 1888 record that Meredith had felt 'obliged' to resign his post as consulting surgeon, and that Thornton had already been engaged in his place. Evidently, Meredith's discomfort in his position had been apparent for some time, if the hospital had already managed to secure another surgeon to replace him. The *Annual Report* for 1887, published in March 1888, noted briefly Meredith's resignation and offered a statement about the 'valuable assistance' he had given 'to the surgical work of the Hospital' over a five-year period.[41] Meredith's 'helping out' here rather than actually undertaking many major operations reveals how keen the hospital was to give the impression that the female staff were taking the lead in clinical work. A protest lodged by Louisa Atkins at the same meeting in which Meredith's resignation was tendered offered a fascinating glimpse into the inner workings of the hospital hierarchy. Garrett Anderson's keenness to uphold the New's purpose as an institution where female medical talents were nurtured was becoming more and more vehement. Proposing that Mary Scharlieb become her clinical assistant at operations, Garrett Anderson encountered a frustrating negative from Atkins, who was not convinced by Scharlieb's surgical competence, and stated unequivocally that she would herself resign if the Committee did not allow her to send serious operation cases to other hospitals if Scharlieb and Garrett Anderson were to work as a surgical team. This dissension from the New's remit as a hospital which supported the clinical ambitions of women doctors presented a shocking ultimatum to the Committee.

It was, however, clearly a step too far, as the next meeting began with Atkins' objections, quoted verbatim in the minutes:

---

[40] *Fifteenth (1886) Annual Report* (1887), p.16.
[41] Minute Books of the Managing Committee of the New Hospital for Women, II, Wednesday 1 February 1888, H13/EGA/20, LMA; *Sixteenth (1887) Annual Report* (1888), p. 6.

37, Gloucester Place

Feb 22/88

To the chairman
Management Committee
Dear Sir,

Referring to the conversation which took place at the last meeting of the Management Committee relative to the present system of operating for abdominal diseases at this Hospital I shall feel much obliged if you will lay my views before the Committee for their consideration.

Hitherto skilled assistance has been applied by Mr Meredith at every serious operation. This assistance is now lacking and I firmly believe that without such assistance the performance of abdominal sections at this Hospital will be injurious to the patients, to the cause of medical women and to the Hospital itself.

Feeling this I could not justify it to my conscience to allow any patient of mine to be operated under the present system. I therefore ask the Committee to consider whether they can allow me either to send my patients to be operated at the Samaritan or to ask Mr Thornton whether he will consent to operate them at the NHW, or, should they consider both these propositions impracticable, whether they can make any other arrangement which will ensure the best interests of the patients.

Otherwise nothing remains for me but to resign my post though I shall do so with great regret for the loss of the post itself and a very real sorrow for the necessary severance from a colleague with whom I have worked amicably for so many years. I am dear Sir

Yours faithfully,
Louisa Atkins.[42]

In this letter, Atkins confirmed the extent to which Meredith had been present at 'every serious operation', implying that Garrett Anderson lacked confidence in operating alone. Such an assessment of the potential disaster awaiting patients at the hands of women surgeons was a stark warning about the paucity of female surgical experience and training.

The Managing Committee responded in an intriguing way. Rather than disregard Atkins' point, they agreed that, although it was not advisable for the reputation of woman doctors and the status of the New itself to send surgical patients elsewhere, they did not want to lose Atkins and would, therefore, ask a reputable witness to comment on Garrett Anderson's surgical technique. It is noticeable that Atkins' original focus

---

[42] Reproduced in the minutes of Wednesday 22 February 1888.

on Scharlieb's capabilities had now disappeared and it was Garrett Anderson who was wholly under scrutiny, suggesting that this was where Atkins' original concern really lay. It is also telling that the idea of submitting Garrett Anderson to independent verification came from Garrett Anderson herself, perhaps both to protect her own surgical standing, as well as, given her doubts about operating, for self-assurance. The receipt of Atkins' complaint further compelled Garrett Anderson to report on every operation to the Committee, as well as, from this point, the recording of every surgical procedure in the *Annual Report* for wider public perusal. Members of the hospital staff and management evidently felt some sensitivity about surgical competence to clarify the facts and figures at the same time as undergoing internal divisions over precisely this issue.

Louisa Atkins was, however, not mollified by such an offer. This controversy had exposed a rift which only widened over the next couple of months. The independent witness, George Granville Bantock, appointed President of the British Gynaecological Society in 1887, refused to undertake an examination of Garrett Anderson's surgery, as he felt that all operations in the hospital should be performed by the all-female staff. Bantock worked with Thornton and Spencer Wells at the Samaritan Hospital in London and was a keen ovariotomist.[43] The support of such an important figure would have been incalculable, but so, because of his defence of the female surgeon, was his refusal. Garrett Anderson continued to operate. By late March 1888, Atkins issued an ultimatum. Either she be allowed to send her patients to a surgeon outside the hospital, as was the norm elsewhere, or she would resign immediately. Atkins' resignation at the beginning of April came after she had, presumably by suggestion, witnessed another operation by Garrett Anderson, which, however,

did not in the least modify my opinion that she is not competent to undertake such operations singlehanded. I deeply regret the course taken by the Committee as it will assuredly confirm the growing opinions that in the minds of the Staff personal or collective advantage takes precedence over the sense of responsibility for the lives of the patients.

---

[43] See, for example, Bantock's article 'Fourth Series of Twenty-Five Cases of Completed Ovariotomy', *BMJ*, 1.1047 (22 January 1881), 112–15 and 'Notes on Three Years' Ovariotomy Work at the Samaritan Free Hospital: Eighty-Two Cases Without a Death', *BMJ*, 1.1435 (30 June 1888), 1375–6. Bantock was also a vehement supporter of non-Listerian methods of antisepsis, preferring absolute cleanliness, as well as an opponent of bacteriology. See 'Notes on Three Years' Ovariotomy Work', 1376, and 'The Modern Doctrine of Bacteriology, or the Germ Theory of Disease', *BMJ*, 1.1997 (8 April 1899), 846–48. For more on antiseptic and aseptic developments in surgery in the late nineteenth century, see Worboys, *Spreading Germs*, especially chapter 5.

This being my own opinion I cannot any longer acquiesce in the existing arrangements and must ask the Committee to appoint my successor at the earliest date possible.

My medical connection with the Hospital being severed you must allow me as a subscriber to express my great surprise that a course of action taken by any members of the Staff which necessitates the resignation from conscientious motives of three members of the Staff should not have been more thoroughly investigated by the Committee; and further to state my opinion which will I believe be shared by all disinterested outsiders that the neglect of the Committee on this point is injurious to the interests of the patients, the Subscribers and the Hospital.[44]

Rather than act professionally in this instance, claimed Atkins, the hospital was compelled to protect and bolster Garrett Anderson in her public image. This meant that the triple resignation, due entirely to 'conscientious motives' and concern for the patients, was obscured from the outside world. To compound this 'neglect', there was to be no enquiry into the reasons for their departure. The Committee was dealt another blow in this meeting, as Mary Dowson also tendered her resignation for precisely the same reason as Atkins. Dowson's letter, less fulsome than Atkins', reflected upon her disagreement with the 'policy now pursued with regard to operations [which] precludes my working in harmony with the Medical Staff'.[45] By supporting Garrett Anderson, as the most senior woman doctor in the hospital and the most renowned female medical pioneer in Britain, the Committee had lost three valuable members of staff in as many months. The cause of medical women and their right to perform surgery had been supported, but only by disregarding the mistakes, which Atkins and Dowson had felt sufficiently serious to merit complaint.

In June 1888, Meredith wrote to clarify his reasons for departure. He 'found that the record of Mrs Anderson's operations at which he had been present shewed too high a percentage of failures', but that he 'should always retain a kindly feeling towards the Hospital and its staff'.[46] Subscribers, as predicted by Atkins, also expressed concern at the evident problems within the 'internal workings' of the hospital, and two wrote for clarification. They were pacified with the knowledge that a difference of opinion had resulted and that staff had resigned rather than

---

[44] Copy of Louisa Atkins' resignation letter from minutes of Wednesday 11 April 1888.
[45] Copy of Mary E. Dowson's resignation letter, dated 3 April 1888, in minutes of meeting held Wednesday 11 April 1888.
[46] Noted in the minutes of Wednesday 6 June 1888.

been dismissed from their posts.[47] The Hospital Letter Book contains the response to Miss A.R.C. Wainwright, which was dated 24 April 1888. Miss Bagster's tone was defensive, but honest:

Dear Madam,

We are having papers printed to send to the subscribers to inform them of the changes in the Medical Staff.

With regard to Miss Atkins's resignation, her own explanation was that she could not consent that her own patients should be operated on in severe cases by one of the Women Physicians.

It was with great reluctance that the Committee accepted her resignation.[48]

However, Miss Wainwright was clearly not yet satisfied with the explanation and the following letter in the book asked her to attend a meeting with the Committee.[49] The fact that this letter was dated three months after the last implied that a brief correspondence was insufficient. A more personal explanation from the Committee themselves must have resolved the issue, as there were no more letters from Miss Wainwright.

In public, the summer of 1888 saw the launch of fundraising for new premises, whereby, in opposition to the surgical controversies of recent months, the phrases 'low death-rate' and 'skill, care and attention' formed a consistent refrain whenever the hospital was mentioned.[50] In June 1888, Garrett Anderson's surgical skills were witnessed and approved by the curious choice of Francis Imlach, a surgeon at the Women's Hospital in Liverpool, and a man who was no stranger to libellous remarks about his own capabilities. Only two years previously a scandal had threatened to end his career, when Imlach had been accused of performing unnecessary ovariotomies, and 'unsexing' his patients. Although he was acquitted of any wrongdoing, both in an internal enquiry and after a complaint from a patient's husband was rejected in court, Imlach's reputation, as well as the cause of radical surgical procedures for the diseases of women, received a setback. Garrett Anderson had been called upon as

---

[47] A letter from Mrs Parish was mentioned in the minutes of Wednesday 6 June. Miss Wainwright's complaint about the ignorance in which subscribers were kept is mentioned in the minutes on Wednesday 13 June 1888. Her concern was addressed in the meeting on Tuesday 26 June.

[48] Letter from Miss Bagster to Miss A.R.C. Wainwright, 24 April 1888 in *Hospital Secretary's Letter Book*, H13/EGA/229, LMA.

[49] Ibid., 14 June 1888.

[50] See the newspaper cuttings reporting upon the public meeting in aid of the Building Fund on 7 July 1888, including extracts from *Daily Chronicle*, *City Press*, *Times*, and *Globe*, ANC.

an expert for the report investigating Imlach's cases, and had concluded 'that the work done during the year is very creditable to the skill and courage of the medical staff of the hospital'.[51] Imlach repaid her loyalty when Garrett Anderson's skills were questioned: '"Have just witnessed as difficult an abdominal section as any surgeon could have to perform; and think that in technical skill and promptness I have never seen anything much more perfect". Francis Imlach'.[52] The 'four or five' procedures originally suggested by Garrett Anderson herself in February, in order to appease Louisa Atkins, had been reduced to just one unidentified abdominal section. Additionally, her competence had been assessed by someone whose own had only very recently been scrutinised.

With the backing of the hospital's Managing Committee and independent verification of her abilities, Garrett Anderson began to perform more complex and risky procedures 'entirely without outside help'.[53] It was also noticeable that she reported on her operations at meetings of the Managing Committee, either for self- or institutional reassurance. Even while the disagreements with Atkins were at their height, Garrett Anderson, in a specific section of the meetings now devoted to her surgical report, made clear her performance of unspecified 'difficult abdominal operation[s]', where the patient was 'so far doing well'.[54] Yet this was also in line, as Sally Wilde argues, with the trend in the 1890s, as procedures developed, for major, new surgery to be performed, which had never been attempted by the surgeon before.[55] Interestingly, soon after the triple staff resignations, oophorecetomies were first conducted in 1888. That year, Garrett Anderson was vindicated, as there was only one operation death out of 54 cases, and now they were listed separately for the first time, this success was even more evident. The following

---

51 As quoted in *Liverpool Mercury*, 12162 (Friday 31 December 1886), 3. The paper contains a number of letters in the second half of 1886 from the husbands of patients who claim their wives have been 'unsexed' by the procedure, which offer a patient-related perspective on this controversial operation. See, especially, the correspondence from 'Justice', who laments that his wife was not informed of 'the consequences of the operation': 'are they told the extent to which the operation known as ovariotomy will incapacitate them?', 12050 (Monday 23 August, 1886), 6.

For more on the 'Imlach Case', see Morantz-Sanchez, *Conduct Unbecoming*, pp. 127–8. The implications of the Imlach case were still rumbling on at the beginning of the twentieth century. See 'The Imlach Controversy', *BMJ*, 2.2129 (19 October 1901), 1176–9.

52 Reported in the minutes of Tuesday 26 June 1888.

53 A letter from Elizabeth Garrett Anderson about two operations carried out on 25 July 1889, quoted in Louisa Garrett Anderson, *Elizabeth Garrett Anderson*, p. 274.

54 Minutes of the Managing Committee, 7 March 1888.

55 Wilde, 'Truth, Trust', 316.

year there was only one death, again from an ovariotomy, this time from a total of 81 cases.[56] Over the next three years, the hospital saw a move away from operations concentrating on the diseases of women and entered new surgical territory, with the introduction of ophthalmic surgery, as well as the performance of a splenectomy in 1890, and nephrectomies from 1891. The latter operation had first been performed successfully in Britain only six years before Garrett Anderson's attempt, by a member of New's consulting staff, Knowsley Thornton.[57] Surgery on the spleen was very rarely attempted, even in the experimental 1890s by the most prominent risk-takers. As Skene Keith noted in 1894: '[t]he general mortality has been so great that an operation which may have to end in the removal of the spleen is one which requires very grave consideration'.[58] Five years later, the American surgeon Charles T. Parkes concluded that splenectomy was 'attended with such overwhelming mortality, that its performance can scarcely be justified'.[59] Despite Thornton's experience, he had sworn after two further failures, where both patients bled to death, and the death four years later of his only successful case, never to perform this procedure again.[60] Thus it appears that Garrett Anderson took the lead here; this was corroborated in a letter to her sister Millicent Garrett Fawcett, which noted the rarity of the procedure:

---

[56] See 'Operation Cases', *Eighteenth (1889) Annual Report* (1890), p. 18.

[57] Knowsley Thornton, 'Two Cases of Splenectomy', *Medico-Chirurgical Transactions*, 69 (1886), 407–417. Spencer Wells had unsuccessfully performed a splenectomy in 1865. Twelve out of the 34 operations had been performed in Britain, with Thornton's the only success; the Italians led the way with four completed procedures (416–17). By 1888, Spencer Wells had been successful: 'Remarks on Splenectomy, With a Report of a Successful Case', *Medico-Chirurgical Transactions*, 71 (1888), 255–63. This operation occurred in December 1887. This had increased to two successes for Wells by the end of 1890. See Wells, 'The Bradshaw Lecture on Modern Abdominal Surgery', *BMJ*, 2.1565 (27 December 1890), 1465–8. These results differ from those noted by Harold Ellis, who attributes the first successes to French and German surgeons, and the first British attempt in 1895. See *The Cambridge Illustrated History of Surgery* (Cambridge: Cambridge University Press, 2009), p. 109.

[58] Skene Keith, *Textbook of Abdominal Surgery* (Edinburgh and London: Young J. Pentland, 1894), p. 310.

[59] Charles T. Parkes, *Clinical Lectures in Abdominal Surgery and Other Subjects* (Chicago: Chicago Medical Book Co., 1899), p. 73.

[60] Knowsley Thornton, 'A Lecture on the Lines of Advance in Abdominal Surgery', *BMJ*, 1.1835 (29 February 1896), 513–17; 514.

In 1886, Lawson Tait also commented that splenectomy was an 'operation which I myself have not yet ventured to perform, and do not think that when performed for disease of the spleen [...] is ever likely to be successful', *Liverpool Mercury*, 12162 (Friday 31 December 1886), 3.

I had a very big operation at the New yesterday and so far all promises very well with the patient [...] [I]f mine recovers it will be quoted for a long time. – I fancy too that [mine crossed out] the tumour in my case was larger than any yet. It was a much overgrown spleen. I tell you this for the <u>sake of the cause</u>.[61]

Unfortunately, the patient died from septicaemia, so Garrett Anderson had achieved neither plaudits for the hospital nor for the female surgeon. Risk had been implemented at the New for 'the sake of the cause'; precisely what had been feared by Louisa Atkins two years previously.

Between 1891 and 1892, six nephrectomies resulted in a 66.7 per cent mortality rate; in 1888, Lawson Tait had recorded, from 12 cases, only two patient deaths.[62] There was an inevitable element of risk in performing new procedures such as this, but, with the surgical profession still acquiring confidence in itself, surgery at the New had to be carried out with an eye to innovation and progression if women were to operate fully.[63] The increase in procedures and specifically in serious abdominal operations was noted by the House Committee at the beginning of 1892. A 'great tax' was being placed on the nursing staff, which had been necessarily supplemented by outside help.[64] The hospital was simply not prepared for an upsurge in operations. By May of that year, however, a dedicated 'Ovarian Ward' had been created, later to be renamed the Louisa Isaac Ward, creating space for the recovery of serious operative cases, as well as indicating the dedication to still-controversial procedures.[65] When Garrett Anderson decided to hand over her post to Scharlieb in autumn 1892, 44 major operations and abdominal sections had been performed, with a mortality rate of 13.6 per cent, more than double the previous year, when there were 84 cases (minus eye operations), but with just under 6 per cent mortality. By the time she passed on her post, Garrett Anderson had been assisting others and performing surgery herself for 20 years. She had not been specially trained in the discipline, but then, as Scharlieb put it, early women medical pioneers were 'never able to be what is called pure physicians or pure surgeons. We

---

[61] Elizabeth Garrett Anderson to Millicent Garrett Fawcett, 22 October 1890, Autograph Letter Collection, The Women's Library, 9/10/111 (ALC/3001).

[62] There were three operations in each year; with two deaths and one recovery: *Nineteenth and Twentieth Annual Reports* for 1891 and 1892 (1892; 1893), p. 20.
    Lawson Tait, 'General Summary of Conclusions from a Second Series of One Thousand Consecutive Cases of Abdominal Section', *BMJ*, 2.1455 (17 November 1888), 1096–100; 1100.

[63] On the surgeon's acquisition of 'confidence' in the 1890s, see Wilde, 'Truth, Trust', 324.

[64] Meeting of 5 March 1892, Minutes of the House Committee of the New Hospital for Women: February 1890–January 1894, H13/EGA/035, LMA.

[65] Meeting of 25 May 1892, ibid.

had of necessity in those early days to be willing to give advice to women as to their health, whether from the medical, surgical or obstetric point of view'.[66] Female medical staff at the New had proved that women could perform complex and difficult procedures. The woman surgeon could exist, and operate no differently to her male comrades, who had received more specialist clinical and surgical training. However, while surgery revealed precisely what women could do, it also highlighted their limitations. The early woman surgeon was forced to contend with her own difficulties, but she was also faced with opposition from her colleagues. If, as Garrett Anderson claimed, one could only become skilful though experience – 'no one can operate well who is not operating constantly' – curtailing and disrupting practice was a regular feature of the first 20 years of the NHW.[67] Although the New was founded to support medical careers, surgery was one area in which male and female members of staff could unite against the progression of the woman doctor.

The 1890s

Controversy was not to leave the woman surgeon in the 1890s, but scandal was tempered with success. This decade saw both ongoing controversy surrounding Garrett Anderson's surgical principles, even when she was not actually practising at the hospital, and, with a new team operating, a formalisation of the NHW's commitment to the cause of female surgeons. The number of operations increased, as indicated in Figure 1.1, yet they did so at a steady rate and ranged more widely than the predominantly gynaecological procedures carried out during Garrett Anderson's reign. This is not to state that the decade which witnessed Mary Scharlieb's management of the New's surgical side saw the primary focus of the institution change nor that the 'cause', as Garrett Anderson would have put it, was in any way discouraged by the operations performed. Rather, Scharlieb's decade-long regime was characterised by the recognition that the individual operator was part of a team of professionals, who acted together for the good of the patient. The period between 1892 and 1902 was one of consolidation at the NHW, where female surgeons were encouraged to carry out a wider range of surgery to enhance their experience. It was also one where, in spite of continuing attacks upon their abilities, women surgeons gained confidence by operating quietly and allowing the statistics to speak for themselves.

---

[66] Scharlieb, *Reminiscences*, p. 141.
[67] Garrett Anderson quoted in Scharlieb, *Reminiscences*, p. 134.

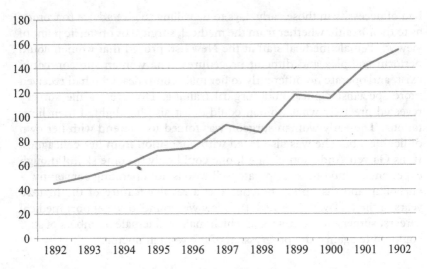

Figure 1.1 Major Operations Carried Out: NHW, 1892–1902.[68]

Within a month of Garrett Anderson's resignation, the Managing Committee received the report of the Medical and Sub-Committees which called for the following resolutions:

1) That members of the Medical Staff should retire at the age of 60.
2) That Mrs Scharlieb and Miss Cock should be appointed to the Inpatient Surgeons.
3) That Miss Webb and Mrs Boyd be appointed to the Outpatient Surgeons for five years.
   [...] 8) Abdominal operations. That Mrs Scharlieb be authorised to perform these operations and Mrs Boyd assist. That no member of the staff be authorised to perform abdominal operations until she has acted as principal assistant in this hospital with at least 12 cases; and that any number of staff may claim the right to assist with their own cases.[69]

The resolutions were put to the vote and passed. What is interesting about the first point is that Garrett Anderson had retired from the New at the age of 56. While the mistakes perceived in the 1880s were never put down to the age of the surgeon, it was clearly a concern for the future. Additionally, of course, retirement when posts for women were still so scarce was fundamental to fulfilling the hospital's mission statement of assisting female members of the medical profession to gain institutional

[68] Statistics calculated from *Annual Reports*.
[69] Minute Books of the Managing Committee, II, 1 December 1892.

experience.[70] Similarly, points 2 and 3 rewarded the experience of Schar-lieb, Cock, Webb and Boyd, while simultaneously restricting the outpa-tient roles of the latter two to five years only. As hospital clinical work was always gained first at outpatients, this allowed both the chance to progress to in-patient roles, but also to permit others, in turn, to take their place seeing temporary cases. The most telling point, given the concerns about surgical ineptitude, was number 8, which demanded at least a dozen assistant roles before abdominal operations could be carried out. If the 1890s was characterised by the growth in experimental procedures, the NHW was urging caution, at least as far as operating-theatre personnel were concerned, and insisting upon some practical experience for its sur-geons. This point also gave members of staff more control over their own cases. That Garrett Anderson had taken the lead in surgery at the hospital was evident when, upon her departure in November 1892, the New was also deprived of its surgical instruments. Some more would be needed, remarked the Secretary, as 'Mrs Anderson would be no longer lending those that she had been in the habit of bringing for major operations'.[71] Without Garrett Anderson exercising manual control,[72] although there was a need for new instruments, there was evidently more freedom to follow patients from consultation to operation, as well as participating in their surgical care. The Managing Committee, in approving the demands made by their medical counterpart, had evidently learnt from the débâcle of the previous decade that rifts could not be healed by placing trust only in one person.

With this change in outlook after Garrett Anderson's departure, it is fruitful to consider how the New dealt with very public accusations of surgical misconduct. Two controversies hit the institution during the 1890s, but they were handled very differently to those of the 1880s. Both stemmed from criticism about the ways in which surgery was performed

[70] In a footnote to this desire to keep the personnel of the hospital moving, it is intriguing to note that some members of staff clearly did not want to lose their posts to others. In 1916, long-standing member of the Managing Committee, Alice Westlake, wrote to the Chairman, A. Gordon Pollock, to complain that not all medical staff were as highly principled as Louisa Aldrich-Blake. Maud Chadburn, who was a founder of the South London Hospital for Women, discussed in chapter 5, came in for particular scorn, as 'selfish' for keeping 'both posts in her own hands, when the younger doctors are so much in want of hospital practice'. See letter dated 30 May 1916 from Alice Westlake to A. Gordon Pollock, Historical Papers, H13/EGA/228/5, LMA.

[71] Meeting of 7 November 1892, Minutes of the House Committee.

[72] On the ways in which surgical instruments allow the surgeon manual control, see Ghislaine Lawrence, 'The Ambiguous Artifact: Surgical Instruments and the Surgical Past', in Lawrence, ed., Medical Theory, Surgical Practice, pp. 295–314; and, more recently, Thomas Schlich, 'Negotiating Technologies in Surgery: The Controversy about Surgical Gloves in the 1890s', BHM, 87.2 (Summer 2013), 170–97; 170–1.

at the New. The first came from a surprising source: Elizabeth Blackwell, the 73-year-old *grande dame* of medical women. Her opinion was sought in connection with ongoing rumblings of discontent about the ways in which hospital patients were abused and experimented upon by blood-thirsty, ambitious surgeons. In May 1894, the *Daily Chronicle* newspaper ran a campaign to expose what it labelled 'human vivisection', a practice, it noted, which was occurring in hospitals throughout Britain. The out-cry was part of a late-Victorian obsession with the increasing power of medicine and the medical profession over defenceless individuals, who were stripped of their liberty by the probing instruments of scientific experimentation.[73] Vaccinators and vivisectors had borne the brunt of public loathing for over a decade; now it was the turn of the surgeon to be subjected to charges of brutality. 'Houses of charity', shrieked the *Chronicle*, were being turned, by younger, ambitious members of the sur-gical profession, into 'butchers shops' [*sic*], whereby innocent, and it was alleged, healthy, individuals were persuaded to undergo unnecessary and dangerous operations. Not for their own benefit, of course, but all for the desire to 'destroy human lives in the interests of science'. Accord-ing to the *Chronicle*'s exposé, the grasping surgeon experimented upon patients solely to keep up with the latest 'surgical fads', while unsuspect-ing patients simply agreed to the operator's demands.

The paper lambasted the Dickensian-sounding youths who made up future practitioners:

The new school consists of [. . .] enthusiasts who have only just passed from the stage at which young men go forth from the hospitals on football or boat-race nights to parade the West End in gangs, knock foot passengers off the pavement, and then, in the interests of what they call sport, destroy the glasses of some more or less innocent proprietor of a West End drinking-bar; and, having returned to their Bayswater or Bloomsbury lodging in the early morning and tried to sleep off the effects of bad whisky and worse cigars, go forth to gloat over men older than themselves destroying human lives in the interests of science.[74]

Louche, irresponsible, idle and careless, these were the people in whose hands lay innocent lives; untrustworthy, clumsy and dangerous youths. The claim that daring operative procedures represented progression was dismissed scornfully, as contemporary surgery was branded uncivilised and barbaric. In a celebratory edition, published for the Diamond Jubilee

---

[73] For an account of the reaction against medical intervention during this period, see, for example, Nadia Durbach, *Bodily Matters* (Durham, NC: Duke University Press, 2005).
[74] 'The *Daily Chronicle* on Human Vivisection', *BMJ*, 1.1743 (26 May 1894), 1143–4; 1143.

of Victoria's accession to the throne, the *BMJ* begged to differ. Labelling the era a 'Renaissance' as far as the advancement of surgery was concerned, the periodical concluded that 'Heaven has given us a new race of men'. It was indeed a 'Golden Age':

The student sixty years ago would see an occasional operation for strangulated hernia, perhaps an ovariotomy; there he would stop. The radical cure of hernia, known to Paré, had fallen into disuse; the surgery of the liver, the gall bladder, and the kidney was unknown. Perforation of the stomach, or the bowels, or the appendix, was left to itself; cases of acute obstruction shared the same fate; so did ruptures of the abdominal viscera from external violence. The general work of abdominal surgery was hardly so much attempted, save perhaps once or twice in a surgeon's lifetime. Of such success as we now obtain there was not a trace.[75]

Where the *Chronicle* saw destruction and frailty, the *BMJ* envisaged exploration and progress: the preservation of health rather than the wilful encouragement of illness. For the latter, the Victorian period had witnessed unprecedented 'success' through the development of procedures previously considered impossible and the conquering of disease in organs and parts of the body assumed inaccessible. Risk was essential to progress.

. It was surgical exploration of and operation upon the abdomen, however, which still caused the greatest outcry at the end of the nineteenth century. The *Chronicle* article had been prompted by a report issued by the Medical Officer of Health for Chelsea, Dr Louis Parkes, who had recently expressed concern about the disproportionate number of fatal operations at the Chelsea Hospital for Women. Hospitals specialising in the diseases of women were, time and again, the focus of public distrust. Some of the most virulent controversy surrounded abdominal surgery on women; the surgeon demonised in popular culture as a human vivisector, experimenting dangerously and without a care upon the defenceless female, robbed of her organs of generation. Ovariotomy was considered both 'the starting point in the modern advance of abdominal surgery', as Spencer Wells put it, and a practice considered initially as 'little short of murder', as Ornella Moscucci has noted.[76] Notorious cases such as that of Francis Imlach and the more recent accusations of Alice Beatty against her surgeon Charles Cullingworth for removing both her ovaries

---

[75] 'The Renaissance of Surgery in the Victorian Age: Abdominal Surgery, 1837–1897', *BMJ*, 1.1903 (19 June 1897), 1527–31; 1527; 1530.

[76] Sir Thomas Spencer Wells, 'The Bradshaw Lecture on Modern Abdominal Surgery', *BMJ*, 2.1564 (20 December 1890), 1413–16; 1413, and Ornella Moscucci, *The Science of Woman* (Cambridge: Cambridge University Press, 1990), p. 134.

without consent helped to keep such controversial surgical procedures in the public mind.[77] With such a history, abdominal surgery, particularly that upon women, was both momentous progress and barbaric regression. The subject was particularly emotive when the popularity of operations to 'unsex' women was contemporaneous with the increasing social anxiety over the high rate of infant mortality.[78]

For some, the risk was unacceptable. The *Daily Chronicle* sought the viewpoint of the first woman to qualify professionally as a doctor by being placed on the Medical Register: the British-born, but American-raised, Elizabeth Blackwell. Despite Blackwell's age, her iconic status meant that the *Chronicle* had secured an impressive scoop. Blackwell had a great deal to say about the alarming, as she saw it, trajectory of the woman who performed daring surgical procedures. She feared that surgery, with its glamorous and daring status, had replaced medicine as a 'cure-all'. The modern-day approach, she felt, was too hurried and too impatient. Blackwell's concerns were not only for helpless female patients, however. She used the *Chronicle* reporter to voice her distrust of those women only too keen to perform 'reckless operations' which 'maim[ed]' their own sex for life. Prompted by what sounded like an attack upon her fellow medical women, the reporter asked: 'Do you consider that women practitioners are less liable to this "operative madness" than men?' Blackwell's response was intriguing:

I have no hesitation in saying that *at present* my own sex is suffering from the epidemic, but it is imparted to them by their surroundings. You see it is very contagious. They learn from men, and live in the atmosphere of surgery. They are over-anxious to do as men do, and so their reverence of creation and their sympathy for the poor and suffering is in abeyance. A woman – and a very clever one – boasted recently that she had just completed her fiftieth operation of a particular and very dangerous kind – a kind such as I think it must have been difficult to find within her reach, fifty cases in which it was necessitated. She had probably been taught that the operation was frequently necessary, and she is no more reckless than those who taught her; but her sense of humanity was, perhaps, for a while in abeyance. I am, however, persuaded that this will pass away so far as women are concerned; the danger is an almost inevitable accompaniment of the early stages of a movement in the ultimate success of which I have the greatest belief – the educating of women so that they may alleviate the physical sufferings of their own sex, not only as nurses, but as physicians and surgeons. I do not believe that the study and practice of surgery necessarily tend to unsex a woman.

---

[77] For more on the Beatty versus Cullingworth case, see my article, 'Risk, Responsibility and Surgery in the 1890s and early 1900s', *MH*, 57.3 (July 2013), 317–37.

[78] See, for example, Anna Davin, 'Imperialism and Motherhood', *History Workshop Journal* (*HWJ*), 5 (1978), 9–65.

It is a noble work, this curing of disease, and must be nobly done, whether by men or women.[79]

Blackwell had intended to devote her life to surgery, but had been infected with purulent ophthalmia by a young patient at La Maternité in Paris, which had left her blind in one eye and incapable of intricate surgical procedures. She was, therefore, unable to become, as she had hoped, 'the first lady surgeon in the world'.[80] So, while Blackwell did not believe that the existence of the woman surgeon was wrong per se, the aping of the infectious masculine swagger of surgical success could only detract from the true 'curing of disease'. It was this discrepancy between the risks involved in opening up a patient and the ultimate restoration of health which was so distressing for this elderly pioneer.

Blackwell drew pointed attention in this interview to a very clever female boaster, who could only be Elizabeth Garrett Anderson. As we have seen in the first part of this chapter, Garrett Anderson was notoriously keen to promote the surgical work done at the NHW for the 'sake of the cause'. Blackwell criticised Garrett Anderson for three things. Firstly, performing unnecessary procedures and therefore ignoring the real cause of illness in order to risk lives for reputation's sake; secondly, for trying to compete with and even outdo male surgeons; and, finally, because a combination of both these reasons meant she was losing her humanity in the process. Indeed, even though Blackwell was still acting – in name, if not literally – as a consultant physician to the New, the Managing Committee of the hospital chose to maintain a dignified silence over these pointed accusations. In the first meeting of the Committee after the article was published, on 31 May 1894, the notes record that the Chairman, Mr Gaselee, will write to Garrett Anderson – evidently the target of the accusations – to prevent her from responding to Blackwell's article or from being interviewed in the Daily Chronicle.[81] The fact that this was passed unanimously revealed how troubled they were by Garrett Anderson's potential to make matters worse, by engaging in public combat with her predecessor. After a decade of internal divisions over surgical procedures, drawing attention to the painful schisms which had existed in the hospital would not encourage its patients to undergo some of the operations at which Blackwell was hinting. Nor would accusations of recklessness, as far as patients were concerned, do

[79] 'Human Vivisection: Interview with Dr Elizabeth Blackwell', Daily Chronicle, 22 May 1894, ANC.

[80] Elizabeth Blackwell, Pioneer Work in Opening the Medical Profession to Women (London and New York: Longmans, Green and Co., 1895), p. 154; p. 157.

[81] Minute Books of the Managing Committee II.

anything for the reputation of the female surgeon. Blackwell was clearly willing, without directly identifying perpetrators, to critique the hospital for which she still acted as consultant. That institution, however, was not willing to involve itself in an unseemly debate which could only sorely inflame public sensibilities and hint that all was not well among 'lady doctors'.

Three years later, in October 1897, another accusation of improper conduct was directed at the NHW. Unlike the *Chronicle* attack, however, this one named the hospital outright, even pinpointing its location. The only saving grace in this latest scandal was that it took place in an American medical publication and much effort was expended in order to keep it on the other side of the Atlantic. A. Earnest Gallant responded to a recent editorial on 'Anaesthesia as a Speciality' in the New York-based *Medical Record* with a corresponding glance at British anaesthetists. To do this, he posed a series of questions about the development of the specialty to his friend George Bell Todd, Professor of Zoology at Anderson College Medical School and well-known Scottish practitioner. In an apparently innocuous article, Bell Todd made a curiously libellous comment. Apropos of nothing, he stated: 'I may here remark that female medical practitioners in this country are peculiarly unfitted to give anaesthetics. That such is the case I know from experience and it is well illustrated at the Women's Hospital, Euston Road, London, which is remarkable for the failures in administering chloroform correctly.'[82] Here Bell Todd unmistakably identified the New, which had, of course, moved to the Euston Road in 1890. Neither did he mention any other institution by name nor critique any other administrator of anaesthetics, so the NHW's prominence, or, it might be said, failure, was more pronounced. Furthermore, Bell Todd did not support his comment with any other evidence. The surgeon was not blamed for any mistakes while a patient was on the operating table, but responsibility was placed squarely in the hands of the anaesthetist. Such focused censure for errors made during surgery may, however, provide an explanation as to why Bell Todd directed such bile at the NHW.

As Ian Burney has remarked, the 1890s witnessed developments in the professionalization of the anaesthetist, but also a corresponding increase in anaesthetic deaths.[83] This, in turn, fuelled the wider publicity during the same period surrounding the danger and unreliability

---

[82] 'Anaesthesia and its Administration in Great Britain and Ireland, with Special Reference · Made to its Being Made a Specialty', *Medical Record: A Weekly Journal of Medicine and Surgery*, 52.20 (13 November 1897), 722–3.

[83] Ian Burney, *Bodies of Evidence* (Baltimore, MD: Johns Hopkins University Press, 2000), p. 140.

of anaesthesia,[84] and, ultimately, the practise of surgery in Britain. In the early 1890s the anaesthetist to the hospital was Mrs Keith, who had been in her post since 1889 and was noted as having given anaesthetics 115 times during 1893.[85] In the autumn of 1893, the House Committee had also called for a book specifically to note the administration of anaesthesia, evidently aware that a record was crucial.[86] Deaths from the process were few, however, in spite of Bell Todd's accusations. Of eight surgical deaths in 1893, only one resulted while under anaesthesia.[87] This death was publicised and the report in the *BMJ* might have given Bell Todd cause for concern. 'Death Under Chloroform' was a regular feature in the periodical, but not one which frequently detailed cases at the New. The dead patient had suffered from goitre and some dyspnoea, but displayed no evidence of cardiac or respiratory disease. There were no problems to begin with, but after ten minutes, the chloroform was removed due to rapid, deep breathing. Breathing then ceased and although artificial respiration was carried out for three-quarters of an hour, the patient showed no signs of recovery.[88] The Hospital Letters Book provides further information about what happened to 43-year-old Mrs Jane Valentine, including a heart-breaking response to her husband, who, whether through superstition or distrust of anaesthesia, had clearly sought to prevent the operation to which his wife had consented. As the secretary writes:

Dear Sir,

It is with the greatest regret I have to tell you that the operation of your wife was begun before I received your letter. She had expressed her wish to have it done and gave her consent.

I feel deeply sorry that we did not hear from you sooner for your wife died under the chloroform. I can only add my sorrow for you in this great trouble.[89]

Notification of the death was also made to the coroner through a letter from the Resident Medical Officer, Annie Anderson, who stated that 'a patient died from the effects of chloroform administered for an operation for removal of part of the thyroid gland'. She continued that death was in no way due to the operation, which had barely begun, and that artificial respiration and circulation were carried on for some time

[84] Ibid., p. 141.   [85] Minutes of the Managing Committee, II, 11 January 1894.
[86] Meeting of 13 October 1893, Minutes of the House Committee.
[87] *Twenty-Second (1893) Annual Report* (1894), p. 20.
[88] 'Death Under Chloroform', *BMJ*, 2.1696 (1 July 1893), 33.
[89] Letter to Mr Valentine, dated 17 July [*sic*] 1893, Hospital Secretary's Letters Book.

after apparent death.[90] The inquest on Mrs Valentine was further noted in the Minutes of the Managing Committee on 13 July.[91] Neither the letter to Mr Valentine, the report to the coroner, nor the acknowledgment of the death in the *BMJ* mentioned the sex of anaesthetist or surgeon; the assumption, naturally, was that both were female.

In fact, while we can assume that the anaesthetist was Mrs Keith, the operator was in fact James Berry of the Royal Free Hospital, consulting surgeon to the New since 1891, and a specialist in the removal of goitres, who had clearly been called in especially for this difficult case.[92] Berry's leading role in this operation revealed inadvertently that the New were still seeking outside help for some procedures. Previously, a goitre sufferer in 1889 had been sent to the RFH, presumably to Berry, two cases in 1891 had been relieved, but not operated upon, while not one goitre patient for the rest of Scharlieb's regime underwent surgery at the hospital, even though there were six cases in 1902.[93] There were clearly some instances when even Garrett Anderson had acknowledged her lack of experience for the benefit of the patient, and Scharlieb evidently followed suit. The onlookers in Mrs Valentine's procedure were Stanley Boyd, Surgeon to the Charing Cross Hospital and consulting surgeon to the New, as well as other NHW staff members. When he wrote about this case in 1900, Berry remarked on a number of points relevant to the decision to operate on 'Jane V.'. Mrs Valentine's goitre was especially dangerous, as it was both parenchymatous, and causing her dyspnoea, which required urgent operative treatment before it killed her. Anaesthesia was, therefore, vital, as the goitre required extirpating rather than a less serious enucleation. However, the death of Jane Valentine caused Berry to rethink his policy as to how a patient suffering from dyspnoea should be treated. He had, before this case, considered a general anaesthetic indispensable, regardless of the patient's condition, but in later procedures Berry adopted morphine, cocaine or encaine. Though only suffering three deaths from the 72 goitre patients upon whom he had performed extirpation, Berry justified his actions even in these fatal outcomes, because of the severity of dyspnoea. He concluded: 'I know of

90 Letter from RMO Annie M.S. Anderson, dated 17 VI [*sic*], Ibid.
91 Minutes of the Managing Committee, II, 13 July 1893.
92 Notification of Berry's appointment can be found in *Nineteenth (1890) Annual Report* (1891), p. 7. For more on Berry's career at the RFH, see Lynsey T. Cullen, 'Patient Records of the Royal Free Hospital, 1902–1912', PhD thesis, Oxford Brookes University, 2011.
93 See *Eighteenth (1889) Annual Report* (1890), p. 16; *Twentieth (1891) Annual Report* (1892), p. 18; and *Thirty-First (1902) Annual Report* (1903), p. 20.
    For more on the thyroid in the late nineteenth and early twentieth centuries, see Schlich, *Origins*, especially chapters 6 and 7.

no class of patients so grateful to the surgeon as those from whom a suffocating goitre has been removed'.[94] Although neither this, nor Berry's change in procedure, was any consolation for the Valentine family, the necessity of the goitre's removal overrode any concerns about the application of anaesthetics.

As the only publicised case of death under anaesthesia at the hospital in the early 1890s, it must have been what prompted Bell Todd's barbed comment. While Bell Todd blamed the anaesthetist in every failed procedure, Berry would surely have advised the member of his operating team dispensing the anaesthetic, especially if specialist care was required. By making the anaesthetist responsible, Bell Todd shifted the fatal outcome onto the shoulders of the dispenser rather than the adviser. Either way, he deemed the anaesthetist incorrect in her application and, therefore, professionally incompetent. If anaesthetic could not be dispensed accurately, neither could operations be carried out successfully: failure characterised the NHW. Although Bell Todd's words were published in late 1897, it was not until February 1898 that the Managing Committee of the hospital became aware of the slanderous accusations levelled at their surgical staff. They wrote immediately to ascertain whether the remarks could be 'rightly attributed' to Bell Todd and upon 'what facts [he] base[d] the statement'.[95] Although Bell Todd responded reasonably quickly to this letter, he did not answer the second question about his sources for the claim.[96] There were no further records of correspondence in the Hospital Secretary's Letters Book, but the minutes of the Managing Committee offered more insight into how seriously the New took this unfounded report. The necessity of 'plac[ing] the matter in the hands of a lawyer' was mentioned at the meeting on 3 February 1898, when the story was first brought to the Committee's attention by the anaesthetist. Bell Todd clearly defended his stance, because on 10 March, legal advice had been sought and Bell Todd was communicated with again, without response this time. The minute concluded with a decision to send a solicitor's letter to state that unless an apology was sent to the hospital the correspondence would be sent to the *BMJ*.[97] Bell Todd evidently backed

---

[94] James Berry, 'Notes on Seventy-Two Consecutive Cases of Removal of Goitre by Operation (Extirpation or Enucleation)', *BMJ*, 2.2062 (7 July 1900), 3–11; 11. He later noted in 1920 that he was using local anaesthesia less and less for goitre operations, as anaesthetic expertise in light ether anaesthesia was preferable. See 'Discussion on Anaesthesia in Operations on the Thyroid Gland', *PRSM*, 13 (1920), 52–5; 55.

[95] Letter to Prof. George Bell Todd, dated 3 February 1898, Hospital Secretary's Letter Book.

[96] Ibid., dated 15 February 1898; Bell Todd's had been dated 10 February.

[97] Minutes of the Managing Committee, III: April 1895–March 1906, 3 February and 10 March 1898, H13/EGA/21, LMA.

down at this point, although it was not until the summer that a solution was sought. A letter was drafted by Greenwell, the New's solicitor, and it was requested that Bell Todd publish it in the original American periodical, as well as the *Lancet* and the *BMJ*. A month later, however, Bell Todd had evidently demanded alterations, which were not accepted. It had also been decided, upon Greenwell's advice, not to submit the apology to the British medical journals.[98] In September 1898, nearly a year after the initial accusations of misconduct had appeared, George Bell Todd's response was published in America.

It is worth quoting the dictated letter in full.

To the Editor of the Medical Record.

Sir: My attention has been drawn to an article which appeared in your issue of November 13th last, under the title of 'Anaesthesia and its Administration in Great Britain and Ireland', by Prof. George Bell Todd, of Glasgow, and in which I am made to say that the Women's Hospital, Euston Road, London, 'is remarkable for the failures in administering chloroform correctly'.

The article in question was a private communication from myself to a friend, and published without my knowledge or consent.

With reference to the extract above quoted I would remark that the information has been furnished to me by the authorities of the said hospital, from which it appears that between January 1, 1894, and December 31, 1897, anaesthetics were administered thirteen hundred times at the hospital, that there were during that period two deaths on the operating-table. Inquests were held in both cases, and in one instance only was a verdict of 'death from chloroform' returned. This shows that the above-quoted statement is unfounded and incorrect, and I regret that the sense should have appeared in the article referred to.

George Bell Todd, MB.
Glasgow, August 25, 1898.[99]

The NHW's success here in ensuring Bell Todd retracted his statement was threefold. Firstly, Bell Todd's public acknowledgement that his comments were both incorrect and without foundation exonerated the hospital from any concrete blame in administering anaesthetics; secondly, that they were made privately revoked any sense of professional objectivity about the state of anaesthetic practice in Britain; and, finally, but most

---

[98] Ibid., 2 June and 7 July 1898.
[99] Letter from George Bell Todd to the Editor of the *Medical Record*, 'Anaesthesia and its Administration in Great Britain and Ireland', *Medical Record*, 54.12 (17 September 1898), 430–1.

importantly for the New, in retracting his harsh judgement, he had been made to print the, in fact, impressive statistics achieved by the surgical team. From initially claiming that women were remarkable for their failures in administering chloroform correctly, Bell Todd was compelled to flaunt their outstanding achievement of a 0.15 per cent death rate on the operating table itself. This was a triumph both for the anaesthetist and, correspondingly, the skill of the woman surgeon and her all-female team. The hospital achieved a further accomplishment through its limited publicity of the case, confining Bell Todd's apology to the original source of the article. Publication in the British press may have led to unwarranted pressure of attention, as well as charges of bragging, something which the New were evidently keen to avoid since Garrett Anderson's departure and Blackwell's warnings in the *Daily Chronicle*. While the New won a moral victory here, this was not the last time Bell Todd would find himself forced publicly to reverse his opinions. In 1912, he was struck off for procuring abortions, a charge for which he had also been tried and acquitted the previous year, and sentenced to a lengthy seven-years' penal servitude.[100]

While the NHW had treated the two controversial events which could have destabilised its reputation with canny calmness, it also sought to honour the commitment of its surgical team in the 1890s. Two years after Garrett Anderson's resignation and nearly seven months after the attack in the *Daily Chronicle*, Mary Scharlieb and Florence Nightingale Boyd were rewarded with new titles. On 6 December 1894, the Managing Committee considered the Medical Council's recommendations and decided Scharlieb and Boyd should be 'termed surgeons'.[101] This was acknowledged publicly in the *Annual Report* for 1894.[102] Although most women doctors were still restricted in what they could achieve institutionally, the recognition of specialty was crucial for progression in surgery and for the New's reputation as a primarily surgical centre. As Scharlieb remarked later, this period saw the start of both an immensely successful partnership and the growth of surgical practice at the hospital:

---

[100] For a sanitised account of his trial, see the *Standard*'s reporting on Monday 3 June, 8, and Tuesday 4 June 1912, 10; for a more precise summation of his charges, see 'Medico-Legal: Penal Servitude for Procuring Abortion', *BMJ*, 1.2685 (15 June 1912), 1407; and for the end of Bell Todd's career, see 'The General Council of Medical Education and Registration', *Lancet*, 180.4658 (7 December 1912), 1593–8. Bell Todd appeared to have ended his days in America, dying in California, on 18 November 1926, at the age of 65. See a very brief obituary, which simply listed his residence, education and key dates, in *JAMA*, 88.6 (5 February 1927), 422.

[101] Minutes of the Managing Committee, II, 6 December 1894.

[102] *Twenty-Third (1894) Annual Report* (1895), p. 6.

surgery became 'a very marked feature'.[103] So thoroughly did Boyd and Scharlieb understand each other's ways 'that is was just like one brain directing two pairs of hands'.[104] From the divisions of the 1880s and the public attacks of the 1890s grew, according to Scharlieb, an understanding with the advantage of one way of thinking, but two skilful pairs of hands with which to operate effectively. In 'taking full charge' of surgery at the New,[105] Scharlieb bypassed the need for absolute reliance on the consulting staff and, with the confidence of the Managing Committee and dedicated assistants, began to operate independently. From 1893, rather than wavering in its performance of risky and controversial operations after the concerns raised about procedures at the hospital, the competence of its staff and the growing public worries about the wisdom of surgery, the NHW determined to prove its success in promoting the woman surgeon and defending her actions.

The *Annual Reports* for the 1890s illustrated the growth of risky operations, including bladder, gastric, kidney, liver and rectal procedures, as well as for the diseases of women. Scharlieb described her final ten years at the hospital as providing 'exacting' and 'very interesting' surgical work, but referred also to the 'peaceful routine' which was established, composed of 'much work, many anxieties, and ample causes for thanksgiving'.[106] While the New catered solely for women and children, it did not consider itself a specialist institution and always insisted on its status as a general hospital, reflected here in the variety of procedures performed. Patients admitted to the New suffered from 'general' complaints, as well as gynaecological ones, and surgical procedures were not confined to specifically female ailments. Experience in surgery was obtained only through practise, and the institution's insistence on multiple attempts before assistance in serious cases helped to hone operative skills. Indeed, the first *Annual Report* to be published after the change in personnel remarked upon the very good results obtained from a large number of major operations, stressing, no doubt with the problems of 1888 still in mind, the rapport the staff had with their male counterparts, who sought advice from the women surgeons and even placed their own patients under female care for operative treatment.[107] The stress on co-operation between the women themselves, as well as the trust of male practitioners, focused attention away from the thrusting,

---

[103] Scharlieb, *Reminiscences*, p. 135.   [104] Ibid., p. 136.
[105] Ibid., p. 133. Scharlieb notes that this was always Garrett Anderson's intention, and that 'outsiders' should give way to the female surgeon, who would be either herself or a chosen replacement, viz. Scharlieb herself.
[106] Ibid., p. 165.   [107] *Twenty-Second (1893) Annual Report* (1894), p. 12.

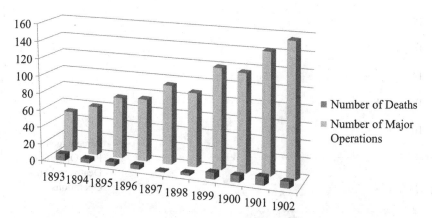

Figure 1.2 Number of Major Operations and Post-operative Deaths: NHW, 1893–1902.

selfish and reckless image of the *fin-de-siècle* surgeon, so beloved of the popular press, and instead towards the fellow feeling existing between professionals and their concern to obtain the best for their patients.

While the hospital had defended itself successfully against the attacks of Blackwell and Bell Todd, deaths following operation, even if they did not occur in the theatre itself, continued initially to rise under Scharlieb. In 1893, the first year of Scharlieb's promotion to senior surgeon, operation deaths were at their highest ever: eight out of 51 major cases. However, for three years – 1894, 1895 and 1897 – there were five deaths out of 59, 72 and 93 operations, respectively; in 1896, there was only a single death out of 74; in 1898, three out of 87; and in 1899, the number had risen to seven out of 118 cases (Figure 1.2).

From 1900, there was a distinct correlation between the number of deaths and the number of patient refusals. In 1900, there were eight operation deaths and nine refusals, out of 130 cases; in 1901, ten deaths and ten refusals, from a total of 149 cases; and in 1902, eight operation deaths and seven refusals in 155 major operation cases (Figure 1.3). In 1902, Scharlieb took a coveted specialist post in the Gynaecological Department of the Royal Free Hospital, the first woman to hold such a senior position in a general institution. By the time she left, there were three times as many major operations carried out at the NHW as there had been ten years earlier, but with the same number of fatalities: an impressively consistent statistic. The growing confidence of Scharlieb as a surgeon and the support of her team contributed to an exponential increase in risky operative procedures, but a steadying hand in controlling surgical

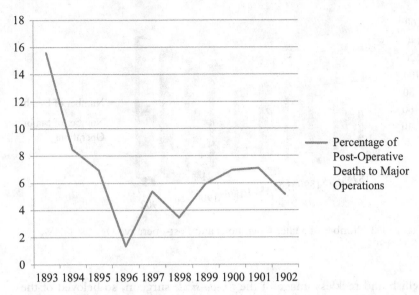

Figure 1.3 Percentage of Deaths to Major Operations: NHW, 1893–
1902.[108]

and post-surgical death. Typically self-effacing about her own abilities,
Scharlieb herself attributed survival rates partly to the development of
pathology at the hospital, which allowed the surgeon greater accuracy of
diagnosis and treatment.

In an 1897 article for the *BMJ* simply titled 'Surgery at the New Hospital for Women in 1896', Scharlieb gave a statistical report of surgical
practice at the hospital for the year when only one death had occurred.
The latter case of chronic intestinal obstruction had been due to the
surgical inaccessibility of malpositioned viscera.[109] In other words, every
operable case survived. Scharlieb's account was remarkable not for its
Garrett Anderson-like 'bragging' about institutional triumph, but for its
attribution of success in a number of cases to pathological confirmation
of disease before surgery was attempted. This was especially vital in the
case of 'Mrs S.', who, at the age of 25, presented the staff with difficulties.
Her youth, a recent miscarriage and lack of evidence from examination
alone would have led any surgeon to an incorrect diagnosis. However,
curettings revealed a more sinister explanation for her symptoms, and
Mrs S.'s cancerous uterus was removed. She recovered rapidly, and was

[108] Statistics calculated from *Annual Reports*.
[109] Mary Scharlieb, 'Surgery at the New Hospital for Women in 1896', *BMJ*, 2.1910 (7
August 1897), 338–9; 338.

still in good health at the beginning of 1897. While the surgical removal of Mrs S.'s diseased womb saved her life, it was the impetus to operate provided by microscopical evidence which encouraged her surgeon to alter her diagnosis and act in time. The individual's clinical expertise and surgical skill was fallible, argued Scharlieb, and could only be improved by scientific confirmation of disease. Resistance to pathological support was still pronounced in the 1890s, particularly among gynaecological surgeons, who trusted their own diagnoses based upon experience in examination above and beyond what could be gleaned from laboratory findings.[110] After detailing a number of 'stormy cases', Scharlieb turned to the 'uniform progress' of ovariotomy cases. Only a few years before this had been a procedure causing the hospital and its surgical staff enormous private and public concern, but Scharlieb characterised it as uncomplicated, routine, often very easy, and entirely uneventful. The article concluded with an examination of kidney cases and a radical hernia cure, which confirmed the hospital's general status, as well as indicating the diversity of procedures women surgeons carried out at the New. In publishing this account, Scharlieb promoted the skilful performance of female surgeons at the hospital, their growing confidence in attempting a variety of procedures, as well as her own belief in the fundamental importance of science in surgery.

'Surgery at the New Hospital for Women' was also notable for its use throughout of patient narrative to illustrate statistics. Although this was, of course, not unusual, the hospital was far keener in the 1890s to turn the gaze away from the woman surgeon and onto her patients. This had the effect of extolling the surgical achievements of the New through the relief and satisfaction of the patient herself. A piece in the *Illustrated London News* on the hospital in autumn 1892 remarked upon the 'pervading presence of the womanly element', from the personal interest in the patients, to attention even to minor troubles and recognition of mental as well as physical needs; sympathy, it argued, was present in the very fabric of the New itself.[111] In the scrapbook of prized newspaper cuttings, a semi-fictional account, also published in late 1892, about 'Mrs Brown's' visit to the hospital stressed that 'What She Saw There' instilled her with

---

[110] See Steven Jacyna, 'The Laboratory and the Clinic: The Impact of Pathology on Surgical Diagnosis in the Glasgow Western Infirmary, 1875–1910', *BHM*, 62.3 (Fall, 1988), 384–406, and, for gynaecology, Ilana Löwy, '"Because of their Praiseworthy Modesty, They Consult Too Late: Regime of Hope and Cancer of the Womb, 1800–1910', *BHM*, 85.3 (Fall, 2011), 356–83. For more on Scharlieb and her colleagues' promotion of pathological enquiry in surgery see chapter 3 of this book.

[111] 'The New Hospital for Women', *Illustrated London News*, 2786 (10 September 1892), 342.

hope and courage.[112] Though she was one of many, Mrs Brown had a great spirit, but poor health; her fear of hospitals and cowardliness in the face of doctors prevented her seeking assistance for ongoing ailments. A recommendation from an evidently middle-class 'visitor' led her to the New, where the anticipation of remoteness was transformed into the pleasant friendliness of the institution's aspect. Though she was early, and the doors were not yet open, a crowd was already waiting to be admitted. The women did not know each other and yet 'a sense of comradeship' was instantly established in the 'common need and hope' they all felt and desired. Mrs Brown's own East-End home was dark and dingy; the New, by contrast, overwhelmed with its light. Its bright cheerfulness created a comfortable, sympathetic atmosphere for the friendless Mrs Brown. The medical staff expressed interest in each patient's history, and they insisted on calling each woman by their first name. Fortified with confidence, Mrs Brown was treated by 'Miss ____' with friendliness, sympathy and patience. Clarity dominated their encounter – both in the (unnamed) diagnosis and in the prospect of a cure once she was admitted. Mrs Brown was shown around the wards, which were similarly airy and cheerful: '"What a nice holiday", she said, "to be here!"'. At the end of the afternoon, Mrs Brown left with 'fresh life', reassured that something could be done to help with her burden.

Mrs Brown was an archetypal, overworked, underfed and ailing prospective patient, and her reaction was, of course, idealised. However, the article deliberately and consistently created fellow feeling – between the patients themselves, between the patients and their surroundings, and between the doctors and the patients. Institutions were inevitably alert to the contemporary public furore about surgical experimentation and sought to reassure that patients would be treated well and everything would be carried out in their best interests. Mrs Brown's 'craven-hearted' reaction to everything medical was reversed by the end of her visit, which instilled her with courage to fight her condition. As the 1890s ended, however, and in spite of the growing surgical confidence achieved at the NHW, there was a corresponding growth in patient complaint and resistance, suggesting that the Edwardian patient was far more willing than her Victorian equivalent to refuse operative interference, despite the increasing safety and success of procedures. Fundamental here to note was that patient refusal had very little to do with the statistical riskiness of the operation, and, indeed, there was no consistent pattern in the kinds of procedures patients will not undergo. In the three years between

---

[112] 'The New Hospital for Women, and What Mrs Brown Saw There. By Her Neighbour', *Queen*, 10 September 1892, *ANC*.

1900 and 1902, there were 26 refusals of surgical treatment for various ailments out of 434 major operation cases, or just under 6 per cent of the total number. Situations where operations were actually carried out for the same conditions reveal that there were only five deaths: two for fibroids; two for tubercular peritonitis; and one for cancer of the uterine body.[113] Over the three years, successful operations numbered 34, three and six respectively. What the patient perceived as a risk-filled undertaking was, on the whole, statistically unlikely to be the sort of operation where death rather than cure or relief resulted. Surgical success, therefore, had very little to do with patient perception of the operation itself.

The Hospital Letters Book contains correspondence with patients who thought twice after the process of undergoing an operation. At the beginning of 1898, a Miss Livesey wrote to the secretary of the New to complain about having been anaesthetised, still a concern for many. A couple of weeks later, another response was recorded. Miss Livesey had clearly responded in an aggressive manner about the whole surgical team. As the secretary wrote:

As those who took part in the operation are prepared to testify that it was done with your apparent consent and that you certainly expressed no objection. If the authorities of the Hospital could see any possible ground of complaint, they would of course investigate it fully, but I cannot see that there is anything they could do in the matter.[114]

Although Miss Livesey's letters have not survived, she certainly objected to her surgical treatment some time after it had taken place. Similarly, in 1903, correspondence was recorded with a Miss Reidford, whose 'various complaints' were addressed by the Managing Committee. As she had attended the New in the first half of 1899, however, they could hardly deal effectively with objections being brought three and a half years after her stay.[115] Neither woman was mentioned again in any context, so both must have given up their pursuit of the hospital for perceived surgical injustice. The Letters Book also contained a number of enquiries requesting further information about what was wrong with a patient, or what had been done to assist them. This, of course, encourages different readings of the reasons why patients complained. As the next chapter will explore more fully, some patients simply did not know what had

---

[113] Statistics calculated from *Twenty-Ninth (1900)*, *Thirtieth (1901)* and *Thirty-First (1902)* *Annual Reports* (1901–1903).
[114] Letters to Miss Livesey, 2 January 1898 and, in response to one dated three days earlier, 15 January 1898, in Hospital Secretary's Letters Book.
[115] Minutes of the Managing Committee III, 8 October 1903; and letter to Miss Reidford, 9 October 1903, Hospital Secretary's Letters Book.

happened during their hospitalisation and were ignorant even of what had been removed during procedures. A Mrs Scott wrote on behalf of her (now dead) daughter in 1906, confused as to why she had been operated upon. The secretary reminded Mrs Scott that she had been informed from the start that her daughter should be admitted for an operation to have a tumour removed. That Mrs Scott had not been told again was because the surgeon 'understood that you agreed to her coming for that express purpose'.[116] Mrs Scott's mistaken impression as to what was wrong with her daughter was not especially unusual, as the next chapter will show. 'What Mrs Brown Saw' and 'What Mrs Scott Was Told' were evidently not as clear and transparent as the NHW believed.

Patient perception of a cure, however, was one area where radical and conservative surgery met and where the woman surgeon could defend her decision to operate. In a fascinating, strikingly modern follow-up of patients from the NHW, published in the *BMJ* in 1899, May Thorne, assistant anaesthetist and former senior house surgeon to the New, interviewed ex-patients to discover the post-operative effect of an abdominal section on the patient's mentality and lifestyle. Ostensibly responding to a paper given by Herbert Spencer at the Obstetrical Society in 1897, which explored post-surgical complications, Thorne examined the after-history of 88 patients from the New between the key years of 1888 and 1897.[117] Of these 88, only five had returned for further surgery. Case 2 had attended the hospital seven years after her first procedure for ovariotomy in 1888 with a ventral hernia, as did Case 59, who had originally been suffering from salpingitis and ovaritis in 1896, while Case 70, who had undergone a Caesarean Section in 1895, had an abdominal hysterectomy the following year. The only other who had returned was Case 34, who was not cured of salpingitis and ovaritis, and had continued pain after her operation; a further procedure was attempted at the New, where her left ovary was resected. This too was unsuccessful; the patient went to another hospital and died a few days later. One further patient, Case 76, was readmitted. She had a protracted convalescence and returned

---

[116] Letter to Mrs Scott, 23 July 1906, Hospital Secretary's Letters Book. Presumably Miss Scott was suffering from cancer, which had not been fully removed during the operation or which had recurred: her 'illness ended fatally'.

See also letters to C. Meyerstein, Esq, 12 December 1889 and 16 December 1889; Mr Valentine (the husband of Jane Valentine, discussed above), 17 July 1893; Miss Rebecca Bloomfield, 24 June 1893; Mr Spanswick, 25 January 1898; the Countess of Portsmouth, 15 February 1898; Mrs Willows, 22 December 1898; Mr Richard O'Saviour, 17 April 1907.

[117] May Thorne, 'The After-Effects of Abdominal Section', *BMJ*, 1.1988 (4 February 1899), 264–5. For more on May Thorne's later career, including her trial for surgical negligence, see 'Risk, Responsibility and Surgery'.

five years later in a moribund state with acute intestinal obstruction, dying soon after admission. Two patients attending for exploratory operations had since died. One of these, Case 65, who left 'unrelieved', had contracted bronchitis a year after admission in 1895, while the other, Case 66, had died in 1897, two years after she had attended the hospital, although the cause was unknown. Case 22, who had undergone a double ovariotomy in 1893, died from cancer of the uterus a year later; Case 89 had also died from malignancy three months after her procedure – in this instance, of the perineum. The unrelieved or those who had continued to suffer were in the minority, however, and the responses given by over 80 patients were overwhelmingly positive in their interpretation of what effects surgery had upon their everyday lives.

This list offered an intriguing glimpse into how female patients viewed operations which might be labelled 'human vivisection' or 'unsexing', such as removal of the ovaries. While the questions asked clearly suggested the restoration of health rather than suffering, the answers were certainly not uniform and many were quoted verbatim, allowing a brief glance at the individual, though anonymous, respondent. Of the 82 surviving patients, who had not returned for further procedures or died of other causes, only ten described their health as poor or 'not good', with just under half of these recurring symptoms probably related to the causes for which they originally underwent an operation. Case 3, for example, was 'never free from pain' in the lower part of her back, implying ongoing gynaecological problems after a single ovariotomy. In contrast, Case 6 had 'no pain' but 'much general weakness', which encouraged her to think of 'all kinds of imaginary illnesses', suggesting, even to the patient herself, a mental cause rather than anything physical. Lack of strength was also mentioned by some, although this was not necessarily linked to the operation. Case 69, who had a hysteropexy, did not have much pain, but did not feel so strong; Case 51, who never felt well, worried about nothing, but did not elaborate as to whether she had always felt like this or whether she attributed it to her abdominal hysterectomy. Menopausal symptoms were also noted by two patients who had both ovaries removed. Flushings were experienced by Cases 24 and 26. On the other hand, a few offered concrete evidence for their recovery of strength. Three former patients mentioned resuming or beginning occupations with a differing variety of physical labour required. Case 5's very good health ensured that she was able to earn her living from mangling. Although weak for two years after her hysterectomy, Case 48 was now a manageress in a busy hotel, while Case 57 worked hard for the Salvation Army.

Even more of a boon for those who carried out controversial gynaecological procedures was the reassurance that fertility was not always affected. Cases 18, 19 and 68 had become pregnant since their procedure, scotching the popular misconception that any form of abdominal surgery upon women resulted in sterility. The first two patients both had single ovariotomies, while the latter had a hysteropexy. It would be hard to insist that unnecessary surgical interference had led to a destruction of their childbearing capabilities. All described better general health, ranging from good in one case to excellent in the other two. Case 19, indeed, described her general health as poor before the procedure, emphasising succinctly how transformative surgery had been for her. Nearly a quarter of the former patients claimed excellent health, and a quarter mentioned the operation itself leading to an improvement in their condition. Indeed, every single one who discussed the operation claimed improvement. Even though this must have been presented as a leading question, asked along the lines of 'How is your health since the operation?', those who enjoyed good or better health attributed their recovery to the surgical procedure and those who still suffered did not suggest that it was a cause in their continued ill-health. The ultimate result, of course, was a magnificent vindication of operations on women by women, especially those involving gynaecological procedures which had dominated debates over surgical experimentation in an institutional setting. Such an article could certainly bolster the New's perception of its surgical success in the past decade, despite its own internal obstructions.

Conclusion

Mary Scharlieb's *BMJ* obituary in 1930 by her former NHW colleague, Jane Walker, drew attention to her surgical skills:

Several obituary notices have called her a pioneer. In my opinion this is an incorrect description of her. Rather did she become a woman doctor to enable her to help the sufferings of her fellow women. In no sense did she attempt to blaze the trail for medical women coming after. She was a most beautiful operator, but it was all done in such a quiet, modest, unassuming, almost commonplace manner that it seemed, even at the very beginning, to be the most ordinary thing in the world for a woman to be doing big abdominal surgery. It is, of course, true that delicacy of touch and the smallest of hands, as well as knowledge and practice of needlework, were a great asset – (whoever has seen Mrs. Scharlieb quietly knitting at a committee of both men and women could doubt that?) – but she had never had an operating knife in her hand till she was turned 40 years of age, and yet very soon she became one of the six great abdominal surgeons of the world. That, think, makes her almost of the nature of a phenomenon.

She brought ordinary common sense and naturalness to all she did. She had no peculiarity.[118]

For Walker, it was Scharlieb's natural abilities which ensured her success as a surgeon. Phenomenal, indeed, but certainly not peculiar. Similarly, Frederick Treves was said to have spent any free time watching Scharlieb operate: 'her movements, her sureness, her delicacy, were invaluable to watch'.[119] In similar fashion to Walker, what drew Treves was Scharlieb's instinctive deftness, her ease of manoeuvre which instructed even as it fascinated. At the NHW in the 1890s and early 1900s, Scharlieb performed difficult, dangerous and risky procedures, not for the sake of the cause, as Garrett Anderson put it, but, so she and others claimed, for her patients. Scharlieb's record at the New stood for itself and contributed to her being awarded the first senior post given to a woman at the RFH in 1902.[120] The Royal Free had been affiliated with the LSMW since 1877, and it was where the students carried out their clinical work. Now, it had extended the hand of fellowship to qualified women surgeons, breaking new ground once more.[121] As we shall see in the next two chapters, Scharlieb, along with Ethel Vaughan-Sawyer, who was appointed as her deputy at the same time, continued her surgical career specialising in gynaecological procedures.

In her 1924 *Reminiscences*, Scharlieb stressed that the book had been written for one purpose:

my object is to convince medical women students and junior practitioners that a successful, happy, and useful career can be, and ought to be, the guerdon of their toil, though, inasmuch as we can never get any more out of any enterprise than we put into it, they are likely to find that success and opportunities of usefulness will vary directly with the vigour that they put into their studies and the love that they bring into professional practice. It is impossible to do the maximum amount of good to one's patients if one attempts to serve their bodies only. The real success and value of medical and surgical work is in proportion to the degree with which physicians and surgeons recognise the threefold nature of those whom they desire to serve.[122]

---

[118] 'Dr Jane Walker writes', appended to 'Obituary: Dame Mary Scharlieb', *BMJ*, 2.3647 (29 November 1930), 935–7; 937.

[119] P.H. 'Women in Medicine', *Lady's Pictorial*, 20 August 1910, *RFH Press Cuttings, IV*.

[120] See *The Seventy-Fifth Annual Report [. . .] for 1902* (Printed by Love & Malcolmson, Ltd, London, 1903), pp. 18–19.

[121] For more on the history of the hospital, see Lynne A. Amidon, *An Illustrated History of the Royal Free Hospital* (London: The Special Trustees for the Royal Free Hospital, 1996).

[122] Scharlieb, *Reminiscences*, p. vii.

It was this steady, commonsensical approach to operating, gaining experience even when taking calculated risks, which the woman surgeon needed to embody if she was to succeed. While the Chelsea Hospital for Women came under scrutiny in the *Daily Chronicle* and other papers in the 1890s, it is telling that the New, despite its promotion of some of the most controversial surgical procedures on women and in spite of Elizabeth Blackwell's critique of the way it performed, continued quietly operating.

2 The Experiences of Female Surgical Patients at the Royal Free Hospital, 1903–1913

In January 1911, Ethel Vaughan-Sawyer addressed the Royal Free Hospital Medical Society on the topic of 'The Patient'.[1] Vaughan-Sawyer's speech encouraged her audience to consider the practical experience of patients, whose reality is far more complicated than a textbook diagnosis will allow. The practice of medicine in the early twentieth century was precise and increased scientific understanding was illuminating the previously obscure; as a consequence, practitioners were more theoretically knowledgeable than ever before. With this superiority, however, came a corresponding distance from the patient's point of view; an inability to bridge the gap between professional, quotidian routine and the sheer torment of a consultation, operation or prolonged hospital visit. Vaughan-Sawyer's interests originally lay in psychology, and this was evident from her stress upon the necessity for patient empathy in the formation of a fully-rounded member of the medical profession, who considers the condition of the individual and not just the individual's condition.[2] The problem, of course, was that patients were frustratingly anxious or verbose, inarticulate and confused, unable to remember clearly the longevity of their own symptoms or the intricacies of their family history. For Vaughan-Sawyer, however, it was patient incoherence which more accurately resembled medical and surgical practice than textbook neatness. Clinical reality was messy, bloody and painful: patients suffered, noisily.

---

[1] 'The Patient', *London (Royal Free Hospital) School of Medicine for Women Magazine*, 7.48 (March 1911), 350–8. Future references to this periodical will be shortened to *L(RFH)SMWM*.

[2] See Louisa Garrett Anderson's letters to her mother, sent in September 1899, from her post at Camberwell Infirmary, about the possibility of taking 'psychology coaching' from Miss Vaughan. Vaughan was considered to be '100 times better at her work' than the letter-writer, 15 September, 19 September, 28 September 1899. The quotation is from the letter of 15 September. See Letters from Louisa Garrett Anderson to Elizabeth Garrett Anderson, 1899–1901, Elizabeth Garrett Anderson Letters and Papers, HA436/1/3/6, Ipswich Record Office.

This chapter will take Ethel Vaughan-Sawyer's advice and explore a ten-year period at the Royal Free Hospital through the gynaecological case notes of Mary Scharlieb (1903–1909) and Vaughan-Sawyer herself (1904–1913), focusing on the patient's experience from admission to discharge and beyond in some instances. Only one patient-based study of the RFH has been carried out before, but that focused deliberately on both sexes seen by male physicians and surgeons, and excluded the female members of staff.[3] By contrast, I want to address a number of fundamental questions about female patients more generally in the early twentieth century, as well as their specific composition at this particular hospital, which had done so much to promote the medical education and employment of women. Who filled the 12 or 13 beds allotted to these two female surgeons?[4] Why were they admitted and what routes had they taken before seeking hospital assistance? How did they characterise their symptoms, bearing in mind that early pioneers of women's right to enter the medical profession had expressed the untold benefits female patients would receive from discussing their problems with their own sex? What was their attitude to surgical procedures, which could include the modern accoutrements of surgery such as the X-ray, blood counts, pathological reports, and, of course, anaesthetic and aseptic measures? What was life like on the wards and what made some patients discharge themselves before their treatment had ended or even before it had begun? In short, adopting Vaughan-Sawyer's focus will give a unique insight into the female surgical patient's experience of pain, suffering and hospital treatment in the early twentieth century.

It is important to recognise from the outset, however, that case notes are controversial sources of information about medical and surgical care because of their very nature as mediated accounts, written by the practitioner (or would-be practitioner) on behalf of the patient. Ironically, while her lecture asked for attention to the finer points of the patient narrative, it is telling that apart from one personal observation, Vaughan-Sawyer's

---

[3] See Cullen, 'Patient Records'. Cullen excludes the patient notes of female staff; her justification concerns the small numbers of records, which would ensure that it would not be possible to 'conduct a fair and representative comparison': 'Moreover, the study would have had to consider not only the relationship between the male member of staff and male and female patients, but also that of a female member of staff to her patients, which would have proved too broad an examination for this study alone to conduct', p. 38.

In this chapter, I have excluded the notes of Lady Barrett, which are initially small in number and do not begin until autumn 1908.

[4] In 1902, there were 12 beds (out of a total of 170) allotted specifically to 'the diseases of women'; this increased to 13 a year later (of 165) and again became 12 in 1914. See the 1902 *Seventy-Fifth* (1903), 1903 *Seventy-Sixth* (1904), and 1914 *Eighty-Seventh* (1915) *Annual Reports* respectively.

examples of the trials of the clinical experience came from poetry. While the poems of W.E. Henley (1849–1903) intended to awaken her medical audience to the other side of the doctor–patient encounter, they were, of course, shaped and stylised to meet the demands of their genre. Terrors and torments might beset this patient, 'waiting – waiting for the knife', 'near[ing] / the fateful minute', but his voice was as precise in its carefully literary organisation of symptoms as any textbook example.[5] It was not only the poet, however, who moulded patient experience. Two years before Vaughan-Sawyer's speech, the magazine in which it is printed had mocked the current tendency for overembellishment of the patient record by the note-taker. While the resulting text became more graphic, exciting and thus 'delightful and entertaining reading', the patient was lost sight of amongst stylised or lengthy literary passages. Two examples will suffice:

Dr C–r, on approaching the bed, exclaimed with pleasure and surprise at the great improvement manifested since he last saw the patient. He realised, he said, that he had been mistaken in his previous treatment, and confessing this before us all, utilised the case as a theme for a prolonged dissertation on the merits and demerits of the drugs employed, passing a profitable hour before passing on to the next bed, asking me innumerable questions, none of which I was able to answer.

Full post-operative note: Surgeon, Mr L–g; Asst. Surgeon, Miss Bl–r; Anaesthetist, Miss W–tts. Mrs V–gh-n S–wy-r was also present and was asked her opinion of the case. Among others present was a distinguished foreigner, and the House Physician looked in, in the course of the afternoon. Time of operation... [No space for more – Ed].

Note next day – P is wonderfully well considering the operation she went through yesterday.[6]

The first extract is novelistic in its approach, composed ornately, but without any attempt at extracting the vital details about how or why the patient was so improved. It is hardly surprising that the writer could not respond to the questions asked about this case or the next. The second account also omitted important surgical information to discuss the operation in the manner of a society event, noting the presence of others, but, in doing so, running out of space to note precisely which procedure was carried out. What the patient 'went through' in either case will never be known.

It is this filtered nature of the patient experience which has concerned recent investigations into the value of patient notes as a source for the

---

[5] Henley, 'Before', ll.1; 6–7, in 'The Patient', 353.
[6] 'From the Notes', L(RFH)SMWM, 44 (October 1909), 167.

historian of medicine. This is hardly surprising when, to illustrate concerns about the compiling of records, one patient, 20-year-old single servant Mary Roots, who was in the RFH for gonorrhoea and resulting miscarriage, was described as having the all-too-familiar 'life of a second or third rate London serving girl'.[7] In 1992, Guenter B. Risse and John Harley Warner extolled the value of the clinical history as key to 'understanding the discourse and practice of medicine', but also warned of the care which must be taken when examining collaborative institutional documents whose inconsistency of approach would be only too recognisable both to Vaughan-Sawyer and to the readers of the LSMW *Magazine*.[8] Jonathan Gillis has drawn attention to the first half of the twentieth century as a point when the patient history was characterised by its dual nature, which comprised both the patient's faulty account and the physician's interpretations of and observations upon that narrative.[9] Such competing voices superseded the dominant format in the second half of the nineteenth century, whereby the physician took control in order skilfully to reveal the facts of the case.[10] The theorisation of surgical case records has received far less attention, but Ortrun Riha has provided a German example from the Göttingen University Hospital, which examines the problems of statistical research when sources are incomplete and advocates a prosopographical approach to patient history.[11] Far less evident in current research are case studies of patient records themselves.[12] The problems anticipated by those who have theorised about patient histories and the lack of surviving documents have combined in another way to silence the patient voice and the complexity of the clinical encounter remains underexplored.

If the historian has been unable to hear the patient voice because of professional reinterpretation, then another dimension is added to their silence when the patient is female. Thirty years ago, Mary Poovey, influenced by Foucauldian cultural history, lamented the passivity and

[7] Mary Roots (MS: 1906; Part I), Dr Scharlieb's Case Notes: Women, H71/RF/B/02/30/004, Royal Free London NHW Foundation Trust, LMA. Patient records will appear throughout in this shortened format to distinguish surgeon, date and number of box. Scharlieb's run from 1902–1903: H71/RF/B/02/30/001–1907–1908: H71/RF/B/02/30/006. Dr Vaughan Sawyer's Case Notes: Women from 1904–1908: H71/RF/B/02/31/001–1919: H71/RF/B/02/31/012.

[8] Guenter B. Risse and John Harley Warner, 'Reconstructing Clinical Activities: Patient Records in Medical History', *SHM*, 5.2 (August 1992), 183–205; 184.

[9] Jonathan Gillis, 'The History of the Patient History Since 1850', *BHM*, 80.3 (Fall 2006), 490–512; 497.

[10] Ibid., 495.

[11] Ortrun Riha, 'Surgical Case Records as an Historical Source: Limits and Perspectives', *SHM*, 8.2 (August 1995), 271–83.

[12] The notable exception being Cullen's 'Patient Records'.

'silencing of the female body', which was at the mercy of the 'super-intendence' of the chloroform-wielding male professional.[13] Poovey concluded that 'the medical representation of woman silenced real women'.[14] In a witty rejoinder to Poovey, Regina Morantz-Sanchez later wondered how the medical men had actually 'g[o]t there', forwarding the possibility that, against type, they had been requested to provide treatment by the female patients themselves.[15] By contrast, Anne Digby has acknowledged the part played by earlier feminist accounts in situating the patient encounter within cultural and sexual politics, but has welcomed instead a more balanced interpretation where *soi-disant* victims and oppressors are not so readily identified along the lines of gender.[16] This latter point is especially important when considering that not all doctors were male and not all patients were female; sometimes, as is largely the case in this book, both were women. In a number of recent articles focusing on surgery in the late nineteenth and early twentieth century, Sally Wilde has advocated reconceptualising clinical encounters in a far more detailed manner than the predictable duality of 'doctor–patient relationship' will allow. Patients were autonomous, made decisions about their treatment, were influenced by a number of factors outside the advice of their practitioners, and gambled upon still faltering procedures working successfully. Professionals, meanwhile, were uncertain about the outcomes of their experimental surgical practice and by no means in control of patients, who requested operative treatment independently of their judgements.[17] While acknowledging that the majority of early twentieth-century female patients had different responsibilities to their male counterparts, an intensive study of case records at the RFH indicates that women were just as capable of being obstinate as far as their health and its maintenance was concerned. They were also choosy about their treatment, whatever the purported medical or surgical benefit. Female patients were willing to listen to advice, but they would not always take it up. In the end, and this is why case histories provide such a frustrating, but also so intriguing a resource, they were more likely to do exactly what suited them as an individual, rather than what succeeded (or not) for the person in the next bed. Rather than flattening out the differences between around 1400 individuals to search for the typical

---

[13] Mary Poovey, '"Scenes of an Indelicate Character": The Medical "Treatment" of Victorian Women', *Representations*, 14 (Spring 1986), 137–78; 154; 146.
[14] Ibid., 156.   [15] Morantz-Sanchez, *Conduct Unbecoming*, p. 139.
[16] Digby, *Making a Medical Living*, p. 259.
[17] See, for example, Sally Wilde, 'The Elephants in the Doctor–Patient Relationship: Patients' Clinical Interactions and the Changing Surgical Landscape of the 1890s', *Health and History*, 9.1 (2007), 2–27 and 'Truth, Trust'.

or the average, this chapter will examine the variety of ways in which female surgical patients, in all their many guises, negotiated their time in the RFH.

The Background of Patients in the Hospital

In order to discover more about the patient base of the RFH, it is necessary to start with an analysis of available statistical records, and continue with an examination of the more narrative details case histories provide so as to situate the patients within a wider institutional framework. Unlike the NHW and other charitable medical ventures, the RFH did not require its patients to possess letters of recommendation. Treatment could be sought by the individual solely, with one exception. Those who were travelling from some distance were required to make written application, stating the details of their case. The hospital was proud to proclaim its usefulness to the 'immediate neighbourhood', some of the poorest areas in the city.[18] It was evident, however, as far as gynaecological patients were concerned, that many would be willing to travel from the other side of the country, and, indeed, from abroad, to be examined by Scharlieb or Vaughan-Sawyer. There was only one fundamental condition of entry: the patient had to be classified as 'sick poor', or 'unable to pay for advice and medicine'.[19] But, in keeping with other voluntary general hospitals keen to attract donations from the wealthy, the RFH regularly insisted upon the worthiness of its patients, who were never admitted simply for rest or refreshment, and the corresponding vigilance of its lady almoner.[20] If, after examination, the patient was found to be incurable, they would, in theory, be discharged. In-patients, if able, had to bring 'a change of linen, towel, knife, fork, spoon, comb, brush, soap, and flannel', as well as providing for 'their own personal washing', so a hospital stay was far from gratuitous for those who might not even possess their own basic

---

[18] See, for example, *The Seventy-Seventh Annual Report for 1905* (London, 1906). This was a particularly interesting year in terms of patient composition, as the number from the local London parishes of St Pancras, Islington and Holborn Union (50) was only one more than the combined number from other London districts and the 'Country' (49). While there were structural improvements being carried out from June 1905, necessitating the closure of 54 beds, it is fascinating to note that, given the insistence on treating the neighbourhood primarily, the RFH was so keen to accommodate its non-local patients, p. 14.

[19] 'Regulations as to the Admission of Patients', *The Seventy-Fifth Annual Report for 1902* (1903), p. 32.

[20] For more on the role of the almoner, see Lynsey T. Cullen, 'The First Lady Almoner: The Appointment, Position, and Findings of Miss Mary Stewart at the Royal Free Hospital, 1895–1899', *JHMAS*, 68.4 (October 2013), 551–82.

items for cleanliness and nourishment.[21] Given the deeply distressing bloody or sanious symptoms experienced by gynaecological patients in particular, the cost of the washing of personal items such as linen must have mounted up, adding another burden to the already weighty nature of their illness.

From 1903, the In-Patient Department of the hospital housed 165 beds and this number remained constant over the decade covered by this chapter.[22] Between 1903 and 1913, the beds allotted to the Diseases of Women were 13, or 7.9 per cent of the total. This was the largest number allotted to a specialist department. Diseases of the eye, in contrast, were given 6 (3.6 per cent) and isolation cases provided with 4 (2.4 per cent). Befitting its status as a general hospital the greatest number of beds were reserved for general medical cases (64: 36 for men; 28, or 38.8 per cent, for women) and general surgical cases (62: 33 and 29, respectively, or 37.6 per cent, for women).[23] In her 1924 *Reminiscences*, Scharlieb lamented what she saw as the 'inadequate number of beds allotted to [her] department', which necessitated turning away very many of the 'serious and interesting cases' discovered at Out-Patients.[24] Statistics concerning the number of female patients seen at Out-Patients confirms this lack of fit between those seeking treatment and places available in the hospital. Given the beds provided, the number of Out-Patients seen by the Gynaecological Department was enormous. From 541 in 1902, the total leapt to 1069 in 1903, reaching a peak of 1568 in 1905, before falling again to 865 by 1913.[25] At its zenith, therefore, there were just over 120 women potentially requiring each bed, revealing the high demand for and use of this special department. The numbers admitted remained fairly constant throughout the decade between 1903 and 1913, as shown in Figure 2.1. From 138 in 1904 to 174 a year later and 159 in Scharlieb's final year at the RFH, numbers averaged out at around 129 for

---

21 'Regulations as to the Admission of Patients', p. 32. The continued call in *Annual Reports* for 'cast off clothing for the use of poor patients on leaving the Hospital' indicated the genuine poverty experienced by some. See, for example, *The Eightieth Annual Report for 1907* (1908), p. 20.

22 This number was very small compared to other metropolitan hospitals. The London, for example, offered 900 beds after its early twentieth-century expansion. See A.E. Clark-Kennedy, *London Pride* (London: Hutchinson Benham, 1979), p. 159.

23 Statistics obtained from *Annual Reports*. See, for example, *The Seventy-Sixth Annual Report for 1903* (1904), p. 11. Accident cases were allotted 17 beds from 1903; this was reduced to 16 in 1909 [*The Eighty-Second Annual Report for 1909* (1910)], and raised again to 17 in 1914 [*The Eighty-Seventh Annual Report for 1914* (London, 1915)].

24 Scharlieb, *Reminiscences*, p. 170.

25 See *The Seventy-Sixth Annual Report for 1903* (1904); *The Seventy-Eighth Annual Report for 1905* (1906); and *The Eighty-Sixth Annual Report for 1913* (1914).

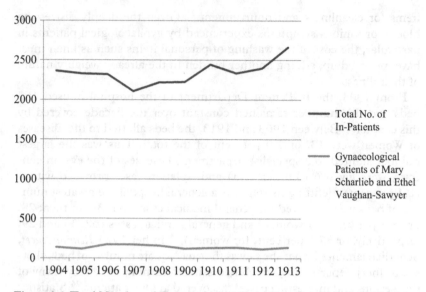

Figure 2.1 Total Number of Gynaecological Patients in Relation to the Total Number of In-Patients: RFH, 1904–1913.

the last five years covered by this study, when Vaughan-Sawyer took on Scharlieb's position.[26]

Given the stated aim of the RFH, namely, to see patients from the immediate metropolitan vicinity and then only from the 'sick poor', it is useful to explore the social and geographical background of those who sought treatment at the hospital (Figure 2.2). Until 1909, the *Annual Reports* listed the residences of only those who were present in the hospital on their census day of 1 January, but from this date it is possible to compare the numbers attending throughout the year. As the statistics reveal, the hospital did indeed serve the immediate neighbourhood more frequently than other parts of London or the rest of the country. When patients from outside the inner metropolitan areas of St Pancras, Islington, Finsbury and Holborn are combined with those from elsewhere in the country, however, the propinquity of the patient base looks less consistent. By 1913, there were only 120 more patients from the areas surrounding the hospital than other London districts and the rest of the country combined. This distribution could point to

[26] Numbers of patients are calculated from the number of case notes. Inevitably, some patients appear more than once, but are treated as separate cases for the purpose of this study. 1903 has not been included here as the records are incomplete.

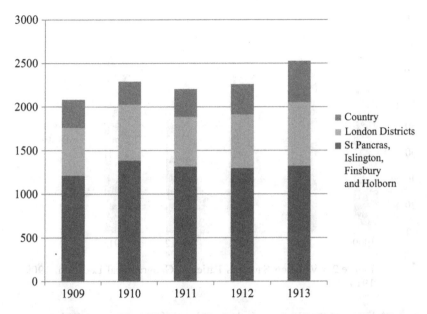

Figure 2.2 Total Number of In-Patients and their Geographical Location, 1909–1913.

the reputation of the RFH and its medical and surgical treatment. As Cullen has noted, surgeons to the hospital, such as Sir James Berry, were internationally renowned for their procedures. Berry's expertise in goitre and in the disfiguring conditions of hare lip and cleft palate would have been particularly welcomed by anyone searching for a surgical solution to these very visible afflictions.[27] Of course, a more cynical suggestion would be that the ease of entry to the hospital, without a letter of recommendation, might attract those who had failed to gain admission elsewhere. The very central location of the hospital, on Gray's Inn Road, might also determine its wider popularity. Either way, the RFH, given its small size, proved an attractive option for a large number of patients, who were not necessarily living near the institution.

A comparison with the in-patients of the Gynaecological Department between 1909 and 1913 reveals that women who sought treatment at the RFH for diseases peculiar to their own sex were, by contrast, largely from the metropolis (see Figure 2.3). This is not surprising given the number of outpatients in relation to the few beds available for specialist

27 See Cullen, 'Patient Records', p. 73. Also chapter 1, for Berry's goitre procedure at the NHW.

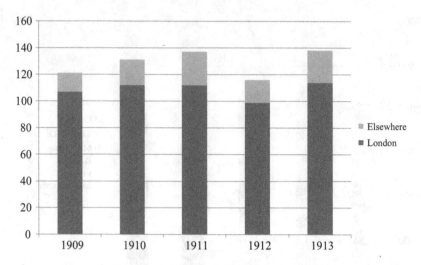

Figure 2.3 Vaughan-Sawyer's Patients: Geographical Location, 1909–1913.

care. Admission to the hospital would require prompt attendance at Gynaecological Out-Patients, which might prove more difficult for those coming from a distance. The large number of metropolitan female patients could also be explained simply by their gender. If the average number of days spent by in-patients in the RFH between 1909 and 1913 was 24.04, this was a long period of time for anyone to be away from employment or family, let alone the large number of children some of the patients had to support, feed and clothe. The recovery time from a serious surgical procedure, as well as any consequences of that operation, such as wound suppuration, the formation of sinuses or reactions to medication, would further delay the return home. Patients were also sent on to Convalescent Homes to complete their treatment through rest and recuperation, and, if operations failed, as they sometimes did, then a further stay in hospital might be the only solution to a final cure. If admission was sought at a nearby hospital then worries about home might be partially alleviated, although proximity to one's troubles could also have the opposite effect, as will be discussed later. Conversely, patient notes from the Gynaecological Department reveal that the RFH attracted women from all four corners of Britain. For example, Florence McClelland came to the hospital from Scotland in 1907; Mary G. Le Brun travelled from Guernsey in 1910 and Elizabeth Cuthbert from Norfolk in the same year; Louie Carren arrived from North Wales in 1913. Others came from even further afield, adding another category to the patient census unrecognised by the *Annual Reports*. Emily Marichean was from St Vincent, Jennie Blanchard had reached the RFH via South Africa and America, Annie Crowl had been a missionary in China for 15 years, while Katie Sykes had lived in Denmark and South Africa. A number of patients were back from India: Winifred Walden, to use only one example, was 'invalided home' in 1909 from her post as a missionary.[28]

While a speedy return to family may have been a priority for both male and female patients, it is important to realise that not all women treated at the hospital were married or occupied with looking after their home or children. Neither a patient's age nor employment, for example, can be discerned accurately by looking at *Annual Reports*, because they do not list background in such detail. The 16 beds allotted solely to 'Accidents' suffered by men, however, and the category of 'Injuries', such as burns, fractures, concussions, visceral and multiple injuries, as well as the 'brought in dead' section, recorded in yearly medical and surgical reports give some idea of industrial occupational hazards. Case histories, with the patient's age, address, marital status, next of kin (in some instances) and employment provide much more precise information about each individual, and allow the historian to fill in the silences left by more public documents. The Gynaecological Department dealt with young and old alike: from newborn babies, such as the unnamed 'Baby Hobbs', William J. Roberts, or Arthur James Brumell to three 77-year-olds – Rebecca Bosher, Kate Turner and Susannah Chapman.[29] Figure 2.4 shows the age distribution of the in-patients seen by Scharlieb and Vaughan-Sawyer between 1903 and 1913. Of the 1403 patients seen by the two in this decade, women in their twenties (419) and, in particular, their thirties (470) dominate the numbers, followed a little way behind by females aged 40 to 49 (309). This differs from Cullen's findings concerning the patient base of other physicians and surgeons at the RFH, where those in their teenage years and twenties dominated surgical practice.[30] The distinction is not surprising, however, as far as the diseases of women were concerned. As obstetrician Thomas Wilson remarked succinctly in 1907, 'women in the full vigour of adult life' were most susceptible to infection and disease: parturition and sexual intercourse still key parts of their everyday lives. Puberty and the climacteric, as indicated by the smaller numbers in their

---

[28] See: Florence McClelland (MS: 1907; Part II); Mary G. Le Brun (EVS: 1910; Part I); Elizabeth Cuthbert (EVS: 1910; Part I); Louie Carren (EVS: 1913; Part I). Emily Marichean (MS: 1908; Part II); Jennie Blanchard (MS: 1904); Annie Crowl (EVS: 1911; Part II); Katie Sykes (MS: 1904); Winifred Walden (EVS: 1908; Part I).

[29] See: 'Baby Hobbs' (MS: 1905; Part I); William J. Roberts (MS: 1907; Part II); Arthur James Brummell (MS: 1906; Part II); Rebecca Bosher (MS: 1904); Kate Turner (EVS: 1910; Part II); Susannah Chapman (EVS: 1911; Part I).

[30] Cullen, 'Patient Records', p. 89.

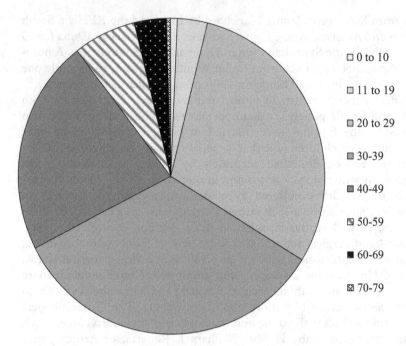

Figure 2.4 Age Distribution of Patients in the Gynaecological Department under Scharlieb and Vaughan-Sawyer, 1903–1913.[31]

teens and fifties, were also stages of potential concern.[32] By the early 1900s, developments in bacteriology and pathology had strengthened the understanding that it was not simply the weaknesses of inherent femaleness which caused women's bodies to ache and to bleed, but often the introduction of external forces which then destroyed from within.

Given the predominance of women in their twenties and thirties, it would be easy to assume that the majority of patients treated by the Gynaecological Department were wives and mothers, who may have been employed in the past, but were now dedicating their lives to home and husband. However, the range of occupations, as displayed in Figure 2.5, shows a far greater variety of situation and status than might be expected. 'House', the RFH shorthand for housewife, dominates, to the extent that

---

[31] This chart includes 1401 of the 1403 patient records, which comprise all of the patients in the files of both surgeons between 1903 and 1913. Only two patients are excluded as their ages have been spread across too great a range in the notes (one patient, Mary Lake [EVS: 1911; Part I] is noted both as 36 and 40; and one, Edith Lewis [EVS: 1912; Part II] is aged both as 51 and 31).

[32] Thomas Wilson, 'On Pelvic Inflammations in the Female', *JOGBE*, 12.1 (July 1907), 3–27; 10.

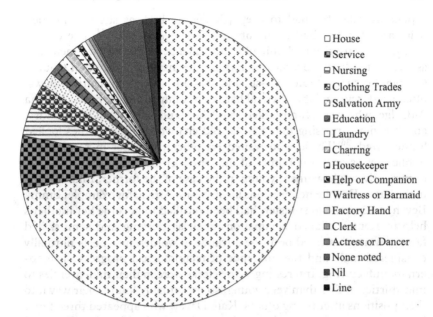

House
Service
Nursing
Clothing Trades
Salvation Army
Education
Laundry
Charring
Housekeeper
Help or Companion
Waitress or Barmaid
Factory Hand
Clerk
Actress or Dancer
None noted
Nil
Line

Figure 2.5 Occupations of Female Patients, 1903–1913.

72 per cent of patients were labelled this way. Situations occupied largely by single women or, less frequently, widows, were the next largest categories. Service included a variety of general servants, but also maids such as chamber, lady's, parlour, as well as cooks in private residences or in institutions, such as hotels or clubs. The nurses in the survey were from other hospitals, mental institutions and asylums, and a specialist maternity nurse. Patients from the clothing trades included tailoresses, an embroideress and a corsetière, and were largely comprised, again, of young single women, widows or those who needed to supplement the family income. One woman, Maria Dearman, who worked at home, and, therefore, could be mistaken for a housewife, was, in fact, running a treadle sewing machine in addition to her household chores: work she described as 'hard'.[33] The number of Salvation Army women is interesting, as the home from which they were sent was in Hackney, East London. As some of these patients' notes contained letters from the matron there, addressed directly to Scharlieb or Vaughan-Sawyer, and described symptoms and suffering, informal connections must have been established between the two institutions. In the case of Martha Parker, for example, Alice H. Halls wrote informally to Sister Milner of the RFH

---

[33] Maria Dearman (EVS: 1911; Part II).

explaining that she 'had to keep [Parker] in bed, as she was in such pain' and that this had been constant for 'seven weeks'.[34] The education sector comprised schoolchildren, students (including two medical), as well as teachers, governesses and, in one instance, a London County Council Lecturer.[35] Laundresses and charladies, predominantly widows, often aged, revealed the physical hardships of their menial posts. Martha Aldridge, who was 64, remarked that 'she stands all day' in the laundry, and it is not surprising that 53-year-old charwoman Eliza Miles looked 'rather tired'.[36] Those who waited on others, whether in restaurants, public houses or in the homes of the lonely or invalids, were again predominantly single women: young in the case of the former, middle-aged in the latter. Despite her previous life in South Africa, for example, Emma Bevan, a 52-year-old spinster, had been recalled to become her mother's help in Kent.[37] Skilled occupations such as clerking and semi-skilled factory work illustrated both the advance of women into posts normally considered male and the influence of technological progress on modern manufacturing. Interestingly, the clerks were in their mid-twenties to mid-thirties, rather than very young, so presumably found their way into their positions after trying others. Kate Davey, who appeared three times in the notes, was first a waitress, then a clerk, and, in her final stay, had returned to service.[38] Occupational mobility was evidently more possible, if not necessary, at this point for a single female who had only herself to support. The range of employment held by patients at the RFH, from the very menial to those requiring training and qualifications, offer a different picture to the official representation of the patient base given by the *Annual Reports* of poverty and necessity.

It was not only the single or widowed who were represented in the gynaecological case notes of the RFH as employed. In *Women in Modern Industry*, published in 1915, B.L. Hutchins made the salient point that 'women's work is subject to considerable interruption, and is contingent on family circumstances, whence it comes about that women may not always need paid work, but when they do they often want it so badly that they are ready to take anything they can get'.[39] Picking up a former

---

[34] Letter from Alice H. Halls to Sister Milner, dated 28 January 1911, attached to the notes of Martha Parker (EVS: 1911; Part I).

[35] The medical students are Kathleen Baylis (MS: 1906; Part I) and Mary Atherton (MS: 1907; Part II); Cora Sergeant is the LCC lecturer (MS: 1907; Part II).

[36] Martha Aldridge (MS: 1907; Part II); Eliza Miles (EVS: 1913; Part II).

[37] Emma Bevan (EVS: 1911; Part II).

[38] Kate Davey (MS: 1907; Part I) and (EVS: 1909; Part II; 1911; Part I).

[39] B.L. Hutchins, *Women in Modern Industry* (London: G. Bell and Sons Ltd., 1915; republished Wakefield: E.P. Publishing Limited, 1978), p. xiv. Hutchins explains that the analysis was completed before the outbreak of war in the summer of 1914 (v), and so provides a useful source for this pre-war study.

trade or beginning a new one when times were hard is evident from the situations of a number of married women attending as in-patients. Annie Hobbs remarked that her husband had been out of work for six months, compelling her, though heavily pregnant and unwell, to work for Eley's, a firearms manufacturer in Edmonton.[40] Lizzie Fife was an in-patient twice in 1904. When she was first admitted in April, suffering from haemorrhage following a miscarriage, she was given the occupation 'house'. By August, however, when she was pregnant again and another miscarriage threatened, she had evidently returned to work, as she was now listed as a milliner.[41] Georgiana Mary Hardcastle acknowledged that she had been a waitress only for the last three months, having been married for five years, with two children under four, but did not explain why she had taken up employment at this point.[42] At 44, Louisa Francis worked as a bookfolder and had to walk five miles to her place of employment; as four of her five children were dead and the survivor was 20, she evidently did not work to support them, but circumstances dictated that she had both to take on employment and walk there.[43] A number of women had continued to work since their marriages, whether they had children or not. Again, the range of occupations was wide. Hard or physically demanding employment was carried out by Ada Bowman, who was a laundress, and Emily Burt, a dairy-maid, when she first visited the hospital as a married woman.[44] Although noted as 'house' on the cover sheet, Elizabeth Smith's work was 'very heavy, with great worry'; hardly surprising given she stated that she was occupied between 7.30am and 12.30 midnight.[45] Beckish Schwartz, although noted as a housewife, claimed that she had 'been working at washing and cleaning up to the present illness', which had contributed to the premature labour of a dead six-months' child.[46] Catharine Bennett's dual existence was emphasised by her roles as 'house and char'.[47] Annie Baddock worked in a factory as a cartridge maker, while Helen Longman, who was yet to have children, had continued her life in service.[48] Sarah Woods combined keeping her own house with the management of another, while the notes of Louisa Whelan did not elaborate any further upon precisely what she did in 'perfumery'.[49] Margaret Llewelyn Davies' introduction to a

[40] Annie Hobbs (MS: 1904). See also (MS: 1906; Part I) and her final visit and death (MS: 1906; Part II).
[41] Lizzie Fife (MS: 1904).   [42] Georgiana Mary Hardcastle (EVS: 1904–1908; 1904).
[43] Louisa Francis (EVS: 1904–1908; 1908).
[44] Ada Bowman (EVS: 1913; Part II); Emily Burt (MS: 1904); (EVS: 1904–1908; 1905). On her second visit, Emily Burt has 'house' as her occupation.
[45] Elizabeth Smith (MS: 1908; Part II).   [46] Beckish Schwartz (MS: 1908; Part II).
[47] Catharine Bennett (MS: 1906; Part II).
[48] Annie Baddock (MS: 1907; Part II); Helen Longman (EVS: 1912; Part I).
[49] Sarah Woods (MS: 1907; Part I); Louisa Whelan (MS: 1907; Part II).

collection of 160 *Letters from Working Women*, published in 1915, offered a salutary consideration of the 'incessant drudgery' experienced by the early twentieth-century working-class wife and mother. Those critical of working married women did not consider the double burden faced by those compelled through circumstances to seek employment: housework differed very little from servitude in Llewelyn-Davies' eyes. She warned: do not 'forget that the unpaid work of the working woman at the stove, at scrubbing and cleaning, at the washtub, in lifting and carrying heavy weights, is just as severe manual labour as many industrial operations in factories'.[50] Female patients who were married and who worked offer a rare insight into the juggling of responsibilities many women were forced into to keep their household in order. When coupled with the pain and suffering of illness, this burden was made even heavier.

An examination of the background of female patients at the RFH would not be complete without exploring the family histories of illness given by the patient which allows us to place the individual within a wider social network. The case notes traced keenly any potential patterns in ill-health between the patient and their wider circle of family members. This was in order to establish the possibility of hereditary disease, as well as dangers of the local environment which could constitute future threats to existing good health from infectious friends and relatives. The most popular queries concerned incidences of rheumatic fever, and, perhaps most importantly for a department dealing with the female generative organs, tuberculosis and cancer, two of the most feared diseases of the early twentieth century.[51] Given the secrecy surrounding infectious diseases such as TB, as well as the terror associated with cancer, the pathology of which was still uncertain, as chapter 3 will explore, it is surprising how much was revealed by patients when asked for the history of their family's health, even if it was not relevant to the current condition. Ada Hanton's circumstances were particularly extreme. Although she was attending as an in-patient for the incomplete miscarriage of her tenth child, she discussed her background with stark frankness, revealing a willingness to talk about illnesses usually stigmatised. Her

---

[50] Margaret Llewelyn Davies, 'Introduction' to *Maternity. Letters from Working Women* (London: G. Bell & Sons Ltd, 1915), ed. Gloden Dallas (London: Virago, 1978), p. 6.

[51] For tuberculosis in the early twentieth century, see Linda Bryder, *Below the Magic Mountain* (Oxford: Clarendon Press, 1988). For cancer more generally in the period concerned, see Ornella Moscucci, 'The British Fight against Cancer: Publicity and Education, 1900–1948', *SHM*, 23.2 (August 2010), 356–73; on cancer and gender, Moscucci, 'Gender and Cancer in Britain, 1860–1910: The Emergence of Cancer as a Public Health Concern', *American Journal of Public Health*, 95.8 (August 2005), 1312–21; and more specifically focusing on cancer of the cervix, Ilana Löwy, *A Woman's Disease* (Oxford: Oxford University Press, 2011).

father died of bronchitis, four of her brothers had 'consumption' and her mother was in Colney Hatch, vernacular for the lunatic asylum located in that area.[52] Rachel Watts' mother died in an asylum, where she had been incarcerated for 14 years, and two of her aunts were also inmates. The risky revelation that there was insanity on the female side was obviously brave in an institutional environment.[53] Louisa Harrington, also in for a miscarriage, had a 'strong family history of consumption'. Harrington's mother died of pneumonia (from which the current patient had also suffered), her father of cancer; all her father's brothers had died from consumption and five of her sisters and one of her brothers suffered from the disease too. The next generation had not been exempt either: Harrington's youngest child had 'consumption of the bowels' and 'suffers with its chest'; the eldest a 'cough'.[54] While her mother died, quite rarely, of nothing but 'old age', the rest of Elizabeth Smith's family background was more complicated. Her father and one sibling died of rheumatic fever, the other siblings died from consumption, heart disease, and Bright's disease. One died from blood poisoning. Additionally, an aunt and a cousin had succumbed to cancer.[55] Rose Law was found to be suffering from inoperable carcinoma of the cervix. Her history showed a remarkable incidence of the disease in the immediate and wider family. Law's mother died of 'cancer of the bladder', her sister at 44 (Law's current age) of 'cancer of the womb', a maternal uncle of 'cancer of the throat', and a paternal aunt of 'cancer of the breast'.[56] The specificity of detail given by patients permits a wider perspective on the prevalence of ill-health in the early twentieth-century family. Similarly, the willingness of some patients to lay bare a possible 'taint' contradicts received wisdom that many found infectious or life-threatening disease a taboo subject.

If openness to inquiry was evident in patient notes, the opposite was also true. Family breakdown and ongoing dissent were apparent, ensuring that a request to detail the condition of relatives was met with a negative or a tirade. Although Louisa Norfolk was one of 13 children, she now knew 'nothing of [her siblings]' and 'has never been ill in her life'.[57] Eighteen-year-old housemaid, Trixie Lucreace, lost her parents when she was a child and, therefore, 'knows nothing about her family history'.[58] Cecilia Chambers was an 'orphan and brought up in an orphanage, so does not know family history'.[59] The splitting

[52] Ada Hanton (MS: 1904).   [53] Rachel Watts (EVS: 1911; Part II).
[54] Louisa Harrington (MS: 1905; Part I).   [55] Elizabeth Smith (MS: 1908; Part II).
[56] Rose Law (EVS: 1913; Part I).   [57] Louisa Norfolk (MS: 1904); (MS: 1907; Part I).
[58] Trixie Lucreace (MS: 1904).   [59] Cecilia Chambers (MS: 1907; Part II).

up of a family through more violent means occurred a number of times in the notes. Alice Dignum had 'no relations' and the only thing known about her parents was that her mother was Jamaican.[60] Lily Burtles' husband was in an asylum, and had been there longer than the child she was carrying had been in existence.[61] When Florence Coleman first visited the RFH, her husband was alive, although she was charring for a living and looked 'distressed'; by 1911, eighteen months later, she was a widow, her husband having been in asylum for a year before his death.[62] Although married, without any mention of separation noted in her history, Annie Stafford did not want to talk about her spouse and remarked that her husband was healthy 'as far as she knows'.[63] Fanny Backshall dated all her many problems to her marriage, explaining that 'her health was good until' this point; now she suffered from a variety of pains, aches and attacks of 'general debility', none of which she had experienced before she wed her husband.[64] Having procured an illegal abortion, Mrs Constance Webb or Mrs Mary Ross, depending upon which name was really hers, falsified information and disguised her background.[65] Other women sought to defend the awkwardness or embarrassment of their situation. Twenty-four-year-old Rose Nash's stoicism characterised her history. She could 'remember no illnesses of any kind' and 'has always been well and healthy'. Although 'circumstances have not been quite so good lately', she insisted that she 'always has enough food and has no great cause to worry'. When asked about her paleness, Nash responded by confirming that she 'always is', clearly anxious not to concern anyone.[66] Alice Reynolds, exhausted after nursing one of her seven children with scarlet fever, had a miscarriage in hospital after days of bleeding. The frustration of the note-taker with Mrs Reynolds' cheery outlook was palpable: 'patient looks very pale and exhausted but expresses herself as feeling very comfortable; the patient says she feels stronger and better every day – but she looks extremely pale. [...] She still looked exceedingly anaemic and ill, but expressed herself as feeling quite well and gaining strength daily.'[67] At times, those examining patients were forced to rely solely on the person in front of them, if they were co-operative, to assist in a clinical diagnosis. Risse has expressed concern over the lack of consideration in the history of medical institutions about the 'isolation from family networks' which

---

[60] Alice Dignum (EVS: 1913; Part II).   [61] Lily Burtles (EVS: 1910; Part II).
[62] Florence Coleman (EVS: 1909; Part II); (Part 1911; Part I).
[63] Annie Stafford (EVS: 1910; Part II).   [64] Fanny Backshall (EVS: 1904–1908; 1908).
[65] Constance Webb/Mary Ross (MS; 1908; Part I).
[66] Rose Nash (EVS: 1908; Part II).   [67] Alice Reynolds (EVS: 1906; Part II).

resulted from a stay in hospital.[68] But, as some of the female patients of Scharlieb and Vaughan-Sawyer implied, the family network might be something from which the patient was keen to distance herself. Placing an individual within a family environment in order to determine susceptibility to specific conditions was not as easy as it sounded when patients could obscure, deliberately or otherwise, their connections to others.

Drudgery and ingrained family suffering were not the lot of every woman between 1903 and 1913. There was another category, split into three in the graph of female occupations, which offered further evidence that the 'sick poor' were not the only patients to frequent the hospital. The sections represented 'None noted', 'Nil' or '–' are worth exploring in more detail. 'None noted' was the most unreliable of the three, as it referred to a blank on the cover sheet, where the note-taker failed, deliberately or otherwise, to fill in the question. While some years have very complete records, others, like Vaughan-Sawyer's for May–December 1913, have 29 blank boxes for occupation, out of a total of 71 patients. Of those, some can be ascertained. Marjorie Crittenden was eight months old; Emma Bull was 14, and could have still been at school, but her history noted that she was a bookbinder; and 23-year-old Ethel Tweed's record stated that she was an assistant in a baker's shop. It was harder to guess whether women in their sixties, such as Emily Higham or Mary E. Piddington, were still employed. As previous paragraphs have shown, it was entirely possible that widowed female patients, like both of these, worked to support themselves. Hagar Walker was in the hospital for the fifth time in 1913 and had been an in-patient on and off since 1906. She had previously been described as 'house', but her occupation was now left blank, either through oversight or familiarity.[69] Some may not have chosen to reveal what they did or the note-taker did not write down 'house', as it was taken as read, given the number seen. More intriguing was 'nil' or '–', which was nearly always attributed to single women and implied that they did not have to work for a living. In some cases this was due to a long-standing medical condition. Elsie Ward, who was 20, had 'some paralysis' since she was a child, and did not walk until she was four.[70] Twenty-three-year-old Isla Logan, who was said to have previously suffered from 'hysteria', and 'fainted several times a day', appeared to be a

---

[68] Guenter B. Risse, 'Hospital History: New Sources and Methods', in *Problems and Methods in the History of Medicine*, eds., Roy Porter and Andrew Wear (London: Routledge, 1987), pp. 175–204; p. 175.

[69] All patients mentioned in this paragraph, unless stated otherwise, are from (EVS: 1913; Part I). Hagar Walker appears originally in (MS: 1906; Part II), and then in (EVS: 1909; Part I); (EVS: 1911; Part I) and twice in (EVS: 1913; Part II).

[70] Elsie Ward (MS: 1908; Part II).

chronic invalid.[71] Edith James was a private patient of Vaughan-Sawyer, and, therefore, must have been able to pay something for her initial treatment. While women surgeons, such as May Thorne, held 'cheap days' in private practice for less well-off patients, fees were not gratuitous and something was contributed, even if it was offered at a discount.[72] The leisure time of 21-year-old Ida Gladys Ord, whose occupation was replaced by a line, was more than evident in her personal history, which was characterised by visiting a dubious set of 'friends'.[73] Charitable or religious endeavours also occupied others, such as Amy Drake, whose occupation was recorded as 'Church Work' and who resided at Harrow Mission, and the number of Salvation Army officers has already been noted.[74] Cullen has remarked upon the incidence of patients who were hardly to be categorised as destitute poor in other departments of the hospital, so the Gynaecological Department was clearly not alone in admitting those who could pay for treatment.[75] The increased aseptic safety of the hospital environment must have overridden any concerns those who did not have to work for a living might have had about life on the ward of an institution largely composed of the sick poor, as we shall see later in chapter 5.

Reasons for Attendance

After exploring the varied backgrounds of female patients who sought treatment in the Gynaecological Department, it is necessary to consider their reasons for attending in the first place. The majority of patients would have been seen at Out-Patients and admitted from there, either immediately, if the case was serious, or when there was a bed free. Others travelled from outside London, having presented a letter from their own practitioner in order to gain admission to a metropolitan institution. Some of these documents were still extant, attached to the case histories, and pointed to the ways in which the profession operated. Correspondence indicated how general practitioners sought the opinion of specialists, or how stumped specialists requested another

[71] Isla Logan (EVS: 1911; Part I). She does state, however, that she has been worn out with 'nursing' and 'worry' the past six months, but, unfortunately, does not elaborate upon the situation.
[72] Edith James (EVS: 1912; Part I); widowed housekeeper, Lucy M. Jones, is also directly noted as a private patient of Vaughan Sawyer (EVS: 1912; Part I). For private operations and the woman surgeon, see my 'Risk, Responsibility and Surgery', 320.
[73] Ida Gladys Ord (EVS: 1910; Part II).   [74] Amy Drake (EVS: 1911; Part I).
[75] Cullen, 'Patient Records', p. 255.

opinion.[76] A decade after a laparotomy performed by James Berry, where abdominal adhesions had been broken down, Kent resident Kate Johnson was admitted under Vaughan-Sawyer for a recurrence of pain in her abdomen. Her doctor, W. Batchelor Taylor of Sevenoaks, wrote:

I should be extremely glad if you give this woman, Mrs Johnson, the benefit of your advice. She was an inmate of the Hospital for some abdominal complaint and had a section done in 1901. She has been having attacks on the other side resembling renal colic, but not quite typical. I think her old notes on the case might help. She is a case deserving of Hospital treatment.[77]

Given the contemporary outcry over misuse of voluntary hospitals, Taylor prudently concluded his request with a reassurance that this was a 'deserving' case.[78] In Devon, Olive M. Goodwin's case confused her local practitioner, who thought she must be seven months pregnant because of the rapid increase in the size of her abdomen and had prepared accordingly. Unsure of his own assessment, he then consulted another medical man in Torquay, who diagnosed an abdominal tumour and sent the patient to the RFH, where she was, indeed, discovered to have an ovarian cyst.[79] The network of communication between general practitioner and specialist did not only function one way, however. There were also copies of notes from within the RFH addressed to patients' doctors, usually in order to elicit further information about the case or to have medical confirmation of something the patient might have suggested. When Alice E. Howes was admitted she stated that she has been treated previously for 'effusions of blood' under the skin of her arms, legs and face by Dr Mellor of Wood Green and this clearly concerned the hospital. Dr Mellor was subsequently contacted for 'information', which he duly provided. 'Madam', he wrote, 'In reply to yr [sic] letter received last night, the statement of Alice Howes is correct. I considered it a case of Purpura. As far as I know there is no history of bleeding in the family.'[80] In this instance, the RFH, troubled by what a patient suggested about their past history (namely, that they might, without using the term, have haemophilia) and the implications it might have for the success of any future surgical

---

[76] For the 'generally good' (p. 294) relationship between general practitioners and hospital specialists or consultants, see Anne Digby, *The Evolution of British General Practice 1850–1948* (Oxford: Oxford University Press, 1999), especially pp. 294–305.

[77] This letter is actually appended to the wrong set of notes, bound two years before Kate Johnson entered the hospital. See Kate Johnson (EVS: 1911; Part II) and the letter, dated 6 November 1911, which is with the file of Emily Saich (EVS: 1909; Part II).

[78] See, for example, Keir Waddington, 'Unsuitable Cases: The Debate over Outpatient Admissions, the Medical Profession and late-Victorian London Hospitals', *MH*, 42.1 (January 1998), 26–46.

[79] Olive M. Goodwin (EVS: 1912; Part I).   [80] Alice E. Howes (EVS: 1910; Part II).

procedure (the possibility of the patient bleeding to death on the oper-ating table), sought further information from the general practitioner so that they could continue with the patient's treatment appropriately. Communication between different members of the medical profession was vital to ensure that the hospital received lay as well as clinical infor-mation about the patient. This meant that the individual's testimony was supported by well-documented medical evidence, but also reveals the sheer importance of listening to patients so extolled by Vaughan-Sawyer.

While such examples showed the necessity of smooth communication between practitioners and between patient, practitioner and specialist, there were also a number of instances in the case histories where failures in these links caused disastrous consequences. Digby has claimed that 'hard-pressed' general practitioners, when faced with 'difficult or time-consuming patients', might utilise the services of a specialist to put an authoritative stamp on the case, either dismissing it as trivial or eluci-dating the condition for colleague and patient alike.[81] Annie Dryden's general practitioner sent her to the RFH, fearing that she had 'cancer of the lining of the womb'.[82] Vaughan-Sawyer agreed that the patient's history of menorrhagia and dysmenorrhoea, along with the increase in the size of her abdomen, appeared suspicious of malignancy. However, she believed the condition was more suggestive of fibroids, and this, in fact, was what Annie Dryden was discovered to have. Here, communi-cation between patient, general practitioner and specialist ensured that Mrs Dryden was seen quickly, her condition considered through her own testimony, physical examination and finally decided by operation. Her doctor's fears were unfounded, but an overreaction led to the discov-ery of a different problem, which was solved through surgery. Likewise, Ellen E. Winborn was sent in for 'carcinoma of the cervix', because she had been bleeding irregularly per vaginam for four months.[83] Luckily for Mrs Winborn, 'nothing to suggest' such a diagnosis was found. Too frequently, however, women's fears, especially when the problem was gynaecological, were dismissed by their own doctors, as we shall see later in the chapter. The series 'Heard about Hospital', a regular feature in the *Magazine* of the LSMW from 1910, mocked the patient body for its absurdities, malapropisms and general ignorance. One anecdote shed a more serious light on the gulf between the patient narrative and profes-sional opinion. In the form of a question addressed to a student by an examiner, the dialogue ran as follows: 'What is the difference between *symptoms* and *signs*? Answer: A symptom is what the patient *thinks* is the

---

[81] Digby, *Evolution*, p. 298.   [82] Annie Dryden (EVS: 1912; Part II).
[83] Ellen E. Winborn (MS: 1908; Part II).

matter with him. A sign is what *really is*.'[84] Symptoms could be described even if they were not felt, but signs were seen, legible only to the medical professional. Symptoms could be ignored; signs never.

'Heard at Hospital' mocked mercilessly the 'symptoms' described by omniscient patients.[85] One claimed they were suffering from '"nervous ability and haricot veins"', while 'Medical Knowledge in the Laity' was revealed to be particularly scanty: '"Yes, poor girl, she's very ill, her eyes bulge right out". "Why is that?" "She has goitres behind them"'. Nor did surgical advances bypass some, as one particularly sage comment made clear in a discussion about treatment: '"Oh nowadays surgeons never give anaesthetics. They just rub a drop or something on the patient's back and he feels nothing till it's all over"'. Cullen notes the ways in which patient and professional characterise the physical signs of ill-health, such as the size of wounds or swellings, in similar lay parlance, but it is also noticeable that the former had their own ideas about where or when their problems originated.[86] Either through sheer ignorance or deliberate obfuscation, Hettie Beck was convinced that abdominal problems caused by gonorrhoea could be attributed to 'a meal of fried fish'.[87] Margaret Clifford also blamed 'fried fish' for pain, diarrhoea and vomiting.[88] Alternatively, Mary Pipe pointed to her consumption of strawberries.[89] Seventeen-year-old Gladys Ward's sister informed the hospital that she had a nose or a mouth bleed every month instead of a period.[90] Edith Dowes blamed her underclothes, in this case having put on damp tights, for causing the cessation of menstruation.[91] In these instances, Sir James Berry's warning in his *Manual of Surgical Diagnosis* (1904) that '[i]t is well to receive with a certain amount of distrust any diagnosis which the patient himself may have made' was only too apt.[92]

Neither did a number of patients comprehend precisely what previous treatment they had received. This could imply that communication between doctor and patient was not as open or honest as might be assumed, especially when the purpose or consequences of an operation were concerned. Or, potentially, it may mean that the patient did not listen to what they were being told about their condition or understand what

---

[84] 'Heard about Hospital', *L(RFH)SMWM*, 8.51 (March 1912), 43; original emphasis.
[85] All the following examples are from 'Heard at Hospital', *L(RFH)SMWM*, 7.49 (July 1911), 438.
[86] Cullen, 'Patient Records', p. 261.   [87] Hettie Beck (MS: 1905; Part I).
[88] Margaret Clifford (EVS: 1910; Part II).   [89] Mary Pipe (EVS: 1909; Part II).
[90] Gladys Ward (MS: 1907; Part I).   [91] Edith Dowes (EVS: 1910; Part II).
[92] James Berry, *A Manual of Surgical Diagnosis* (London: J. and A. Churchill, 1904; Philadelphia: P. Blakiston's Son and Co, 1904), p. 14.

had happened to them. Professional language might perplex a lay person or confusion may result from how the procedure related to their own bodies. Katie Sykes knew she had an anaesthetic at the Soho Hospital and subsequently 'some operation', but she did not know which.[93] Henrietta Bray was aware that 'something' had been wrong with both of her children; that one had 'something removed from the back passage' and the other 'something from above the eye', but she was unable to articulate what exactly had been removed from each.[94] At either the German or the Homeopathic Hospital, Frances Fidler had 'something' 'passed up into lower passage and the stomach became smaller but not as small as it used to be', while Annie Cohen dated her problems from the time she was examined by a doctor 'who did some manipulation with an instrument'; since then she had 'never been well'.[95] A number of confused accounts were related to conditions surrounding pregnancy. It is not clear whether this was because the female patient evidently had other things to worry about at this point, and, therefore, might not remember in detail what had been said, or because miscarriages and parturition were experienced as an inevitable routine by both doctor and patient. Bessie Barrett knew that 'afterbirth had grown to the womb and had to be taken away', while Martha Aldridge was 'told by a doctor at University College Hospital' that passing clots after going 'beyond your time', which she had done 12 or 14 times, meant a miscarriage.[96] Margaret Robertson's muddled account of her previous RFH operation was compounded by the fact that her old notes from 1892 could not be found. She was informed, she stated, that there was a tumour in her pelvis as large as an apple, and in the tumour there was an abscess and from this she had 'got blood poisoning'.[97] By contrast, Louie Barnard remarked that she had been curetted twice at St Mary's Hospital, but when she was opened up, her right ovary and fallopian tube were absent, something which she had not previously mentioned. Vaughan-Sawyer was left to 'surmise' that these had been removed at St Mary's.[98] Eliza Croft stated categorically that she 'was not told what her previous operation was for' at Marylebone Hospital for Women. It was noted in the margin of her notes that the left ovary had been removed.[99] The late nineteenth and early twentieth century saw increasing agitation at the way hospital patients were treated, with the formation of organisations such as the Society for the Protection of Hospital

---

[93] Katie Sykes (MS: 1904).   [94] Henrietta Bray (MS: 1905; Part I).
[95] Frances Fidler (EVS: 1912; Part I); Annie Cohen (EVS: 1912; Part I).
[96] Bessie Barrett (MS: 1905; Part II); Martha Aldridge (MS: 1907; Part II).
[97] Margaret Robertson (EVS: 1913; Part II).   [98] Louie Barnard (EVS: 1912; Part I).
[99] Eliza Croft (EVS: 1910; Part I).

Patients.[100] It is easy to see when reading some accounts of past procedures why groups were calling for more clarity in the clinical encounter. While the language used by patients to describe their symptoms revealed their lack of knowledge about clinical terminology or their imprecision about exactly what was wrong with them, quoted phrases from the notes indicated the extent of the pain suffered. Berry remarked on the patient tendency to compose narratives from reading about a condition rather than experiencing it, especially if the sufferer was middle class: a 'glib' and imaginative line of symptoms resulted.[101] Some of the gynaecological patients of Scharlieb and Vaughan-Sawyer were no exception. Edith James, for example, a private patient of the latter, had the 'unhealthy appearance of a chronic invalid' and her narrative was lengthy and extremely detailed, explaining every symptom felt and hospital stay undergone over the past 15 years.[102] Many others, however, were only able to characterise their suffering through bald, visceral description, without attempting to make their vocabulary anything other than understandable to all. These phrases, placed in inverted commas in the patient records, succeeded in drawing the attention of the note-taker to the individual with the condition, rather than the condition itself. The patient voice was not suppressed here, but only too audible. Women utilised familiar, often household analogies or metaphors to discuss the reality of their situation. Knife imagery featured a great deal. Ellen Elliot's sharp abdominal pain was 'like a knife in the womb' and another Edith James described her pain as 'sharp like knives'.[103] Elizabeth Bennett's pain on defecation was also 'sharp like a knife'.[104] Violent actions, like a kick or a punch, illuminated the ways in which some ached. Annie Bodley's abdomen hurt 'as if she had a blow on her back', for example.[105] The majority of patients, whether they were mothers or not, sought to use the language of childbirth to compare with their present suffering: 'bearing-down pains' characterised many gynaecological cases at the RFH.[106] The sheer unpleasantness of passing clots or heavy bleeding per vaginam reminded some of cuts of meat or offal. Mabel Frost suggested her discharge contained 'thick pieces like liver' and Elizabeth Trewhella

---

[100] See, for example, my 'Risk, Responsibility and Surgery', 330–2 for the Beatty versus Cullingworth case which led to the formation of this society.
[101] Berry, *A Manual*, p. 14.   [102] Edith James (EVS: 1912; Part I).
[103] Ellen Elliot and Edith James: both (MS: 1904). For a recent exploration of how patients describe pain, see Joanna Bourke, *The Story of Pain* (Oxford: Oxford University Press, 2014), especially pp. 53–87.
[104] Elizabeth Bennett (MS: 1905; Part I).   [105] Annie Bodley (MS: 1908; Part II).
[106] Two of very many examples will suffice: from a single patient, Eva Foster (EVS: 1912; Part II) and a married one, Elizabeth Collett (MS: 1905; Part II).

also found 'lumps of liver' within her blood.[107] Graenia M. Johnso
compared the mess caused by a miscarriage as like passing 'brain'. Rut
Barden was less specific, simply noting the 'pieces of flesh coming away
The amount of blood lost, whether from coughing or vaginally, was fr
quently measured in chamber pots. Sarah Handford expressed her lo
in half-chamber pots, while Ruth Barden explained an episode wheret
she brought up a 'chamber-full' of blood from her lungs.[108] By contras
Amelia Young's rectal discharge appeared more innocent than the bloo
iness of other images: 'like the white of an egg'.[109] Its innocuous natu
belied the seriousness of her condition: carcinoma of the sigmoid. Ot
ers were far more idiosyncratic in their choice of description, especially
symptoms or signs were not easily evident on the patient's body. Elizabe
Mackinney's example of her abdominal swelling feeling as if there was 'a
egg rolling about in her stomach' was a particularly individualised way
label what turned out to be an ovarian cyst.[110] Caroline Williams' dai
chores provided her with an ideal way to depict the internal trouble sl
had been having. While using a wringing machine, she felt as if her 'insic
had been twisted'.[111] Gertrude Figg, by contrast, could only point to
sinking feeling 'as if her inside was dropping from her'.[112] After her fir
confinement, Emma Storrie explained that her 'insides were outside'.[1
These patients, the majority uneducated housewives, could not easi
replicate lists of symptoms learned from books or have recourse to lite
ary language, as Berry claimed more middle-class persons could. The
examples were illustrated through comparisons with what they knew
the home, cooking, childbirth – but were none the less potent for th
familiarity.

Some of the more outlandish reasons for illness so mocked in tl
'Heard at Hospital' series and the ignorance apparent in the patie
records themselves obscured the more precise knowledge which sever
patients showed regarding their condition. Such a grasp of sympton
and signs tended to stem from experience, which allowed a patient
recognise when there was something wrong with them because they hav
been through the same process before. Martha Penry's case provide
an excellent example of a patient's quick thinking in seeking hospit
treatment because she was familiar with her condition. Mrs Penry w
admitted twice in 15 months.[114] The second time she arrived at tl

[107]   Mabel Frost (EVS: 1913; Part II); Elizabeth Trewhella (MS: 1908; Part II).
[108]   Sarah Handford (EVS: 1912; Part I); Ruth Barden (MS: 1908; Part I).
[109]   Amelia Young (EVS: 1904–1908; 1907).   [110]   Elizabeth Mackinney (MS: 1904)
[111]   Caroline Williams (MS: 1905; Part I).   [112]   Gertrude Figg (MS: 1905; Part II).
[113]   Emma Storrie (EVS: 1913; Part I).
[114]   Martha Penry (EVS: 1911; Part I) and (EVS: 1912; Part II).

hospital she knew what was wrong with her and informed the doctors. Sudden pain and a heavy feeling in her abdomen alerted Mrs Penry to the fact that she was haemorrhaging internally. Although she had not been feeling well for weeks, it was the speed with which the pain came on that told her she had experienced another ruptured ectopic gestation. Similarly, in some instances, a family member's or friend's awareness of particular signals, which pointed to something they recognised or understood, was also evident. Frances Graves' mother told her 'that there was something the matter with the womb'. It turns out that Mrs Graves' mother was correct, as her daughter was discovered to have an eroded cervix.[115] Overreaction, especially to bumps and swellings, also suggested that fear of cancer, as already noted, led some women to be more concerned about possible sources of disease. Although she had only a cyst of Bartholini's Gland, Annie Stafford came to the RFH because she was terrified that the lump might turn into a 'tumour'.[116] Wider awareness of the potential causes of pain, whether that was from personal experience, family connections, or greater publicity of diseases in the early twentieth century, all prompted some patients to seek treatment as quickly as possible to end both physical and mental suffering.

There were numerous circumstances where both symptoms and signs were ignored by the professional, with consequences only for the patient. If public trust in medicine was increasing at the end of the nineteenth and the beginning of the twentieth century, some patients might have had cause to think the opposite.[117] Some were lucky. Vaginal examinations were not performed by the doctors of Julia Randolph and Esther Chapman, but the former's practitioner advised her to go to hospital and the latter was given initially successful medical treatment by hers.[118] A few cases in particular showed a more disastrous failure to consider patients seriously enough: all of these were dismissed as instances of the menopause. As American gynaecologist Howard Kelly urged, 'every week of delay in radical treatment [. . .] is precious time lost'. He had no qualms about blaming the general practitioner for 'a fault which makes him responsible year by year for the loss of many lives'.[119] In May 1904, Ellen Mead was admitted with extensive, inoperable carcinoma of the cervix. Three months before she had been to a Dr Roberts of Cambridge Gardens, who had given her medicine and told her that the excessive bleeding she was experiencing, her loss of weight and extreme

---

[115] Frances Graves (MS: 1904).   [116] Annie Stafford (EVS: 1910; Part II).
[117] On trust, see, for example, Wilde, 'Truth, Trust'.
[118] Julia Randolph (EVS: 1910; Part I); Esther Chapman (EVS: 1910; Part II).
[119] Howard A. Kelly, *Medical Gynecology* (New York: D. Appleton and Company, 1908), p. 155.

weakness were due to 'the change of life'; her painful, persistent backache, he decided, was caused by sciatica.[120] When Mrs Mead came to Out-Patients, she was admitted at once. Although Scharlieb believed her cancer might be operable, when the patient was opened up, it was discovered to have spread to the iliac vessels and was irremovable. As a note appended to her history reveals, Ellen Mead died ten weeks after leaving hospital. Sarah Timpson, a 46-year-old steam-laundry worker, experienced similar treatment.[121] She had been bleeding for three months and had seen a Dr Wyborn of York Road. He informed Mrs Timpson that it was 'the change of life', which he deduced without any examination of his patient. When Sarah Timpson came to Gynaecological Out-Patients malignancy was feared and she was admitted and underwent a panhysterectomy for carcinoma of the fundus uteri. By 1907, there was a recurrence and the cancer became inoperable. A self-confessed 'very strong' woman who did hard physical work as a laundress, the last time she appeared in the notes, she was compelled to walk on crutches because of the pain. Mary Hilier was not examined by her doctor, Dr Stokers of the New Kent Road, despite vaginal bleeding. He did give her medicine and told her to stay in bed for two weeks and the bleeding stopped. She went to the RFH, where she was diagnosed as having carcinoma of the fundus uteri; she refused hysterectomy and was discharged.[122] Jane Thomas also had a detailed history of irregular bleeding.[123] She too visited a doctor, who gave her medicine and told her to stay in bed until she was better. When, after a month, she was so weak 'she felt she could not continue her daily life without help', she consulted Dr Edith Sargeant, who sent her immediately to the RFH. Mrs Thomas had an abdominal hysterectomy for cervical cancer. There was a recurrence at the beginning of 1907, and she died four days after admission. Agnes Wade had experienced vaginal bleeding for a year and had consulted a doctor, who informed her that she was undergoing 'the change of life' and 'treated her accordingly'. The pain became worse, so she consulted another doctor, who advised her to seek further advice. She was treated at the RFH for carcinoma of the cervix, but, a year later, it had spread, become inoperable, and she died in hospital.[124] Finally, Florence M. Spanghton was told by her doctor that she had miscarried because of blood loss and passage of large

---

[120] Ellen Mead (MS: 1904). She also appears as Emily on the front cover.
[121] Sarah Timpson (MS: 1905; Part I) and for the recurrence (MS: 1907; Part I).
[122] Mary Hilier (MS: 1905; Part I).
[123] Jane Thomas (MS: 1907; Part I); recurrence and death in hospital also (MS: 1907; Part I).
[124] Agnes Wade (EVS: 1909; Part II); (EVS: 1910; Part I).

clots.[125] As she informed the RFH, she was very much aware that she was not pregnant, so knew something was wrong. Mrs Spanghton was cachetic, evidently extremely ill, therefore, and was subsequently found to have inoperable carcinoma of the cervix. The failure of these five medical men to provide adequate initial consultation, in spite of patient concerns, ensured that vital symptoms and signs were missed, effective treatment was given too late, and conditions became inoperable.

That there was an obvious gender division here between the reaction of the one medical woman mentioned and the male general practitioner warrants discussion. This is not to suggest that all medical men were unable to spot malignancy or that female doctors were preternaturally aware of such conditions. Maud Davis' male doctor, for example, gave her medicine to stop haemorrhage, but, concerned about her health, encouraged her to seek further advice as soon as possible.[126] Women doctors treated women; male general practitioners treated both sexes and were perhaps less used to seeing such conditions or hearing similar concerns. Although very few of the gynaecological patient base used the services of medical women, as we shall see, those who did were referred quickly to specialists when anything suspicious arose. This might be because the female medical network was small and therefore particularly tightly interrelated; many women doctors had passed through the LSMW, for example, and maintained connections with it, the RFH, the Association of Registered Medical Women, and other female-run institutions.[127] The case of Ethel Joud illustrated the extent of international links between medical women. Joud had been married for five years and lived in India for the same length of time. Three years previously, she had seen a male doctor there; later, six months before her admission, she had seen a 'woman doctor', who recommended the RFH. On her return to London, she had visited Scharlieb, who referred her for admission under Vaughan-Sawyer.[128] Even more fascinating was the number of women who had been sent to the RFH from female general practitioners. The total was surprisingly small. Not all patients named their local doctor, neither did note-takers always write down the first name of the practitioner, and so it was not possible to be precise on the actual figures involved. However, of 1403 patient records examined, only 73 women named a general practitioner of the same sex. Nearly half of those patients mentioned Mary

125 Florence M. Spanghton (EVS: 1907; Part I).
126 Maud Davis (EVS: 1911; Part II).
127 For connections between medical women, institutional or otherwise, see Elston, "'Run
     by Women'".
128 Ethel Joud (EVS: 1909; Part I).

Scharlieb, who, even after retirement from the hospital in 1908, continued to act as Consultant to the Diseases of Women and regularly sent her own patients there.[129] Ethel Vaughan-Sawyer had previously seen seven of these women. So, out of the 73, 39 patients had already seen the two female surgeons at the RFH. The relatively few seeking out treatment by medical women may be the result of their lack of prominence in areas where patients lived, or perhaps because there was still a stigma about female doctors. Certainly, while women were willing to see several different general practitioners, they nearly always sought male advice. The only exceptions were teachers. Some 50 per cent of Scharlieb's patients who described themselves as teachers had sought her advice privately beforehand; this was true of a third of Vaughan-Sawyer's cases, who had also been to see Scharlieb.[130] It could be suggested then that more of the educated and single chose to visit women doctors than their working-class counterparts. Interestingly, though, one patient, Alice M. Turner, first saw a male doctor, and it was he who pointed out that she had a swelling in her abdomen; she only decided to see Scharlieb when the problems became worse.[131] This pattern was similar to many other narratives encountered in the notes of women from all backgrounds. As the case of Harriet Stanford made clear, some female patients had been searching for years for someone to help them, moving from doctor to doctor in the hope that one would eventually and successfully effect a cure.[132]

Whether through the desire to obtain a male opinion or a decision to go straight to a hospital where women's diseases were treated and bypass a general practitioner, the case notes of the Gynaecological Department revealed that the majority of women patients saw medical men before coming to the hospital. The speed with which female general practitioners sent their patients to the RFH, however, generally exceeded that of their male colleagues. Not one patient, however, of the 1403 seen by Scharlieb or Vaughan-Sawyer between 1903 and 1913 made reference to embarrassment at or feeling uncomfortable by a male practitioner's examination. One of the key arguments women had utilised to claim their suitability to practise medicine was simply not relevant to the RFH's female patients.

---

[129] *The Eighty-First Annual Report for 1908* (1909), p. 19.
[130] Patients of Scharlieb: Alice A. Turner (MS: 1907; Part I); Margaret Barker (EVS: 1909; Part II); Fanny Freeman (EVS: 1911; Part I); not patients: Ellen Kinsey (MS: 1908; Part II); Gypsy Andrews (EVS: 1911; Part I).
[131] Alice A. Turner (MS: 1907; Part II).
[132] Harriet Stanford (EVS: 1904–1908; 1908). Since the birth of her first child, Mrs Stanford had undergone a number of procedures to repair a perineal tear; none had been successful.

The time it took a patient to seek either male or female medical advice was a vital part of the case history. It allowed the specialist to track the progress of an illness, and determine, especially in gynaecological cases, the likelihood of malignancy even before tests were carried out or laparotomies performed. Cullen has drawn attention to those who wait, dismissing symptoms and allowing the historian an 'insight into how patients judged the seriousness of their own ill-health in relation to the cost of missing work or disrupting their family lives to receive treatment'.[133] Economic considerations were of importance to the female patients who worked, but the majority of housewives would have been concerned primarily with the effect any absence through hospitalisation would have on the family. Women did not always seek treatment as soon as they 'understood their bodies to be ailing'.[134] Additionally, due to the very nature of the conditions witnessed, even if a problem had been thought solved, as in the case of Harriet Stanford's ongoing perineal tear, repeated childbearing could literally reopen old wounds. The patients who waited the longest for treatment were those who had prolapses or torn perineums; neither of which would have made daily life very comfortable. It is possible that both conditions were considered peculiarly female, and, therefore, something which women, by their very nature, had to expect. As one writer began, when dealing her maternal 'sufferings' for the 1915 collection of *Letters from Working Women*: 'I thought, like hundreds of women do to-day, that it was only natural, and you had to bear it.'[135] 'Bearing it', though, was a messy, bloody, often filthy business for the women involved. Edith Abrahams, who was in the RFH four times between 1903 and 1906, had suffered from vaginal haemorrhages since her first and only confinement in 1890.[136] Although she had sought professional advice several times, including treatment at St George's Hospital for a decade, Mrs Abrahams' situation had been worsening, the bleeding coupled with epileptic fits and loss of consciousness. After 20 years of dysmenorrhoea following catamenia at 14, single clerk Ethel Court put into words the suffering many women must have gone through by claiming succinctly that the pain was so bad that she would frequently 'contemplate suicide'.[137] Miss Court was the only patient to

---

133 Cullen, 'Patient Records', p. 137.
134 Regina Morantz-Sanchez, 'Negotiating Power at the Bedside: Historical Perspectives on Nineteenth-Century Patients and their Gynaecologists', *Feminist Studies*, 26.2 (2000), 287–309; 300.
135 'Letter 21: How a Woman May Suffer', in *Maternity*, pp. 48–9; p. 48.
136 Edith Abrahams (EVS: 1910; Part I); see also twice (MS: 1906; Part I). There is no extant record for her 1903 stay in the hospital.
137 Ethel Court (EVS: 1912; Part I).

phrase her suffering in such a shocking tone, but the sentiment would be understood by many. Torn and retorn perineums were dealt with by Mary Surtees and Eliza Miles for 18 years, Caroline Leggatt and Alice Munday for 15 (the latter including four years of 'difficulty in holding the motions'), and Elizabeth Mitchell for 12.[138] Emma Spooner's perineum was torn seven years before, and again five months previously, but she had incontinence of faeces ever since the first incident.[139] Similarly, Eliza Skate suffered from faecal incontinence for 12 years following childbirth. Prolapses had been experienced by Louisa Watson for 17 years and Mary Blogg for 15.[140] One of the most disturbing prolapses was that experienced by 43-year-old Lily Langley, who, on admission, was discovered not only to have a misplaced uterus, but also bladder, appendages and coils of intestine.[141] Although not as forthright in her description of her feelings as Edith Abrahams, Margaret Gray simply 'hasn't been right' since a miscarriage 18 years before.[142] Emily Ineson's discharge was so profuse that she 'always wears a pad', as did Margaret Dingwall; while Agnes Martin soaked '5 or 6 in half an hour'.[143] By contrast, when Jane Turner's menstruation became so heavy normal pads would not suffice, she was forced to utilise 'bath towels'.[144] The case histories did indeed give an indication of what women were willing to support before they sought treatment. In doing so, however, they drew attention to the very real, vile, profuse, foul-smelling discharges which needed to be stanched and the physical discomfort which must have dogged the lives of already hardworking, hard-pressed women.

As Jane Turner's case revealed, women patients were not averse to controlling their conditions by doing something about it themselves. The cost involved in seeing a doctor, the time wasted sitting in hospital outpatient departments, or even the distress at the possibility of hospitalisation may have been preferable to seeking professional advice. Additionally, the sheer unpleasantness of a situation they would rather keep to themselves or, in some instances, illegal measures, could also prevent medical consultation. Women who suffered from prolapse were quite used to

138 Mary Surtees (MS: 1904); Eliza Miles (EVS: 1913; Part I); Caroline Leggatt (MS; 1907; Part I); Alice Munday (MS: 1908; Part II); and Elizabeth Mitchell (EVS: 1912; Part II).

139 Emma Spooner (MS: 1906; Part II).

140 Louisa Watson (MS: 1905; Part I); Mary Blogg (MS: 1904).

141 Lily Langley (MS: 1905; Part I).

142 Margaret Gray (MS: 1908; Part I), and later (EVS: 1913; Part I).

143 Emily Ineson (EVS: 1911; Part II); Agnes Martin (EVS: 1904–1908; 1908); Margaret Dingwall (EVS: 1912; Part II).

144 Jane Turner (EVS: 1913; Part I). This was misfiled, as Mrs Turner actually attended as an in-patient between 12 August and 13 September 1912.

replacing their own uterus; indeed, for many, the easiness of this rendered treatment worthless. Lily Langley had successfully returned her womb for five and a half years; it was only once she was unable to do so that she sought outside help.[145] Similarly, Prudence Cooper, who had to carry out very heavy work in a laundry, had suffered from prolapse for 15 years. It has 'never caused any pain; the only trouble is the continual discomfort and inconvenience', made worse, of course, by her employment. Only recently had she been unable to replace it properly. Three weeks before her admission, Mrs Cooper finally admitted defeat and went to Clapham Maternity Hospital; as they were unable to replace it, she was sent to the RFH, where her womb was with difficulty replaced. She was later admitted as an in-patient under Vaughan-Sawyer. For 15 years, Prudence Cooper 'never had any treatment'.[146] Less physically demanding self-treatment included measures so 'bowels open regularly'. Most women guarded themselves against constipation, utilising innocent aperients such as senna or liquorice powder; something which Cullen has similarly noted of patients in her study.[147] Piles were also a problem experienced by a number of women; most were ignored until they became intolerable, but Rebecca Shopin stated that she used 'Vaseline' for internal ones.[148] Clara Hughes treated herself with 'Turps', rubbed on to her abdomen in order to ease the abdominal pains she had been experiencing; unfortunately, all that resulted were sores and blisters.[149] Alcohol or drugs were other measures to which some turned in order to numb the pain. Miriam Silverston, a nurse, was a morphomane, and, despite several attempts at treatment, was still addicted to the drug.[150] Interestingly, she also gave her address as Hammond Lodge: a home for female alcoholics.[151] Dorothy Temblett, formerly a popular stage actress (see Illustration 2.1), had drunk regularly for five years, mostly whisky, and had also been taking morphia, 'off and on', since an accident in which she suffered bad burns to her arms from a gas stove explosion.[152] Charwoman Minnie Rogers had 'frequently been drinking heavily', to ease the pain of decade-long sacral backache.[153] Conversely, Hannah Jones and Eliza Jackson were aware that they were unwell, because both were

---

[145] Lily Langley (MS: 1905; Part I).   [146] Prudence Cooper (EVS: 1911; Part I).
[147] Cullen, 'Patient Records', pp. 120–121.   [148] Rebecca Shopin (MS: 1908; Part II).
[149] Clara Hughes (EVS: 1909; Part II).   [150] Miriam Silverston (MS: 1905; Part II).
[151] Silverston's residence in King's Lynn was, by 1907, one of five for female alcoholics run in Britain by the Church of England Temperance Society. See Stephanie Olsen and Gerald Wayne Olsen, 'Church of England Temperance Society (CETS) Inebriate Homes', in Jack S. Blocker, Jnr., David M. Fahey, and Ian R. Tyrell, eds., *Alcohol and Temperance in Modern History. Volume I* (Santa Barbara, CA: ABC-CLIO, 2003), pp. 157–8; p. 158.
[152] Dorothy Temblett (MS: 1908; Part II).   [153] Minnie Roger (EVS: 1913; Part I).

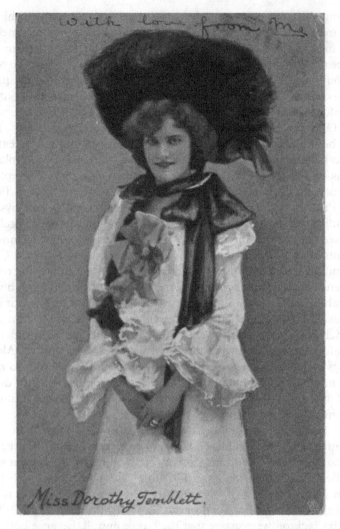

Illustration 2.1 Dorothy Temblett in better days (postcard dated 21 July 1904), Author's Collection.

currently unable to enjoy their daily pints or occasional little whisky, as alcohol caused unpleasant sensations or vomiting.[154]

There were, of course, 'accidental' instances of self-treatment. A couple of falls appeared in the notes, which resulted in bizarre vulval

---

[154] Hannah Jones (EVS: 1911; Part I); Eliza Jackson (EVS: 1913; Part I).

or vaginal injuries. They usually occurred after unlikely household incidents. Maria Blackmore fell off a chair and injured herself 'in the genital area' nine years before admission; she had not been pregnant for seven years after this fall.[155] Annie Hammond was admitted under the influence of drink, having stepped from a table onto a chair for reasons unexplained. Her inebriation was such that she did not need an anaesthetic to have her labial laceration repaired.[156] Unlike Mrs Hammond, Polly Cole explained her strange positioning after a fall. When reaching to pull down a blind, she had fallen and the 'rail of the bedstead passed between her legs'. Profuse haemorrhage resulted. Curiously, the phrase 'removal of a 4½ months foetus' was crossed out, but still visible.[157] While either woman's actions may have been deliberate attempts to bring on a miscarriage, there were other cases in the patient records of the Gynaecological Department where a successful abortion had been carried out. One of the oddest stories involved sitting in the wrong place at the wrong time. Maud Hazell, a 24-year-old single dancer with two children, had suffered two miscarriages in eighteen months, after the birth of her last child. While she was insistent that she had still been menstruating, the private doctor she had seen before she came to the RFH had removed clots and suggested she had miscarried a three months' foetus. She then proceeded to mention that she had accidentally, a month before this alleged miscarriage, sat on a crochet hook, which had entered her vagina and had been difficult to remove.[158] Four years before admission, Nellie Claxton stated that she had brought on a miscarriage with a penholder.[159] Both Agnes Herr and Annie Morris described situations involving 'syringing for [vaginal] discharge', a treatment frequently recommended by both female surgeons for cleanliness, when something went wrong. Herr's douche was simply soap and water, she noted, but she had a miscarriage half-an-hour after 'treatment'.[160] She had been married for eight years and had three children under six; vaginal douching, she insisted, was something she had done for years. Morris, conversely, was aware that she had 'hurt herself'; she had been sent to the RFH by a private doctor and subsequently miscarried in hospital.[161] In contrast to Mrs Herr, Annie Morris was a single, 25-year-old housemaid. Both, however, used the same accident while legitimately carrying out recommended medication to explain their circumstances.

---

[155] Maria Blackmore (EVS: 1910; Part I).   [156] Annie Hammond (MS: 1904).
[157] Polly Cole (MS: 1906; Part II).   [158] Maud Hazell (MS: 1908; Part II).
[159] Nellie Claxton (EVS: 1913; Part I).   [160] Agnes Herr (MS: 1908; Part II).
[161] Annie Morris (MS: 1908; Part II).

Agnes Herr and Annie Morris were frank enough about what had happened to them while treating themselves, but there were a number of other cases where women spoke very openly about contraceptive practices to prevent pregnancy. In public women might have been 'very reluctant to proclaim that they had attempted abortion which was regarded by respectable opinion with the same horror as infanticide',[162] but private consultation with medical and surgical practitioners elicited a very different narrative and offered a stark insight into the desperate lengths some women were prepared to go to regulate their families. While Knight has claimed that before 1914 women generally used drugs rather than instruments to procure abortion, the patients of the RFH employed both methods.[163] Gertrude Blacksley, a 21-year-old married woman, explained succinctly that she was 'in the habit of using sponges in the vagina to prevent pregnancy'.[164] As she was unable to remove the sponge this time, she utilised a button hook; in so doing, however, Mrs Blacksley lacerated her vaginal wall with the hook, caused profuse haemorrhage, and had to come to hospital to have the tear repaired. Sarah Barnett had been married for four years, already had four children and most certainly 'did not wish for another'. She calmly noted that she passed a glass syringe into her vagina to induce abortion. This resulted in a panhysterectomy, because of the peritonitis caused by her actions.[165] Lilian Walker was told of her pregnancy at Gate, the RFH's Casualty Department.[166] She promptly returned home and passed a knitting needle two or three times into her vagina. Additionally, she took five or six different drugs in gin 'with intent to produce abortion'. Although she had only one child, Mrs Walker had tried unsuccessfully to abort it as well. She neither lived with her husband of a decade nor saw him; although the dead foetus and their last meeting three months before appear to have coincided. Emily Franklin, who was 33 and married with six children, admitted taking a couple of pennyroyal pills, known abortifacients, just before she miscarried.[167] She further acknowledged having taken the same number when she lost another child the year before. Two years ago, she had brought on a premature birth at six months by lifting

---

[162] See Pamela Knight, 'Women and Abortion in Victorian and Edwardian England', *HWJ*, 4 (Autumn 1977), 57–69. Also Davin, 'Imperialism and Motherhood'.

[163] Knight, 'Women and Abortion', 60.   [164] Gertrude Blacksley (MS: 1907; Part I).

[165] Sarah Barnett (EVS: 1912; Part II).   [166] Lilian Walker (EVS: 1910; Part I).

[167] Emily Franklin (EVS: 1913; Part I). Pennyroyals appear in Knight's list of easy available cheap remedies, which include 'colocynth (commonly known as "bitter apples"), hiera picra ("hikey pikey" in popular terminology), tansy, [. . .], apiol (combined with steel), gin and gunpowder (the latter bought from the ironmongers), gin and salts, iron and aloes, caraway seeds, turpentine, washing soda and quinine'. See 'Women and Abortion', 60.

heavy weights: the child died. Kate Davey placed the blame for five years of pelvic pain on an abortion induced at three months by an injection into the uterus, which had resulted in peritonitis.[168] Others did not give as much information about their background, but their physical condition led to a diagnosis. Fear of the consequences of an attack by a patient perhaps encouraged Dorothy Neal, a nurse at Colney Hatch, to introduce a long, narrow, sharp and pointed instrument into her vagina.[169] Before she was examined, the note-taker expressed frustration at this 'slightly hysterical' woman, who 'burst into tears when questioned about the accident', which had involved a patient apparently kicking Miss Neal in the abdomen. Only closer inspection under anaesthetic revealed internal injuries inconsistent with an external blow. Others were unable to discuss the reasons behind their circumstances because their actions were lethal. Two cases where treatment had been procured but not properly administered stand out to warn of the dangers of self-medication.[170] Although she did not want to prevent conception, long-standing invalid Annie Cox, who was 'very delicate and has always lived at home', sought to ease her pain by inserting a menthol cone inside her vagina. An abscess formed around the cone and Miss Cox died of septic peritonitis after surgical removal of the object. The most shocking case was that of 'Constance Webb', whose notes queried a criminal abortion. When she was opened up by Mary Scharlieb, twin foetuses were discovered, covered in a white powdered substance, which also appeared in the vaginal vault. Mrs Webb's abdomen was described as 'almost gangrenous', offensive gas escaping as she was operated upon. Despite the removal of her uterus and right ovary, Constance Webb died of acute toxaemia and peritonitis. Bruising was later found on her arms and right hip, suggesting that she was held down while this procedure was performed. While self-treatment might save doctors' fees or personal embarrassment, or even another mouth to feed on limited funds, some of the cases seen by Scharlieb and Vaughan-Sawyer indicated that not everyone who tried to medicate themselves was successful in achieving their ends. Even if they did ensure that conception would no longer be possible, as in the case of Constance Webb, whose generative organs were surgically removed, they might not live to experience or benefit from the consequences of their drastic actions.

Some were prompted to seek treatment due to remarks made by others about their changing physical appearance. More often than not, the

---

[168] Kate Davey (MS: 1907; Part I). See note 38 for more references to Miss Davey in the notes.
[169] Dorothy Neal (MS: 1904).
[170] Annie Cox (MS: 1904); Constance Webb/Mary Ross (MS: 1908; Part I).

patient herself was the one who noticed problems with her own body. In some cases, however, it was someone else, and it was the opinion of that other which propelled the patient to seek medical attention. Many women first noticed symptoms after sex; dyspareunia being a common sign of gynaecological problems and especially malignancy. For example, Emma Hanchett and Elizabeth Goode were diagnosed with carcinoma of the cervix; both became aware that something was wrong after coitus resulted in pain, bleeding and an unpleasant odour in the latter's case.[171] Of just over 1400 patients examined, however, only one man encouraged his wife to see a doctor. Emma Binns explained that it was her husband who noticed her 'getting thinner' and 'has been anxious for some time that [she] should seek medical advice'.[172] For other patients, especially those who were single or widowed, physical changes were observed by friends and relatives, whose comments cast a shadow over a previously good reputation. The gradual enlargement of the abdomen, accompanying fibroids or ovarian cysts, could resemble pregnancy even to the medical man, as confusion over the case of Olive M. Goodwin made clear. At first glance, therefore, even the most virginal could appear otherwise. Edith James, a 38-year-old single governess, had felt her abdomen enlarging for the past six or seven years without obvious cause.[173] The reactions of others determined her next move. At first, friends reassured her that she must simply be suffering from flatulence, and so she did nothing about her condition. Then, however, her abdomen became 'large enough for people to remark about it'; the switch here from friends to people suggested that strangers had made insinuations about her circumstances. The discovery that Miss James had multiple uterine fibroids immediately restored any damage to her reputation and surgery returned her waistline to one more suitable to her situation. Widowed actress Dorothy Temblett was less delicate than Miss James in her description of the accusations she had thrown at her. Her increasing abdomen, due, it was discovered to an enormous ovarian cyst, which reached to her ribs, had led to slurs that, in spite of what she argued, she 'must be pregnant'.[174] Such outside interference in the progress of a patient's illness certainly conceptualises 'clinical interactions', as Sally Wilde has suggested, 'in a more complex and realistic fashion' than the simplicity of the doctor–patient relationship.[175] Often, as the histories of some of the patients imply, there was a well-meaning (or otherwise) intermediary

[171] Emma Hanchett (EVS: 1913; Part II); Elizabeth Goode (MS: 1904).
[172] Emma Binns (MS: 1906; Part II).
[173] Edith James (MS: 1904). This is a different woman to Vaughan-Sawyer's patient of the same name detailed in note 72 above.
[174] Dorothy Temblett (MS: 1908; Part II).   [175] Wilde, 'The Elephants', 22.

in the case, providing a wider picture of the reasons why patients sought or waited for treatment. If women delayed their search for a cure to their ailments through a mixture of denial and stoicism, they could be provoked into seeking help more swiftly if their reputations were attacked publicly or a loved one urged them to act quickly to remedy the effects of evident ill-health.

In the Hospital

So far the composition of the patient base and the reasons for attendance at the RFH have been explored in this chapter in order to determine what brought female patients to the hospital to seek treatment in the first place. When women were admitted into the Gynaecological Department's beds, they were examined, re-examined and conclusions made as to whether or not their case was an operative one or whether rest might lead to recuperation. The period before and after operations, the minutiae of daily hospital life were all recorded in the notes, as were patient reactions to their treatment. Vaughan-Sawyer's 1911 lecture about the patient asked for consideration to be given to what 'bulk[s] large in the patient's eyes', the 'source of great trepidation' which the 'ordeal' of hospitalisation represented.[176] The initial courage summoned up to seek medical opinion was only the beginning of the patient narrative and an examination of the time spent on the ward is essential to understanding the experience of women who passed through the Gynaecological Department between 1903 and 1913.

Case notes were initially divided into a number of sections, which broadly followed the description of circumstances by the patients themselves. After a history of symptoms, the physical examinations by medical and surgical personnel were detailed. The differences in the ways patients responded to this part of the process proved fascinating. Such reactions were especially important because, as we have already seen, most women would not have been examined by a practitioner of the same sex before. As Mary Ann Elston remarks: '[q]ualified female professionals, it was argued, would bring great benefit to women whose modesty precluded them from seeking treatment from middle-class men'.[177] If the majority of patients had not sought female medical help before, it could be imagined that all would respond favourably to the chance to be examined by someone who 'understood' or 'knew' what it was like to experience such symptoms. While many faced examination calmly, this was by no means the case with all. Cullen has suggested that '[p]hysical examinations,

---

[176] Vaughan-Sawyer, 'The Patient', 352.   [177] Elston, '"Run by Women"', p. 78.

particularly the invasive (such as gynaecological examinations conducted with a speculum), demonstrate the growing acceptance of patient discomfort (both physically and emotionally) as an inevitable side-effect of clinical medicine.'[178] Yet, in the gynaecological records, it was precisely the non-acceptance of physical discomfort and the problems attending what should have been straightforward examinations which dominated patient histories. At the RFH, women might have been privileged to be 'under' their own sex, but they still objected to and resisted the ways in which they were treated if it did not meet their expectations. A gynaecological examination was necessarily invasive and mostly instrumental, beyond the usual palpation and percussion, so it is not surprising that many were disgruntled by the process, even if it was carried out by a medical attendant of their own sex.

Twenty-year-old general servant Eliza Love's reaction to examination was mentioned as being very quiet, allowing herself to be examined without rigidity.[179] This was an unusual response to a vital part of understanding the cause of gynaecological complaint. More often than not, patients resisted, either deliberately or because their circumstances ensured that examinations were extremely difficult. The consequences of being unable to examine a patient initially should also be considered, as well as the practices to which the surgeon was compelled to resort to understand more clearly the origins of the symptoms described by the patient. Physical resistance was encountered frequently by those treating the patients at the RFH. Touch, even when carried out delicately, caused some to react strongly. The palpation of Elizabeth Taylor, who had a large abdominal tumour eventually discovered to be a collection of uterine fibroids, caused her 'sickening pain'.[180] Maria Asirti's pre-eclampsia altered her personality and she became violent, continually fitting, which, of course, impeded examination, and refused to allow anyone to touch her when she was still.[181] She was described as very unruly and quite unconscious of what was going on around her, but she managed to resist treatment and could not be made to swallow anything. This ensured that she had to be fed nasally, to which she reacted with extreme violence. When her condition improved, Mrs Asirti became more manageable. Nineteen-year-old servant Maud Burge, however, who was suffering from an abscess of Bartholini's Gland, had no clinical excuse for her behaviour. Her brief stay was accompanied by rudeness, especially about Vaughan-Sawyer, who had been treating her at Out-Patients since the middle of 1903, as well as the RMO, Miss Denny, and the nurses of the ward upon which

---

[178] Cullen, 'Patient Records', p. 249.   [179] Eliza Love (MS: 1904).
[180] Elizabeth Taylor (MS: 1908; Part II).   [181] Maria Asirti (MS: 1904).

she was placed. Although she was in great pain, Miss Burge would not permit anyone to treat the abscess, which was described as needing incision. She hesitated, but finally would not allow anyone to touch her. Unsurprisingly, she was discharged the following morning.[182] Florence Bromley, a 22-year-old married woman, was so 'very intolerant' of examination that she resisted both at Out-Patients and then when admitted to the ward. As a consequence, 'examination was incomplete' and the patient discharged to be watched at Out-Patients.[183]

While some resisted deliberately, others could not be examined for various physical reasons which prevented closer inspection. It was not just vaginal explorations which caused problems. Kate Rocca, for example, had no radial pulse in her right arm as her wrist had been damaged by being put through a broken window.[184] Helen Silver's vaginismus ensured that vaginal examination caused pain and muscle spasm: reactions she was incapable of controlling.[185] Likewise, Tamar Hillyard's body was hard to examine because of a 'vibrating' and 'pulsating' abdomen, which was due to nervousness.[186] Maud Hazell was very constipated when she was admitted, which made both vaginal and abdominal examination unsatisfactory and difficult.[187] Some patients were so thin or so fat that exploration was impeded by the shape of their bodies. Single nurse Ethel Hennessey admitted to having lost a considerable amount of weight over the previous nine months, due to adhesions forming after an appendicectomy, and was described as 'very thin and rather pale'.[188] As she was 'so thin', Miss Hennessey's ovary and fallopian tube could not be felt on the right side; an indefinite mass only presented itself to the palpating hand. Conversely, Elizabeth Lawson was 'extremely fat', ensuring that examination was 'of little value'.[189] Elizabeth Newell's excessive 'stoutness' was blamed for an inability to palpate the fundus of the uterus, while Caroline Radford's heart sounds could only very faintly be heard because of the thickness of her chest wall.[190] The blame in Susan Carter's case for her being 'extremely difficult' to examine was attributed both to the 'amount of fat present' on her abdomen, but also to the fact that she obstructed vaginal exploration by 'hold[ing] her thighs tightly' together.[191]

---

[182] Maud Burge (MS: 1904). This was not the last time Maud Burge appeared in the records, however. She must have thought better of her attitude towards the staff as she was admitted twice over the next nine years: (MS: 1906; Part I) and (EVS: 1913; Part II).

[183] Florence Bromley (MS: 1905; Part I).   [184] Kate Rocca (EVS: 1912; Part I).

[185] Helen Silver (MS: 1907; Part II).   [186] Tamar Hillyard (EVS: 1913; Part II).

[187] Maud Hazell (MS: 1908; Part II).   [188] Ethel Hennessey (EVS: 1910; Part I).

[189] Elizabeth Lawson (EVS: 1910; Part II).

[190] Elizabeth Newell (EVS: 1910; Part II); Caroline Radford (MS: 1905; Part I).

[191] Susan Carter (EVS: 1910; Part II).

Examining a squirming or rigid patient was not an easy task. The fact that women in-patients were being seen by their own sex did not make a difference to those who were resistant, either deliberately or through no fault of their own, to clinical exploration.

For some patients, it was the prospect of further examination, potentially under anaesthetic, which led to a swift discharge from the hospital even before any real treatment, let alone operative measures, had been carried out. As we will see, surgery was both facilitated and stymied by anaesthetics. Those who resisted exploration while awake were often anaesthetised in order to facilitate diagnosis. As Scharlieb and Vaughan-Sawyer's RFH colleague, James Berry put it, '[g]eneral anaesthesia, by producing relaxation of the muscular wall, is of great assistance in deep palpation of the abdomen'.[192] It was precisely this 'relaxation' which troubled a number of women patients in the Gynaecological Department. Even though examination was being carried out by members of their own sex, the 'fear of unconsciousness', as Snow has noted, was enough to put an end to hospital treatment for several patients, who would rather discharge themselves than undergo exploration where resistance was not possible.[193] The 'confidence' identified by historians of medicine of the patient in the surgeon was certainly not apparent for every one of the 1403 cases seen in the reality of day-to-day life on the wards of the RFH. Anaesthesia in particular, even in the early twentieth century, still caused particular dread.[194] Refusal to be put under any form of anaesthetic was one of the most prominent reasons for premature discharge from the hospital. In *Surgical Anaesthesia* (1909), H. Bellamy Gardner reassured his readers that 'the sex and age' of those undergoing vaginal procedures ('between twenty and forty-five'), rendered them 'comparatively easy to anaesthetise', but this was not borne out by the reaction of Scharlieb and Vaughan-Sawyer's patients.[195] Neither would the possible seriousness of the patient's condition prevent departure if the only way that anything further could be done for them would be under sedation. Mary Gunn, a 43-year-old widowed cook, was one example.[196] She was diagnosed as having suspected carcinoma of the uterus, because of her cachetic appearance, as well as irregular bleeding, abdominal pain and loss of flesh. Initial exploration had proved difficult because the patient was so

[192] Berry, *A Manual of Surgery*, p. 128.
[193] Stephanie Snow, *Operations Without Pain* (Basingstoke: Palgrave Macmillan, 2006), p. 94.
[194] See Wilde, 'Truth, Trust' and Burney, *Bodies of Evidence*.
[195] H. Bellamy Gardner, *Surgical Anaesthesia* (London: Ballière, Tindall and Cox, 1909; New York: William Wood and Company, 1909), p. 217.
[196] Mary Gunn (MS: 1908; Part II).

ill and too tender to touch. Consequently, Scharlieb wanted to perform an examination under anaesthetic in order to ascertain whether or not her initial suspicions were correct, and simultaneously remove curettings from the uterus, which could be sent to the Pathology Department to determine diagnosis microscopically. What Mrs Gunn objected to was not the operation per se, but, as was specifically noted, 'examination under anaesthetic'. She left without any solid diagnosis being made.

Marian Freed was in a similar situation, although her queried carcinoma of the cervix had been caught early at Out-Patients by Vaughan-Sawyer, and was, therefore, potentially operable.[197] However, she too refused an anaesthetic and left the hospital after one day without further examination. Betty Schmottken had a mysterious tumour and abdominal pain, which was considered potentially a life-threatening ectopic pregnancy.[198] Scharlieb deemed it impossible to make certain diagnosis in her case without proper exploration under anaesthesia. The patient refused and discharged herself immediately. Rachael Eagle, a 29-year-old housewife admitted for endometritis and a torn perineum, had been attending Gynaecological Out-Patients for the previous two months.[199] She had initially refused admission because she had wanted to wean her baby, but when she did become an in-patient, she supported an initial examination. On being informed that there would be a further investigation under anaesthesia a day later, however, Mrs Eagle made sure that she discharged herself before this could occur. When told that she was pregnant, Gertrude Figg, who had 'felt as if her inside was dropping from her', took the news in and then agreed to undergo an exploratory examination under anaesthetic for a small adenoma of the cervix the following day.[200] Overnight, however, Mrs Figg felt 'foetal movements' and refused to have the procedure, evidently concerned about the possibility of miscarrying her unborn child. The specialist would suggest that 'pregnancy forms no contra-indication to operation', but Gertrude Figg would not take the risk, and discharged herself.[201] Twenty-year-old single tailoress, Bertha Finkelstein, was the most contrary patient as far as the acceptance of anaesthesia was concerned.[202] Initially, she objected to any examination without anaesthesia, but when the time came for her to undergo investigation, she refused any anaesthetic and was discharged. A further attack of pain changed her mind and she was readmitted, finally accepting both examination and anaesthetic.

---

[197] Marian Freed (MS: 1905; Part I).   [198] Betty Schmottken (MS: 1908; Part II).
[199] Rachael Eagle (MS: 1907; Part I).   [200] Gertrude Figg (MS: 1905; Part II).
[201] Howard A. Kelly, *Operative Gynecology. Volume I*, second edition (New York: D. Appleton and Company, 1906), p. 421.
[202] Bertha Finkelstein (EVS: 1911; Part I).

Anaesthesia did, however, have another function in the examination of female patients. It allowed women, particularly the single and thus (largely, though not exclusively) virginal, to be examined without feeling immodest or shamed by the situation on the one hand, and, on the other, to ensure that examination was indeed possible where tight or unruptured hymens prevented access to female generative organs in the first place. The American surgeon, Howard A. Kelly, of Baltimore, visited the RFH in the middle of 1905 and the autumn of 1910 and was present at a number of operations on gynaecological patients, as well as carrying some out.[203] In his textbook *Medical Gynecology* (1912), Kelly extolled the virtues of anaesthesia when approaching those physically and morally sensitive to examination:

There should, of course, be no hesitation in the case of married women, or in cases of inflammatory disease. But there are many instances of young women who suffer from dysmenorrhoea pure and simple, when the question of examination must receive careful consideration. It is always best to exhaust all general therapeutic measures before making it [. . .].

With this precaution, an examination can be made without injury to the hymen, while, should any simple operation such as dilatation and curettage be indicated, it can be performed at the same time. Such a course enables the physician to dispense with the endless local treatments which are so objectionable in young women.[204]

In a number of cases examinations per vaginam were simply not made initially or without anaesthetic because the patient was 'unmarried'. This was noted, for example, in the records of Lizzie Hammant, Nellie Culling, Gertrude Rippon, Lucy Marsden, Alice Jones, Agnes Henman, and Emma Bevan.[205] The latter three were 46, 48 and 52, respectively, so age was no barrier to ensuring the treatment was appropriate to the patient's marital status. In a further nod to delicacy, Clara White was not explored with a speculum, but with a far less intrusive finger 'to avoid tearing her hymen as she is single'.[206] Others could not be examined physically without an anaesthetic precisely because of their virginal state. Twenty-eight-year-old Salvation Army officer Margaret Dingwall's

---

203 In 1905, Kelly operated on Mary Stapleton, Emma Beauchamp and Mary Ann Coleman (MS: 1905; Part I). On his second visit, in 1910, Kelly took 'stereoscopic photos throughout' the Caesarean Section performed on Alice Hollingshed by Ethel Vaughan-Sawyer. Miss Hollingshed had 'markedly deformed legs' and a scoliotic curve to her spine (EVS: 1910; Part II).

204 Kelly, *Medical Gynecology*, p. 112.

205 Lizzie Hammant (EVS: 1913; Part II); Nellie Culling (EVS: 1911; Part II); Gertrude Rippon (EVS: 1911; Part II); Lucy Marsden (MS: 1904); Alice Jones (MS: 1905; Part II); Agnes Henman (MS: 1904); Emma Bevan (EVS: 1911; Part II).

206 Clara White (EVS: 1913; Part II).

hymen was too tight to permit examination per vaginam. Under anaesthetic, however, Vaughan-Sawyer was able to obtain some curettings
through a 'small orifice'.[207] Housemaid May Groome's 'intolerance of
manipulation' was overcome when anaesthetised, while 20-year-old Elsie
Ward proved 'impossible' to examine satisfactorily without anaesthetic,
as both James Berry and Mary Scharlieb discovered.[208] Similarly, Kate
Branfield's hymen, which was intact, became 'very dilatable' under anaesthesia, revealing how the body changed when unconscious.[209] For one
patient, the geographical location of the examination was what mattered,
perhaps offering the only example of the 1403 cases where a patient
placed trust in the institution to provide proper care. Four days before
her admission, 21-year-old Jane Moore had given birth to her first child,
but had suffered from a rising temperature ever since.[210] Mrs Moore
refused exploration of her uterus under an anaesthetic at home, but
expressed willing to have the identical procedure performed in the RFH.

While anaesthesia facilitated diagnosis, it also cured in a few instances.
Margaret Smith was 'hysterical' during anaesthetic induction and
when she came round, but her anaesthetisation had allowed RMO
Miss Edmonds to remove a cervical polypus which had been causing
eighteen months' pain and discharge.[211] Single governess Edith James
was deliberately given gas as an anaesthetic, because she was considered
extremely nervous.[212] In *Surgical Anaesthesia*, Gardner reminded the
medical profession that it was well to put oneself in the position of the
patient before giving an anaesthetic. '[W]ithout any previous experience
of anaesthetics', he stated, 'most people would prefer to be put to sleep
without passing through a long stage of semi-consciousness, by some
vapour or gas which has as little taste as possible, and produces no sense
of suffocation during the inhalation.'[213] The 'selection of the anaesthetic
appropriate' to the patient was vital in ensuring the best possible
outcome for patient, anaesthetist and operator alike, especially when the
patient was of a nervous temperament.[214] Kate Williams, Beatrice Hart
and Ethel Hoskins were anaesthetised with the prospect of discovering
conditions which would warrant further procedures.[215] Miss Williams
had pain in her back and a swollen, 'markedly distended' abdomen since
a confinement the year before admission. Mrs Hoskins was supposed

---

[207] Margaret Dingwall (EVS: 1911; Part II).
[208] May Groome (EVS: 1913; Part I); Elsie Ward (MS: 1908; Part II).
[209] Kate Branfield (EVS: 1911; Part II).   [210] Jane Moore (MS: 1908; Part II).
[211] Margaret Smith (EVS: 1913; Part I).   [212] Edith James (MS: 1904).
[213] Gardner, *Surgical Anaesthesia*, p. 26.   [214] Ibid., p. 28.
[215] Kate Williams (EVS: 1910; Part II); Ethel Hoskins (MS: 1908; Part II); Beatrice Hart
(EVS: 1913; Part I).

to be suffering from an abscess of Gartner's Duct, while Mrs Hart described nine months of amenorrhoea during which she thought she was pregnant. In all three instances, the induction of anaesthesia encouraged the swelling to subside. As Gardner noted, abdominal conditions such as those causing inflammation or toxicity and leading to contraction or rigidity often 'relax in the surgical degree of anaesthesia'.[216] Kate Williams left hospital consequently with a 'flat abdominal wall'. There were instances where the induction of anaesthesia had the opposite effect, and actually failed to assist the operator or help the patient. Ellen Magor's previous operation at the Hampstead Hospital a year before her admission to the RFH and the evident relaxation of her body at the time had ensured that a formerly lax vagina was made so tight during a perineorrhaphy that the patient subsequently experienced dyspareunia.[217] While most relaxed under anaesthesia and gynaecological examination was more easily carried out, two patients resisted. Thirty-two-year-old single woman Edith Edwards' very tight hymen was torn laterally when a Hodge pessary was inserted under anaesthesia by RMO Miss Mccredy to ease backache and profuse menstruation.[218] Her reaction, if she was informed of the tear, was, unsurprisingly, not noted. Unlike Kate Branfield's anaesthetic yielding, Mary Horton, 'a very healthy and well-developed' 28-year-old nurse, still resisted.[219] Her athleticism and strong physique permitted the administration of a deep anaesthesia, but this was 'pushed so far' that she stopped breathing for a bit and had to be given artificial respiration. In similar fashion to Miss Edwards, a slight tear had to be made in the mucous membrane as Miss Horton's hymen was still so tight. From the description of such cases, it is understandable why some preferred, especially if they were single, to refuse an anaesthetic rather than worry about what any potential future husband might imagine.

Deaths from anaesthesia still occurred at the beginning of the twentieth century and popular mistrust would have made patients nervous about the administration. Burney has commented upon the 'ambiguous position of anaesthesia' at the turn of the twentieth century. It was 'more institutionally grounded than ever before, but at the same time vulnerable to the charge that, a half-century of experience notwithstanding, it remained a dangerous and unreliable practice.'[220] Only one patient died from the effects of anaesthesia in the decade explored by this chapter: 15-year-old Gladys Perks, from chloroform poisoning.[221] Others were, however, legibly affected by anaesthesia or the operative process itself and

---

[216] Gardner, *Surgical Anaesthesia*, p. 208.   [217] Ellen Magor (EVS: 1913; Part II).
[218] Edith Edwards (EVS: 1910; Part II).   [219] Mary Horton (EVS: 1911; Part I).
[220] Burney, *Bodies of Evidence*, p. 141.   [221] Gladys Perks (EVS: 1910; Part I).

this must have caused some consternation to those awaiting their own procedures on the ward. Gardner in *Surgical Anaesthesia* and Burney more recently have focused on the most serious consequences of surgical shock and the treatment of emergencies, but there were smaller, although still troubling, reactions to an operation. Most patients, for example, were sick after an anaesthetic, often when they had been returned to the ward to be heard, if not observed, by others. Fifteen-year-old Minnie Earle, who suffered from a regurgitation of mucous during her operation for the removal of tubercular fallopian tubes, ended up with ether bronchitis.[222] 'Rather neurotic' Annie Gilkes disproved Gardner's theory about nervous patients being more troublesome during and after anaesthesia by taking two hours to come round post-operation and remaining apathetic for a further three days.[223] Physical injuries were suffered by others. Jane Marshall, Kate Branfield and Annie Dryden were all burnt by the anaesthetic; the first on her cheek and the second more generally on her face, while the last had a blistered chin.[224] Conjunctivitis affected Olivia Risley after her surgery, while Ellen Wilson suffered from a sore tongue, as did Annie Dryden, and Louie Carren, whose lips and eyes were also affected.[225] Saline infusions also caused problems after an operation, which added secondary suffering to the original site. Cora Sergent had very tender breasts at the location where saline was infused during her procedure, and painful swelling emerged.[226] Similarly, Alice Grenville noticed a sore lump under her breast where saline had been administered.[227] Such small, slight injuries might not be significant in comparison with major surgery, but they would have caused women additional suffering during a time of recuperation, as well as worrying others on their ward about the process they were about to experience.

Resistance to surgical intervention was frequently caused by the patient themselves, whether deliberately or involuntarily, but sometimes delays in alleviating disease, pain or ill-health were attributed to the very poor general condition of the patient in the first place. A number of women were simply 'unsuitable' cases for surgery. There were a variety of reasons why, despite the necessity for surgical treatment, patients were often sent away without a vital operation or kept in for a while before they became suitable candidates to undergo the strains of a potentially lengthy procedure.

[222] Minnie Earle (EVS: 1912; Part II).
[223] Annie Gilkes (EVS: 1913; Part I). Gardner, *Surgical Anaesthesia*, p. 63.
[224] Jane Marshall (EVS: 1910; Part II); Kate Branfield (EVS: 1911; Part II); Annie Dryden (EVS: 1912; Part II).
[225] Olivia Risley (EVS: 1910; Part I); Ellen Wilson (EVS: 1913; Part I); Louie Carren (EVS: 1913; Part I).
[226] Cora Sergent (MS: 1907; Part II).   [227] Alice Grenville (EVS: 1910; Part II).

As already mentioned earlier, Alice E. Howes' tendency to bruise easily encouraged the hospital to communicate with her own doctor for fear of haemophilia affecting her treatment. Laura Helsdown was admitted twice in 1908 and acknowledged that she bled easily when she cut herself and was liable to spontaneous bruising; several large purpura were present on her limbs. She returned after the removal of a cervical polypus had led to non-stop bleeding since her initial discharge. After rest, the bleeding stopped: no further operation was advised because of her possible condition.[228] Edith Peacock bled subcutaneously during her operation, while Gertrude Rippon, who had previously suffered from bleeding gums after dental extractions, was further discovered to have a haematoma beneath the skin after her procedure.[229] Haemophilia in women was considered 'sufficiently uncommon' for a case to be recorded as a memorandum in the *BMJ* in May 1910, but the RFH saw four potential cases over a period of five years.[230] In the late nineteenth century, surgery was to be avoided for haemophiliacs unless it was for a life-threatening condition and a conservative approach was recommended at all times, but Scharlieb and Vaughan-Sawyer were willing to give their possibly haemophiliac patients a chance, allowing them operative treatment when necessary.[231]

Some patients suffered from problems with their heart. Annie Richardson was diagnosed as having double mitral disease and a breakdown in compensation, making the prospect of childbirth life-threatening, while Nellie Brown, despite claiming that she had 'always been strong', had mitral stenosis, which complicated surgery for carcinoma of the cervix.[232] With rest, Mrs Richardson was able to have her first child, and Mrs Brown a (likely) palliative operation, with the anaesthetic carefully tailored to assist her breathing during the procedure. Sometimes, anaesthetists at the hospital were young and inexperienced (male and female) house surgeons, learning all aspects of the surgical trade. Knowledge of this prevented an operation on Alice Attridge, whose mitral obstruction

---

[228] Alice E. Howes (EVS: 1910; Part II); Laura Helsdown (MS: 1908; Part II). However, Mrs Helsdown was operated upon in 1909 and in 1912 when symptoms reoccurred (EVS: 1909; Part I) and (EVS: 1912; Part II).

[229] Edith Peacock (EVS: 1913; Part II); Gertrude Rippon (EVS: 1911; Part II).

[230] E.W. Squire, 'Haemophilia in a Female', *BMJ*, 1.2576 (14 May 1910), 1168. This case, like all three at the RFH, also showed no family history of the disease. For a contemporary view exploring a family where women were carriers (and 'free from the disease'), but never bleeders, see Ernest W. Hey Groves, 'A Clinical Lecture upon the Surgical Aspects of Haemophilia', *BMJ*, 1.2411 (16 March 1907), 611–14.

[231] J. Wickham Legg, *A Treatise on Haemophilia* (London: H.K. Lewis, 1872), especially pp. 113–14.

[232] Annie Richardson (MS: 1908; Part II); Nellie Brown (EVS: 1911; Part I).

needed to be supervised by a skilled administrator.[233] Respiratory conditions, such as phthisis or bronchitis, frequently rendered a patient's condition 'inoperable'.[234] Scharlieb and Vaughan-Sawyer both made decisions about whether to perform surgery in these circumstances or not based on the recommendation of their colleague J. Walter Carr, a general physician with interests in diseases of the chest and of the nervous system.[235] This was the case for Florence Sutherland, whose tubercular lungs counted against surgical success if her tuberculous anal ulcer was removed under anaesthetic. With her present lung condition, surgery would be a 'serious matter', Carr concluded.[236] Minnie Carr was not anxious to have an operation for salpingitis, but her phthisis rendered it impossible anyway; exactly the same happened two years later when she was admitted again.[237] Esther Berensohn left without an operation being performed for dysmenorrhoea, anteverted uterus and sterility, because there were signs of phthisis in her lungs.[238]

On the whole, the older the patient the more likely they were to suffer from conditions which made surgery an increasingly risky business. As Mary Connor was 'somewhat senile and feeble-minded', 'very feeble and old for her [65] years', and troublesomely prone to removing vaginal plugs intended to improve her overall condition before operation, she was sent 'to the Infirmary' for further treatment.[239] Catherine Fountain was 56, but 'prematurely aged and degenerate' with marked emphysema, making her a bad subject for anaesthesia. Gardner warned that '[o]ld people and those who are past middle age must be treated, if anything with greater care than the very young, because impairment of thoracic expansion and commencing degeneration of all parts of the system turn the balance against them in recovery from conditions of collapse'.[240] Fifty-nine-year-old Elizabeth Tranter was 'not considered a good subject for operation' by Carr, but delaying the procedure, to ensure her bronchitis improved, gave her a better chance of undergoing

---

[233] Alice Attridge (EVS: 1908; Part II). In October 1912, to give one example, anaesthesia was given by Mr Howell, a house surgeon. See *The Eighty-Fifth Annual Report for 1912* (1913), p. 8.

[234] Interestingly, Gardner did not suggest calling off an operation because of respiratory problems. See pp. 66–87; especially pp. 74–5.

[235] For Carr's expertise, see Cullen, 'Patient Records', especially pp. 72–3.

[236] Florence Sutherland (EVS: 1909; Part I). Miss Sutherland had previously been operated on by Scharlieb in 1906 for the same anal ulcer, as well as an ovarian cyst, but her condition had rapidly deteriorated since this point, along with her ability to be anaesthetised successfully. She was named as Florrie Sutherland in this note (MS: 1906; Part II).

[237] Minnie Carr (MS: 1907; Part II); (EVS: 1909; Part II).

[238] Esther Berensohn (EVS: 1913; Part II).   [239] Mary Connor (EVS: 1909; Part I).

[240] Gardner, *Surgical Anaesthesia*, p. 61.

an operation for cancer of the cervix. There was indecision over her case, but her own 'anxiety to be operated on' overrode doubt and throughout the operation, her condition was described as excellent.[241] For Henrietta Hall, a combination of bad bronchitis and malignant disease of the ovary ensured that she did not even have the chance to improve her chest condition, dying before an operation could be performed.[242] Other patients were able to have an operation, but, as in the case of Nellie Brown, with carefully controlled anaesthetic conditions. Eliza Larkins' long-standing poor chest problems, primarily due to asthma, did not prevent surgery, but she was deliberately anaesthetised with chloroform, while Olivia Risley's bronchitis was not severe enough to stop an operation for uterine fibroids, but her circumstances affected the timing and type of anaesthetic administered.[243]

A life of poverty and hard work etched itself upon the bodies of many patients. Lack of care for themselves, whether through impoverishment or resulting from self-sacrifice for family members such as husbands or children, physically marked those seeking treatment. Premature ageing has already been mentioned, but appalling oral hygiene was endemic and often delayed operation. Teeth were so infrequently described as 'excellent' between 1903 and 1913, whatever the age of the patient, that the mouths of 20-year-old tailoress Bertha Finkelstein and 16-year-old collar binder Bessie Ellis drew attention less to themselves and more to the 1401 whose teeth were far from perfect.[244] Indeed, a large number of patients had teeth removed while on the ward. Twenty-four-year-old Marie Widden, for example, had fifteen stumps removed from her upper jaw, while Alice Self, who was 29, had eight teeth removed on one of her many visits to the RFH.[245] Simple items such as mouthwash and toothbrushes were recommended for some patients awaiting operation. Their appearance in the margin of the records, where treatment details were usually placed, stated their importance for surgical preparation, but also the fact that they were not familiar to every patient and, as such, constituted 'medicine' for many. Charlotte Kendall (36), who was admitted for an incomplete miscarriage, had teeth extracted and her septic mouth treated; she was also prescribed a toothbrush.[246] Elizabeth Thompson (39) and Helen

---

[241] Elizabeth Tranter (EVS: 1913; Part I). Mrs Tranter's death from heart failure four days after her operation suggested that her state was otherwise.
[242] Henrietta Hall (MS: 1905; Part II).
[243] Eliza Larkins (EVS: 1910; Part II); Olivia Risley (EVS: 1910; Part I).
[244] Bertha Finkelstein (EVS: 1911; Part I); Bessie Ellis (EVS: 1911; Part II).
[245] Marie Widden (MS: 1905; Part II); Alice Self (EVS: 1911; Part I). See also: (MS: 1906; Part I) (MS: 1906; Part II); (MS: 1907; Part II); twice (EVS: 1911; Part I).
[246] Charlotte Kendall (MS: 1908; Part II).

Pinner (21) were given sanitas mouthwash and toothbrushes.[247] As Riha has noted, patient records provide several 'clues to social problems', including poor teeth and dirtiness: 'there seems to be no connection between these categories and living conditions: middle class housewives neglected the care of their bodies, domestic servants working in upper class households walked around with their heads infested with lice, and simple workers had their teeth kept in order'.[248] Such a finding can be applied similarly to the case notes of Scharlieb and Vaughan-Sawyer. Of course, the very nature of gynaecological complaints ensured that it was difficult to guard against uncleanliness. In addition to a cachetic physical appearance, the dying often had a strange smell about them, and so unpleasantness was actually helpful in this instance. Sixty-one-year-old Ellen Parkins, for example, who was riddled with cancer and suffering from general wasting and weakness, had 'a peculiar odour of breath suggesting malignant disease' even before she was given an exploratory laparotomy and the diagnosis confirmed.[249] Dirt was evidently a constituent part of working-class life, but, as Riha makes clear, dirtiness was not confined to the lowest, nor cleanliness to the highest. As we have already seen, the best teeth belonged to two working-class women. Although she had just come out of Holloway Prison, street hawker Elizabeth Langley fascinated because she had an unusual and unidentified skin complaint, not associated with her lifestyle. No mention was made of dirtiness, despite her occupation and circumstances.[250] Other patients had septic conditions unrelated to their gynaecological concerns. Both Annie Ward and Elizabeth Seaton had septic fingers, although no mention was made of how either came to have such an injury.[251] Dirtiness also had another meaning. Annie Gold, whose vaginitis and endocervicitis appeared to stem from masturbation, was claimed to be 'dirty in her ways'. To make sure she did not reactivate her problems, Mrs Gold had her hands bandaged while in the ward as a preventative measure.[252] The patient who was in the worst physical shape was a surprising one, especially given her profession. Dorothy Temblett (see Illustration 2.1), who had been 'on the stage' for nearly a decade since the age of 15, entered hospital in appalling physical circumstances, her head infested with lice. A vestige of self-respect evidently remained, as, while she agreed for it

---

[247] Elizabeth Thompson (MS: 1908; Part II); Helen Pinner (MS: 1908; Part I).
[248] Riha, 'Surgical Case Records', 278.   [249] Ellen Parkins (EVS; 1912; Part I).
[250] Elizabeth Langley (MS: 1908; Part II). It was surmised that she was covered in mollusca or fibromas; the description of her skin dominated the notes.
[251] Annie Ward (EVS: 1913; Part I) and (EVS: 1913; Part II); Elizabeth Seaton (EVS: 1912; Part I) twice; also: (EVS: 1911; Part II).
[252] Annie Gold (EVS: 1912; Part I).

to be cut short, she would 'not allow it to be shaved'. Her operation for an ovarian cyst was postponed until she could be 'got into a suitable state'.[253] As Riha also discovered, lack of care was not simply confined to the poorest, and, as the female patients of the RFH revealed, dirt and dirtiness were not always to be found where most expected.

This section so far has explored the objections patients made to the examinations they were to undergo and the problems experienced by staff in dealing with the various complaints brought up and brought in by their patients. For some, the reality of life upon the ward, as well as the looming prospect of surgery became too much. There were two other key reasons why women discharged themselves from the gynaecological beds: dissatisfaction with their surroundings and the desire not to be operated upon. To take the former concern first. While the RFH was not supposed to admit those who sought 'rest', a few gynaecological patients expressed their gratitude for the peace and quiet their hospitalisation had afforded them. Although nothing abnormal was wrong with Annie Williams, for example, she was allowed to stay in hospital for general debility, weakness and backache. As a consequence, she was 'much improved by rest and feeding' for a fortnight.[254] One patient objected to the 'feeding' given on the ward. Lottie Green's Jewish faith did not permit her to eat hospital food, other than bread and butter, and so she survived on vegetable soups brought in by her sons.[255] For some patients, however, it was the lack of privacy and the sheer noise of a female ward which caused them to seek treatment in more congenial surroundings for which they would, of course, have to pay. Beatrice Allen, a 41-year-old widowed dressmaker, described as 'extremely nervous', discharged herself to go to a private home as she could not stand the noise, which worried her.[256] Similarly, Mary Kenny discharged herself to seek treatment in a private nursing home.[257] Those with very young babies would have their children admitted with them, which must have added to the strange sounds; however, this was too much for the unnamed mother of 14-day-old William Peaseton, who was sent out because she 'does not like having it here': 'it distresses her'.[258] Sleep was disrupted for a number of other reasons, making hospital stays uncomfortable for some. Ruth Barden was only in for one night, because she slept badly, and discharged herself as soon as she could.[259] Annie Solomons experienced bad dreams on the ward, and Nellie Fowler wandered in her sleep and talked about going to work.[260]

[253] Dorothy Temblett (MS: 1908; Part II).   [254] Annie Williams (MS: 1908; Part I).
[255] Lottie Green (EVS: 1910; Part II).   [256] Beatrice Allen (MS: 1907; Part I).
[257] Mary Kenny (MS: 1908; Part I).   [258] William Peaseton (MS: 1906; Part II).
[259] Ruth Barden (MS: 1908; Part I).   [260] Annie Solomons (EVS: 1913; Part I).

Julia Oulds was upset by a thunderstorm and the prospect of the dentist coming in the morning to remove her carious teeth, and Annie Hobbs also was unable to sleep before her operation.[261]

The Central London location of the hospital affected those unused, like Norfolk resident Amelia Powles, to such 'strange surroundings'.[262] Annie Rondle, from East Ham, discovered that her sleep was disrupted by the metropolitan traffic.[263] The 'great heat of the weather' in May 1913 was cited as affecting the recovery of washerwoman Mary A. Broyden, exacerbating her sheer exhaustion.[264] Suffering and worry must have caused disruption to sleep, as well as the medication being taken by patients for the pain. It would not be only the individual disturbed, therefore, but others, influenced by illness, or drugs to which they were unused, calling out or moving around. Lily Connor's combination of chorea and pregnancy had resulted in mental impairment, which gave her wild delusions and she repeatedly tried to leave her bed.[265] Phoebe Smith was also delusional after her operation and heard voices.[266] Miriam Silverston, a morphine addict, took the drug and tried to commit suicide by biting on the mercury of a thermometer in the ward.[267] While some experienced a rest from everyday life, for others the general atmosphere of the hospital, with its strange noises and odd behaviour was insupportable.

Some patients refused further treatment and discharged themselves because they felt cured already. This might have been either an attempt not to undergo an operation, or an unwillingness to spend any further time on the wards. Emma Slater's cyst burst, so, as far as she was concerned, she was well again and refused any more interference.[268] Annie Goldstein was very averse to anything further being done for her. Having been given medicine for old peritonitis at Out-Patients she was reluctant to become an in-patient. When she did agree to come in, she said that she was feeling very much better and so was discharged.[269] Four-times repeat patient, Maria Blackmore, though in great pain from bladder problems, had clearly had enough when she refused to allow a bladder sound to be passed and discharged herself.[270] J. Augusta Smith was in a similar situation to Mrs Blackmore. She had a vesico-vaginal fistula, which continually evaded repair and was the result of a previous operation in which her uterus and appendages were removed. As a consequence, she was miserably incontinent: 'water constantly dribbles away'. The realisation

[261] Julia A. Oulds (EVS: 1911; Part II) twice; Annie Hobbs (MS: 1904).
[262] Amelia Powles (EVS: 1911; Part I).   [263] Annie Rondle (EVS: 1913; Part I).
[264] Mary A. Broyden (EVS: 1913; Part I).   [265] Lily Connor (EVS: 1910; Part I).
[266] Phoebe Smith (EVS: 1913; Part I).   [267] Miriam Silverston (MS: 1905; Part II).
[268] Emma Salter (MS: 1904).   [269] Annie Goldstein (EVS: 1911; Part II).
[270] Maria Blackmore (EVS: 1912; Part II).

that treatment was not working caused Mrs Smith to refuse all further interference and discharge herself. She had clearly had enough.[271] Some, away from their husband and children perhaps for the first time, thought better of their desire to seek treatment and returned home, indicating the pressure women were put under, even when seriously ill, to attend to their home and family. Nellie Hayes was convinced of the necessity for an operation, rather than risk a second attack of pain stemming from pelvic peritonitis, but she decided to go out 'for home reasons', and come back. She did not, however, appear again in the notes.[272] Scharlieb tried to encourage Priscilla Hawgood to remain in hospital while she was carefully observed for irregular bleeding, loss of flesh and backache, but she discharged herself two days later 'for family reasons'. She too was not seen in the future.[273] If husbands encouraged their wives to leave hospital, whether deliberately or because women felt obligated to return home, they also had a more serious role. In a few instances, they were the ones who prevented women from having any form of operative interference. The consent, or otherwise, of a husband was rarely recorded, but objections stemmed exclusively from surgical procedures aimed to cut growths from female generative organs or the organs themselves. There was only one exception. Leah H. Greenwood's husband would not consent to an operation on her breast, for eczema of the right nipple, though he did not seem to mind about the procedure to remove her right ovary and fallopian tube.[274] Interestingly enough, and whatever her husband ordered, the notes ended with a claim that Mrs Greenwood would return soon for the forbidden surgery.[275] An accident during an operation would mostly have to be corrected on the spot to save the patient's life. Fifty-four-year-old Mary Seabrook, whose uterus was perforated when a sound was passed into it, did not have a necessary hysterectomy because she was weakened by the exploratory examination, as well as the RFH not yet having obtained her husband's consent.[276] This was duly provided and the procedure was performed the next day. Two refusals came, however, from the most serious and life-threatening conditions. Mary A. Newland, who was 58, and suffering from extensive carcinoma of the cervix, informed Scharlieb from the outset that 'if she had cancer she would not be operated on as her husband would not allow it'. Annie Tompkins,

---

[271] J. Augusta Smith (MS: 1907; Part I). The original procedure was in (MS: 1906; Part II).

[272] Nellie Hayes (EVS: 1909; Part II).   [273] Priscilla Hawgood (MS: 1906; Part II).

[274] Leah H. Greenwood (EVS: 1909; Part I).

[275] Although, again, there was no record that she did come back to Vaughan-Sawyer for this other procedure.

[276] Mary Seabrook (EVS: 1904–1908; 1907).

meanwhile, sought to share the responsibility for refusing a procedure with her spouse. Mrs Tompkins had a malignant ovarian cyst and was unwilling to have any operation performed. She later altered this to 'she and her husband were unwilling that she have any operation'. While the examples of spousal refusal were few, the fact that they appeared at all limits the claim that the individual patient was able to make a choice about her health.[277] In some cases, the necessity of considering others' opinions subsumed personal desires and suspicions about surgery. This was especially so for malignancy of the female generative organs, as we shall see in the next chapter, which ensured that some patients went untreated.

While consideration was afforded to close family members, other women expressed very clear opinions about what they did and did not want done to them. Elizabeth Tranter's 'anxiety' to be operated on has already been noted. Sterility was one condition where women frequently demanded that everything should be done to help them conceive. As Emily Harris explained, she was 'anxious that all should be done to make it possible for her to have children'.[278] Many saw an operation in the RFH as the solution to all their problems. Katherine Miller, for example, came to see Vaughan-Sawyer for advice about becoming pregnant and was so 'excited' at the prospect of an operation allowing this that she was unable to eat or drink.[279] The accounts of surgery performed by Scharlieb and Vaughan-Sawyer between 1903 and 1913 made frequent reference to patient requests such as these. Jennie Meek was very keen to have children and so made clear, from admission, the necessity of conservatism in any surgical procedure which she might undergo.[280] Similarly, Annie Neal was treated conservatively for reduction of a double hydrosalpinx; an artificial ostia was subsequently formed as the patient was 'anxious for children'.[281] Alice Self, from Aldeburgh, Suffolk, one of 20 children, travelled to the RFH 'on her own initiative' because she was very anxious to have a living child and, desperately, had 'never known what it is to feel well'. Between the period covered by the notes, she attended five times: thrice under Scharlieb and twice under Vaughan-Sawyer. A Caesarean Section finally provided her with her desire in 1911 ('a fine

---

[277] For 'patient choice', see Cullen, 'Patient Records', especially pp. 111–48 and Wilde, 'The Elephants' for the need to consider other factors affecting the doctor-patient relationship.

[278] Emily Harris (MS: 1904).

[279] Katherine Miller (EVS: 1913; Part I). Mrs Miller's cervix was widened to facilitate conception, but Vaughan-Sawyer doubted she would go on to conceive because of the position of her uterus.

[280] Jennie Meek (EVS: 1910; Part II).   [281] Annie Neal (EVS: 1911; Part I).

boy'), although the notes also indicated that she was not thriving and later underwent sterilisation.[282]

Conversely, those who expressed a desire not to have any more children were also considered during surgery. Alice Oxford already had five children and 'was not especially anxious to again become pregnant'. During an operation for removal of her right fallopian tube and most of her right ovary, it was remarked that the left side looked 'fairly' healthy, but that 'no efforts were made to improve the condition' because of her previous comments.[283] Patients were also presented with choices: whether to have another simple procedure or undergo more serious surgery. Multiple patient Hagar Walker was a good example of such an offer. Although she had been curetted twice, in 1903 and 1906, she was still suffering from very profuse menstrual losses and pain. The curetting had helped to some extent, but the improvement lasted only for eighteen months and the problem began again, each time more severely than the former. Effectively, she was incapacitated for a fortnight in every month. As such, Vaughan-Sawyer asked her if she would prefer to undergo another dilatation and curettage or have the fundus uteri removed. Mrs Walker chose the latter.[284] One of the more sickly patients, Edith Fenn, who, at the age of 24, had a long history of illness and gynaecological suffering, was told that a double oophorectomy would be the only cure, as previous palliative operations had been unsuccessful in alleviating her pain. Miss Fenn's 'willing[ness] to undergo it' showed precisely how much she desired a cure, as she was effectively 'disabled from following any occupation' by her problems.[285] At times, and in spite of the dangers or risks associated with a major operation, female patients saw it as the best option, one which would restore long-absent health, after years of un- or partially successful medical treatment.

Sarah Macey's statement that she was 'anxious to go home' would probably resonate with the majority of patients in the gynaecological wards.[286] Many expressed their gratitude after treatment. Olivia Risley felt 'wonderfully strong' after her operation, while Priscilla Greenaway was 'very much better for the operation and is already regaining her

---

[282] Alice Self (MS: 1906; Part I); (MS: 1906; Part II); (MS: 1907; Part II); (EVS: 1911; Part I) twice. Her notes ended abruptly and the comments about sterilisation were on the front page, but not noted inside.

[283] Alice Oxford (EVS: 1910; Part I).

[284] Hagar Walker (EVS: 1911; Part I). Unfortunately, when Mrs Walker returned to the hospital in 1913, she had carcinoma of the cervix. For her other RFH in-patient stays, see note 69.

[285] Edith Fenn (MS: 1908; Part II). See also (MS: 1907; Part II) twice.

[286] Sarah Macey (EVS: 1904–1908; 1908).

colour and getting fat' after the removal of her uterus.[287] Margaret Nixon labelled herself 'very fit', having become plump and gained colour by the time she left hospital.[288] Eighteen-year-old Agnes Darley delighted in instant improvement after surgery for a multilocular ovarian cyst 'the size of a man's head', which had made her very sick and unable to eat properly for a year.[289] Annie Rondle's sentiment that it had been good to be 'off her feet' would also have been understood by a number of hard-pressed patients.[290] Time to themselves was relished, in spite of the institutional surroundings. Alice Lyles and Nellie Brown were observed reading, while Henrietta Bray sewed.[291] After aborting an unwanted fifth child with a syringe and having her uterus removed as a consequence, Sarah Barnett was described as reading the paper and looking quite happy.[292] For many rest would continue at a Convalescent Home, but others, like Louisa Aldred, said they felt well enough without further recuperation.[293] Discharge from hospital did mean some alteration in the lives of patients. Women were warned to take things easy, and often not to return to work yet or to limit their household tasks. Annie Nash, for example, was encouraged to rest a great deal, sit with her feet up, and eat good food.[294] Given the number of times a patient disobeyed a doctor's orders in the notes, often, like Emily Stolz, being told to rest for ten days after a miscarriage and doing so only for three, advice like this was not always followed.[295] The cost of surgical supports could also prevent women from carrying out prescriptions. Annie Ambler was told to wear an abdominal belt, but could only have one when she could afford it.[296] For Annie Bell, a belt fitted over a truss for hernia caused problems and ensured her corsets had to be altered.[297] Inconveniences such as these show that life after surgery had to be adapted as best as the patient could manage.

Neither were cures guaranteed: the number of multiple attendees over a decade attested to this. Other than a recurrence of malignant disease, this was due primarily to the duties of wifehood and motherhood. Female surgeons could advise, as in the case of Frances Graves, who had been married for nine years, had given birth to nine children, eight of them now dead, that she was 'to avoid pregnancy', but such a suggestion

---

[287] Olivia Risley (EVS: 1910; Part I); Priscilla Greenaway (MS: 1906; Part II).
[288] Margaret Nixon (EVS: 1911; Part I).
[289] Agnes Darley (MS: 1905; Part II).   [290] Annie Rondle (EVS: 1913; Part I).
[291] Alice Lyles (EVS: 1911; Part I); Nellie Brown (EVS: 1911; Part I); Henrietta Bray (MS: 1905; Part I).
[292] Sarah Barnett (EVS: 1912; Part II).   [293] Louisa Aldred (EVS: 1906; Part II).
[294] Annie Nash (MS: 1908; Part II).   [295] Emily Stolz (EVS: 1909; Part II).
[296] Annie Ambler (EVS: 1911; Part II).   [297] Annie Bell (EVS: 1911; Part I) twice.

required the co-operation of husbands as well. Plastic operations to repair tears occurred again and again between 1903 and 1913, often on the same women. Elizabeth Osborne and Florence Cruse were just two examples.[298] The former had her perineum repaired in 1906, the stitches giving way, and a year later another operation was performed, while the latter also underwent surgery in 1906, only to return in 1907 because union was not complete. Both had suffered for many years with the consequences of tears sustained through childbirth. A rare letter from the patient themselves was with the file of Laura Toghill, written a year after Vaughan-Sawyer had removed her uterus for fibroids:

I am sorry to have to trouble you again, But [sic] I should be very gratefull [sic] if you could make it convenient for me to come and see you. I have been feeling very unwell for some months past, frequently loosing [sic] blood and I also feel giddy and faint with it at times you performed an operation on me twelve months ago last, April, 7th for tumour on the womb.

Her own doctor had recently died, and she did not like 'to go to a strange, Doctor' [sic], prompting this unusually direct correspondence with her surgeon in an attempt to regain her health.[299] On the whole, though, patients were usually referred to the Out-Patient Department so that their surgeons could 'keep an eye on them': Sarah Wilhelmy and Amy Cook were both observed this way in case malignancy developed.[300] While discharge from the hospital meant the end of treatment for some, for many others repeat visits, either to Out-Patients or again to the Gynaecological Department, were to be made over the years. As we shall see in the next chapter, the following-up of former in-patients was key to the way in which female surgeons operated.

Conclusion

This chapter has explored a decade in the lives of gynaecological patients under Mary Scharlieb and Ethel Vaughan-Sawyer at the Royal Free Hospital. Between 1903 and 1913, over a thousand women were seen, treated, and the majority operated upon. Female patients were from all backgrounds, of all ages and of varying willingness to be treated. The reaction of the actual patient to surgery is rarely considered in the history of medicine, and such a case study certainly permits a refutation

---

[298] Elizabeth Osborne (MS: 1906; Part II) and (MS: 1907; Part II); Florence Cruse (MS: 1906; Part I) and (MS: 1907; Part II).

[299] Laura Toghill (EVS: 1904–1908; 1908). Mrs Toghill did not appear again in the notes, so perhaps saw Vaughan-Sawyer privately.

[300] Sarah Wilhelmy (MS: 1908; Part II); Amy Cook (EVS: 1911; Part I).

of the old tale that women were 'passive and preyed upon' by male surgeons, as Morantz-Sanchez notes.[301] But, as has been shown here, not all female patients wanted to be helped surgically, regardless of the sex of their surgeon. Indeed, more often than not, this would have been the first time the majority had experienced the care of a medical woman. Despite arguments about women's suitability for examining female patients, the 'special sympathy' that was said to exist between them,[302] very few sought out assistance from their own sex until they entered institutions. When they had spent time on the wards, however, many returned, either through geographical propinquity, or, as in the case of Laura Toghill, because the surroundings, as well as the personnel, were by now familiar. Some sought rest in the RFH, but for others it was a source of fear and torment. The variety of response to illness and treatment has been considered and general patterns drawn without flattening out the individual reactions to hospitalisation in the early twentieth century. Case notes, though composed in another hand, allow the patient's voice to be heard, often loudly and clearly, through their opinions about their health, their account of the trajectory of illness, and all the idiosyncrasies expressed throughout their time in hospital. They also permit a more personalised insight into how the layperson viewed the medical profession and, specifically, their reaction to the surgical advances which had characterised the previous half-century.

[301] Morantz-Sanchez, 'Negotiating Power', 292.
[302] Dally, *Women Under the Knife*, p. 204.

3   Women Surgeons and the Treatment of Malignant Disease

On 7 April 1904, 29-year-old May Beecham was admitted to the Gynae-cological Department of the Royal Free Hospital under the care of Mary Scharlieb.[1] Nine days before, she had experienced a 'flooding', noticing dark red lumps, which Mrs Beecham described as resembling 'pieces of liver', coming away when she passed water. Since this point, she had lost large clots, 'nearly half a pint at a time', daily. Sufficiently concerned about her symptoms, May Beecham visited the Out-Patient Department at the RFH on 2 April, and was informed that she must see Ethel Vaughan-Sawyer, Scharlieb's assistant, at Gynaecological Out-Patients, for a more specialist opinion on her condition. At the next relevant oppor-tunity, four days later, Mrs Beecham came back, saw Vaughan-Sawyer and was told she must come in immediately. She became an in-patient the next day. In a little over a week after experiencing any symptoms, and never having suffered any pain stronger than some bearing-down sensations before the floodings, May Beecham was informed she required an urgent operation for a rapidly growing carcinoma of the cervix.

Eight patients admitted to the RFH in 1904 under Scharlieb were suffering from cancer.[2] Four of these were diagnosed, like Mrs Beecham, with carcinoma of the cervix; one from epithelioma of the vulva and another from malignant disease of the liver. May Beecham was different in a number of ways. Firstly, she was the youngest, by a considerable margin; her nearest contemporary was 41, while the other six were aged between 45 and 77. In a textbook first published in 1908, Johns Hopkins University's Professor of Gynaecological Surgery, Howard Kelly, noted that uterine and cervical carcinomas were diseases of the over-forties, with few of the latter occurring before 40 and after 60. While not impossible, diagnoses in those aged between 20 and 30 were

---

[1] May Beecham (EVS: 1904–1908; 1904).
[2] The others were Eliza Fenwick, Rebecca Bosher, Ellen Meade, Ann Gobby, Elizabeth Goode, Ellen Baker and Annie Southwell (MS: 1904).

'exceptional'.[3] Secondly, May Beecham's symptoms had been largely painless and extremely recent. This was not unusual for her condition, where pain frequently indicated that the disease had been caught too late.[4] However, unlike many who suffered similarly, she had sought medical help as soon as her symptoms began, as well as returning promptly for appointments made by the various doctors she saw. Such adherence to life-saving advice would have cheered a profession troubled by patient delay in seeking treatment for suspicious growths, unexpected and intermenstrual bleeding.[5] Thirdly, and most importantly, the combination of her youthfulness and swift reaction, coupled with the willingness of her surgeon to take a risk on her patient's chance of survival, ensured that she was the only cancer patient who left the RFH's Gynaecological Department in 1904 having undergone surgery for her condition. After initial examination and, in some cases, exploration of the extent of the disease, the other seven were deemed inoperable and sent home.

Mrs Beecham's notes recorded the dilemmas which faced her surgeon when considering the severity of her disease and the debate Vaughan-Sawyer entered into when deciding whether or not to try and save her patient's life surgically. Upon initial examination per vaginam, the whole of Mrs Beecham's cervix was seen to be hard and infiltrated with a large friable mass protruding through it; the vaginal wall was also diseased and the base of the left broad ligament was suspected to be involved too. Contemporary opinion, such as that contained in gynaecological surgeon John Bland-Sutton's second edition of *Tumours Innocent and Malignant* (1901), inclined to the melancholic when faced with the spread of the cancer beyond the confines of the cervix itself. Even if it was not too late for operative interference, which it was in around 90 per cent of cases, recurrence was extremely likely and life expectancy poor.[6] Four days after admission, Vaughan-Sawyer was inclined to take this perspective, as re-examination pointed to infiltration occurring rapidly, rendering surgery hopeless. Although expressing doubt about whether a panhysterectomy was justifiable, due to the extent of the growth, Vaughan-Sawyer wavered in her decision, concluding finally that the patient's youth made her anxious to give her a chance. May Beecham was operated upon the

---

[3] Kelly, *Medical Gynecology*, p. 517.

[4] See, for example, H. Macnaughton-Jones' Presidential Address 'Pain Associated with Disorders of the Female Genital Organs', *PRSM*, 3 (1910) 1–10.

[5] See, for example, Herbert Spencer, 'A Discussion on Measures to be Recommended to Secure the Earlier Recognition of Uterine Cancer', *BMJ*, 2.2434 (24 August 1907), 431–4.

[6] John Bland-Sutton, *Tumours Innocent and Malignant*, second edition (London: Cassell and Company, Ltd, 1901), pp. 340–1. *Tumours* was first published in 1893.

next day. The growth was curetted and then her uterus, fallopian tubes, ovaries and the upper half of her vagina were removed in a procedure lasting a lengthy two and a quarter hours. Surgery revealed that there was no infiltration of the broad ligaments, and while the posterior and left lateral fornices were affected, the rectal mucous membrane was not involved. Pathological enquiries further confirmed that the growth was a squamous-celled epithelioma, but the glands present and the vaginal wall were healthy. May Beecham recovered well from her procedure, despite a little wound suppuration, and left the RFH on 24 May 1904, barely two months after her first symptoms.

Optimistically, May Beecham was discharged as 'cured' and, indeed, did not appear again in Vaughan-Sawyer's case notes, which covered the period between 1904 and 1919, nor those of Mary Scharlieb, which finish in 1909.[7] As a firm believer in the need to keep track of patients, Vaughan-Sawyer frequently added follow-up comments to the notes or attached letters from the patient's own practitioner informing her of their progress, but no further remarks were made about the future of May Beecham.[8] Vaughan-Sawyer's response to May Beecham's case and her 'anxiety' to do something to help her patient raise a number of questions about women surgeons and their treatment of malignant disease in the first two decades of the twentieth century. Rather than leaving her to die, in similar fashion to the other seven cancer patients who were admitted in 1904, Vaughan-Sawyer insisted on risking a radical surgical procedure – namely, an abdominal hysterectomy and the removal of all appendages – in order to give her patient 'a chance' of survival. Recent research by Ilana Löwy and Ornella Moscucci on gender and cancer has offered conflicting interpretations of women's involvement in radical surgical procedures. While Löwy has claimed that '[s]upport for hysterectomy as a cancer cure was not limited to male doctors. Women surgeons also actively advocated radical surgical approaches', Moscucci has focused on the '"ineffable freemasonry of sex"' between women doctors and their patients, which, stimulated by a 'long history of feminist opposition to gynaecological surgery', determined to find and support alternative, less

[7] 'Cures' were considered those who had not had a recurrence after five years. See Comyns Berkeley and Victor Bonney, 'Results of the Radical Operation for Carcinoma of the Cervix Uteri based on a Three Years' Basis, more especially with regard to its Life-prolonging Effects', *JOGBE*, 24.3 (September 1913), 145–8; 145.

[8] As well as RFH case notes, such as those, for just one example, of Minnie Fuller (EVS: 1909; Part I), see Vaughan-Sawyer's obituary which confirms this diligence: 'Obituary: Ethel Vaughan-Sawyer, MD', *BMJ*, 1.4602 (19 March 1949), 503–4; see also a postscript by Dr Lina M. Potter about her relationship with her patients who 'adored her to the extent of tolerating whatever she prescribed', *BMJ*, 1.4604 (2 April 1949), 595.

'"mutilating"' non-surgical means to treat cancerous growths.[9] Löwy's article ends in 1910, but both this and *A Woman's Disease* point to a similar trajectory as Moscucci's, noting that from 'the 1910s onwards the treatment of cervical cancer was dominated by the rays rather than by the scalpel'.[10] Both argue that non-surgical treatment appealed from the second decade of the twentieth century to the compassionate nature of women surgeons, keen to speak for their sex and offer less invasive procedures.

Neither Löwy nor Moscucci, however, consider directly the position of the British woman surgeon in the 1910s, seen by both as a key decade of change in attitudes. As this chapter will show, in two different general metropolitan hospitals with prominent female surgeons, the Royal Free and the women-only New Hospital for Women, risky surgery was still performed, and, indeed, was the dominant treatment for cancerous growths throughout this decade. This is not to claim that women surgeons entirely ignored or refused to attempt other forms of contemporary 'cure', such as the newly discovered properties of X-ray or radium therapies, but recourse was had to both as a last resort and only for inoperable cases: surgery came first. Moscucci has suggested that it was 'die-hard' male surgeons who were keen to 'preserve the pre-eminence of operative treatment' for cervical cancer,[11] but at both these institutions radical abdominal procedures were the norm, carried out, altered and perfected for patients with malignant disease from 1900 to 1919. The wealth of extant case notes at the RFH also makes it possible simultaneously to explore the reactions of female cancer patients to the progress of their disease, as well as their responses to proposed and actual treatment over the first two decades of the twentieth century.[12]

Unlike many of their contemporaries, women surgeons' confidence in radical operative procedures was supported by their belief in the value of a diagnostic trajectory in which surgery was the end point, but not the only part. Rather than relying solely on clinical skills founded on experience, women took advantage of modern technology, such as pathological reports, to aid judgement and prove diagnosis scientifically. Löwy has

[9] See Ilana Löwy, '"Because of their Praiseworthy Modesty"', 371; also *A Woman's Disease* and *Preventive Strikes* (Baltimore, MA: Johns Hopkins University Press, 2010). Moscucci, 'The "Ineffable Freemasonry of Sex"', 140.

[10] Löwy, *A Woman's Disease*, p. 51; '"Because of their Praiseworthy Modesty"', 379.

[11] Moscucci, '"The Ineffable Freemasonry of Sex"', 163.

[12] For a series of essays concerned with a later period, see Carsten Timmermann and Elizabeth Toon, eds., *Cancer Patients, Cancer Pathways* (Basingstoke: Palgrave Macmillan, 2012).

remarked that the majority of surgeons and gynaecologists still 'relied above all on direct observation and reading of clinical signs', believing that this was more 'reliable than microscopic observations'.[13] This was applicable even in the early twentieth century, with some older surgeons denying the usefulness of pathology in solving surgical problems. Indeed, as a leading Professor of Obstetrics and Gynaecology, William Japp Sinclair, declared in an address to the BMA in 1902: 'What is not surgical is futile – it is hardly knowledge.'[14] Additionally, as already noted in the case of Vaughan-Sawyer, women surgeons were committed to following the progress of their patients after they had left the hospital through personal correspondence, as well as monitoring the conditions of those who lived nearby through the outpatient system. If, as Moscucci notes, women surgeons wanted to compete professionally with their male counterparts by offering more compassionate forms of cancer care than radical surgery by the 1920s, in the first two decades of the twentieth century such a meticulous programme of affirmation and confirmation of diagnosis, surgical treatment and ultimate results would speak for female skill in operative procedures for malignant disease. Operations for cancer were difficult, dangerous and had to be continually adapted for each patient's particular condition and the extent of the disease.[15] Yet, as with Vaughan-Sawyer's decision to operate on May Beecham, giving patients a 'chance' of survival through the best means available ensured that the women practitioners considered here supported surgical intervention above all else, in spite of the risks involved.

This chapter will ask three key questions about women surgeons and the treatment of malignant disease in the decade and a half between 1904 and 1919. Firstly, what conditions did they treat and how did they operate? Secondly, whom did they treat and why, and, finally, what was the experience of those patients treated? While the first two sections will refer to both hospitals already mentioned, the final analysis will be of the extensive RFH gynaecological case notes, where patients diagnosed between 1904 and 1914 can be followed through to possible five-year 'cures'. Patient reactions to cancer and its treatment were dominated by lay perception of a disease which was beginning to rival tuberculosis as

---

[13] Löwy, '"Because of their Praiseworthy Modesty"', 374. See also Jacyna, 'The Laboratory and the Clinic'.

[14] William Japp Sinclair, 'Carcinoma in Women, Chiefly in its Clinical Aspects', *BMJ*, 2.2170 (2 August 1902), 321–7; 324.

[15] For a wider analysis of surgery in the early twentieth century, which draws specifically on modification and experimentation, see Wilde and Hirst, 'Learning from Mistakes'; and Wilde, 'See One, Do One, Modify One, Prostate Surgery in the 1930s', *MH*, 48 (2004), 351–66.

the era's greatest public health concern.[16] Why potential sufferers did not request medical advice sooner and the response of the general practitioner to a possible cancer will additionally be considered, alongside the perception of what delayed seeking treatment. However, I will also take into account the professional pessimism towards cancerous growths in the early twentieth century and the initial reluctance to operate on potentially 'hopeless' cases by a number of surgeons. This, in turn, fuelled public suspicion of surgical value when faced with this still poorly-understood disease.

Cancer Treatment at the New Hospital for Women, 1900–1919

Although previous research has primarily focused on gynaecological experience,[17] women surgeons at the RFH and the NHW operated on a variety of cases, as befitted the general status of these institutions. That the latter only admitted women and children (and boys below a certain age) did not mean that it treated exclusively gynaecological nor even female-only malignancies, nor carried out surgery solely on these conditions, as we have already seen, as regards the New, in chapter 1. The NHW, indeed, was compelled to make its general status clear in 1905 to the charitable King Edward's Hospital Fund for London, which had been under the impression that the hospital was 'solely for Gynaecological cases' and the 'diseases of women'.[18] While the RFH staff dealt primarily with the diseases of women, as their job titles suggested, they were also confronted with other abdominal complaints and disorders, which were not always passed over to colleagues who dealt with surgical cases of both genders. As neither of these institutions were specialist centres and the treatment of cancer in the early twentieth century took

---

[16] See John V. Pickstone, 'Contested Cumulations: Configurations of Cancer Treatments through the Twentieth Century', BHM, 81.1 (Spring 2007), 164–96; 174; Moscucci, 'Gender and Cancer'.

[17] Löwy and Moscucci focus on gynaecological cancer, especially carcinoma of the cervix, which was one of the most frequently seen cancers in women, as we shall see. Löwy has also explored the treatment of breast cancer (not by women surgeons) in France and America for a later period. See 'Knife, Rays and Women: Controversies about the Uses of Surgery versus Radiotherapy in the Treatment of Female Cancers on France and in the US', in Timmermann and Toon, eds., Cancer Patients, pp. 103–29; also 'Breast Cancer and the "Materiality of Risk": The Rise of Morphological Prediction', BHM, 81.1 (Spring 2007), 241–66.

[18] See the letter from Chairman of the hospital's Managing Committee, A. Gordon Pollock, to Hon. Secretaries, King Edward's Hospital Fund, July 27 1905, KE/248/4, LMA. For more on this charity, see F.K. Prochaska, Philanthropy and the Hospitals of London (Oxford: Clarendon Press, 1992).

place predominantly in general hospitals,[19] it is helpful to ascertain how frequently women surgeons were confronted with malignancy, as well as how often surgery was performed on those suffering from the disease. The first section of this chapter will go on to focus specifically on rectal surgery at the NHW, both because of its prevalence at this institution and because it was a field in which women, such as the hospital's Senior Surgeon Louisa Aldrich-Blake, were contributing to the development of contemporary surgical procedure.

Public understanding of the increase in cancer cases was stimulated by frightening statistics, which also contributed to medical pessimism about the inability, even in an age of improved antisepsis and asepsis, to halt the progress of this disease surgically. At the BMA Annual Meeting in 1907, Herbert Spencer, of University College Hospital, quoted the *Sixty-Eighth Annual Report of the Registrar-General of Births, Deaths, and Marriages in England and Wales* to highlight the current state of affairs.[20] Between 1901 and 1905, there had been just over 73,000 deaths from the most common forms of female cancer. Malignant disease of the uterus, breast, stomach, liver and gallbladder killed over 10,000 women each; uterine cancer killing nearly twice that many. By 1909, deaths ascribed to new malignant growths numbered 34,053 that year alone, and there was a 4 per cent annual increase in cases between 1910 and 1922.[21] Women, and especially working-class mothers, were seen to be particularly susceptible to cancer. Some medical opinion claimed that with their harsh, poverty-stricken lives, filled with overfrequent strain from childbearing, these women's bodies were rendered fertile ground for the development of malignancy.[22] As we saw from the previous chapter, it was precisely this type of early twentieth-century patient with whom the Royal Free, and the other hospitals considered here, primarily dealt. It was also the reluctance of this particular group of women to acknowledge the presence of obvious symptoms which medical professionals blamed for consulting too late to improve the rate of cure. Often the disease had spread so that nothing could be done except send patients home to die, as in the case of seven-eighths of the cancer cases under Scharlieb and Vaughan-Sawyer in 1904. While women did not necessarily consult

---

[19] For this development, see Caroline Murphy, 'A History of Radiotherapy to 1950: Cancer and Radiotherapy in Britain, 1850–1950', PhD thesis, University of Manchester, 1986, especially chapter 1.

[20] Spencer, 'A Discussion', 431.

[21] E.F. Bashford, 'Cancer, Credulity, and Quackery', *BMJ*, 1.2630 (27 May 1911), 1221–30; 1223. Murphy, 'A History of Radiotherapy', p. 63.

[22] For more on this perceived susceptibility, see Moscucci, 'Gender and Cancer in Britain' and Karen Nolte, 'Carcinoma Uteri and "Sexual Debauchery" – Morality, Cancer and Gender in the Nineteenth Century', *SHM*, 21.1 (April 2008), 31–46.

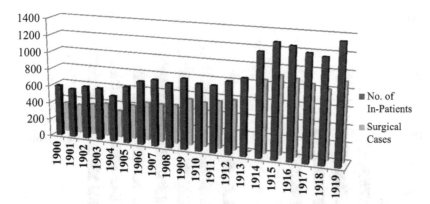

Figure 3.1 Number of In-Patients and Surgical Cases: NHW.[23]

their own sex for ill-health in the first instance, as the previous chapter's study of patients at the RFH revealed, it is vital to consider whether or not female modesty extended to examination and treatment for life-threatening malignant disease by practitioners of the same sex. Whether, indeed, the 'freemasonry of sex', as Moscucci has put it, was evident at women-run hospitals or in female-led Gynaecological Departments.

Over the two decades from 1900, the NHW witnessed a steady increase in the number of patients seen. Indeed, twice as many in-patients occupied the hospital in 1919 as they had done in 1900. As noted in chapter 1, the NHW was established and took pride in itself as a primarily surgical institution and this continued to be reflected in the number of operations carried out in the first two decades of the twentieth century (Figure 3.1). While in 1900, just over 50 per cent of in-patient cases were surgical, by 1919, this had increased to over 65 per cent, with a peak in numbers rising to around 70 per cent consecutively between 1911 and 1915. Although the 1910s have been considered a key decade in the gradual replacement of radical surgery with other, less invasive modes of treatment, the New actually saw a rise in the numbers of major operations being carried out.

Similarly, the *Annual Reports* of the hospital from 1906 make reference to the numbers frequenting the newly established Electrical, or X-Ray, Department, with the patients divided into those attending for diagnosis and those for treatment (Figure 3.2).

---

[23] Numbers collated from those given in *Annual Reports* for the years 1900–1919, LMA, H13/EGA/05/005–H13/EGA/08/006. Unusually, there are no separate surgical, medical or ophthalmic figures given in the reports for 1907 and 1913, so the comparison between overall and surgical in-patients has not been made for these years.

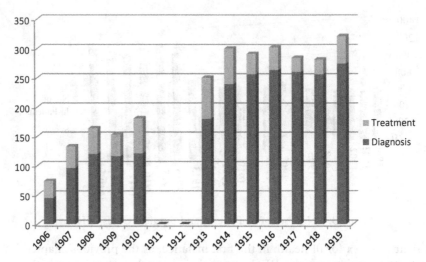

Figure 3.2 Use of the Electrical Department: NHW, 1906–1919.[24]

In both years where a precise list of conditions diagnosed and treated by X-ray were provided, the former made up 72 per cent of the Electrical Department's resources. The sheer variety of conditions treated unsurprisingly bear witness to a new technology being used enthusiastically and experimentally (see Figures 3.3 and 3.4). Neither were the conditions treated gynaecological, as befitting the specialism's scepticism about radiotherapeutic means. In an article published in the *Journal of Obstetrics and Gynaecology* of August 1914, Cuthbert Lockyer was still trying to convince his fellow British gynaecologists of the need to keep up with medicine's evolution by betaking themselves 'to the study of radiology', so far undervalued in comparison with Europe's rapid adoption of techniques.[25] As Joel D. Howell has noted about the American hospital system's adoption of the X-ray, while machines were purchased by and for hospitals soon after Röntgen's discovery of the rays in 1895, usage of the equipment was primarily for diagnostic reasons and even then was utilised far more infrequently than medical literature would have one imagine.[26] Figure 3.2 reveals that, at the NHW, after about a 60:40 split in usage between diagnosis and treatment in the earliest years of the Electrical Department's existence, by 1918, fewer

---

[24] Ibid. There are no statistics provided for 1911 and 1912.
[25] Cuthbert Lockyer, 'The Future of Radiology in Gynaecological Practice', *JOGBE*, 26.2 (August 1914), 92–100; 99.
[26] See especially chapter 4 of Howell, *Technology in the Hospital*.

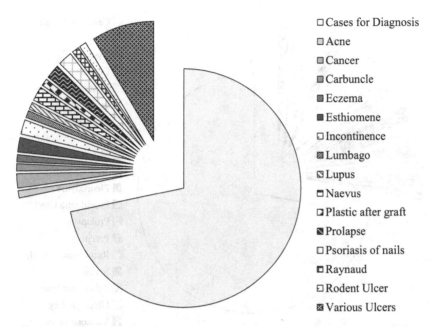

Cases for Diagnosis

Acne

Cancer

Carbuncle

Eczema

Esthiomene

Incontinence

Lumbago

Lupus

Naevus

Plastic after graft

Prolapse

Psoriasis of nails

Raynaud

Rodent Ulcer

Various Ulcers

Figure 3.3 X-Ray Usage, With Breakdown of Conditions Requiring Treatment, 1906.[27]

than 9 per cent of cases received X-ray treatment. Where the surgeons of the NHW could operate, they did.

The number of operations carried out over the first 20 years of the twentieth century at the New shows almost a threefold increase from 328 in 1900 to 883 in 1919, with a peak of 914 in 1916. Similarly, the number of major procedures increases over fivefold between 1900, when there were 115, and 1919, when 600 were performed; again, the greatest amount of serious surgery took place in 1916, when operations peak at 604 (Figure 3.5). In 1900, as the graph reveals, minor procedures dominated, but, as the decade ended, the numbers began to reach parity, until major operations were more than three times as many in 1919 than less serious surgery. The surgeons' confidence in their ability to operate in difficult and risky ways by 1919 provided a stark contrast to the controversy and indecision which dogged the NHW in the first 20 years of its existence, as detailed in chapter 1. Although the 1910s may have witnessed the start of the search for ways of treatment other than surgery, for women surgeons at the New it was a decade where

[27] Statistics for the Electrical Department in *Thirty-Fifth (1906) Annual Report*, p. 25.

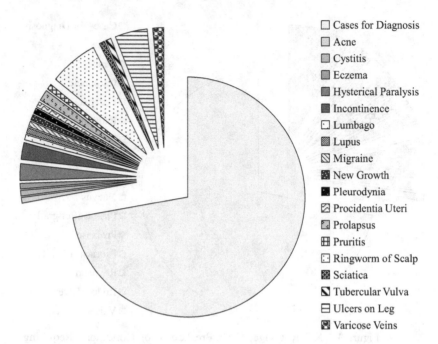

□ Cases for Diagnosis
▨ Acne
▨ Cystitis
▨ Eczema
■ Hysterical Paralysis
■ Incontinence
▢ Lumbago
▨ Lupus
▨ Migraine
▨ New Growth
■ Pleurodynia
▨ Procidentia Uteri
▨ Prolapsus
⊞ Pruritis
▨ Ringworm of Scalp
▨ Sciatica
◣ Tubercular Vulva
⊟ Ulcers on Leg
▨ Varicose Veins

Figure 3.4 X-Ray Usage, With Breakdown of Conditions Requiring Treatment: 1907.[28]

increasing numbers of serious operative procedures were carried out. By 1919, indeed, major surgery was far more likely to take place at the NHW than minor.

A decline in alternative, new technologies such as radiotherapy and the corresponding increase in difficult, time-consuming, risky surgery meant that an in-patient at the hospital was more likely to be operated upon under general anaesthetic than treated medically. Through the death of Miss Rosa Morison, who bequeathed the New a large sum of money in her will, the hospital established what it called a House of Recovery or Continuation Hospital at New Barnet in 1912 (Illustration 3.1).[29] This was not, the New insisted repeatedly to its subscribers, a Convalescent Home, but, rather, an extra limb of the hospital, which freed up space in the main premises for those about to undergo procedures or receive

---

[28] Ibid., in *Thirty-Sixth (1907) Annual Report*, p. 29.
[29] See *Forty-First (1912) Annual Report*, p. 10. Rosa Morison had been the lady super-intendent of women students at University College London for forty years and was a pioneer in women's higher education. See, for example, 'Portraits and Personal Notes', *Illustrated London News*, 3800 (Saturday, 17 February 1912), 230.

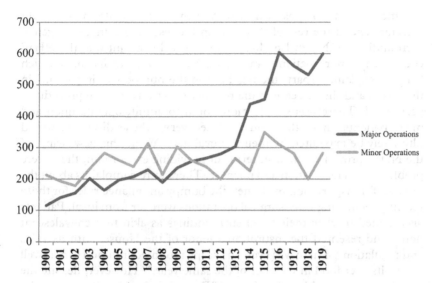

Figure 3.5 Major and Minor Procedures: NHW, 1900–1919.

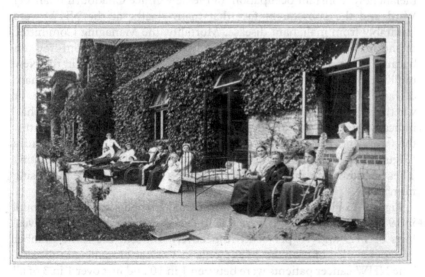

Illustration 3.1 Garden Terrace, Rosa Morison House, New Barnet (c.1916), CMAC SA/MWF/C.44, Wellcome Library, London.

treatment. Some of those who had already been operated upon could therefore spend the rest of their stay in the less urban, more congenial surroundings of North London. In practice, this meant that the NHW could admit more patients and add 20 more beds to its total, which helps to explain, in part, the rise both in the numbers of in-patients in the 1910s and the increase in the number of serious surgical procedures performed. There was simply more room to admit, operate upon and move patients on to the House of Recovery, whose discharge would ultimately be expedited by their removal here. While this new 'wing' of the NHW proved efficient in terms of providing extra room, there were problems with its location and purpose. There were complaints about the modes of transportation to Barnet; the bumpy ambulance rides for those recently recovering from surgical operations were far from ideal. Patients also tended to view their novel surroundings as akin to a convalescent home and resented the institutional tenor of the House, with its rules and regulations. There was even an escape mounted in June 1915 as well as revolts over food in October of the same year.[30] However, despite the initial teething troubles, the House of Recovery played a vital part in the expansion of surgical work at the NHW.

The *Annual Report* for 1900 had drawn subscribers' attention to the melancholy 'constant occupation' of the new Grace Chadburn (Cancer) Ward and the subsequent fact that many deaths at the NHW were inevitably from malignant disease. Mortality, the Managing Committee of the hospital warned its supporters, would be higher from now on because those suffering from various cancers often remained in the New until they died. That year, out of 23 deaths, 6 had been from malignant disease. Whether the alarm was due to public concern about cancer, or whether the hospital felt the need to defend itself in advance now it had indicated its decision to award malignant disease special ward status, this worrying prediction was not proven over the next two decades (Figure 3.6). The other new addition to the building, an Operating Theatre, however, certainly proved useful in dealing with the increasing numbers.

Figure 3.6 shows a peak in deaths from malignant disease at the hospital in 1914, when 36 per cent were due to cancer, yet 1903 and 1917 reveal lows of 11.5 and 10 per cent, respectively. Indeed, the same number of patients died of broncho-pneumonia in 1917 as of malignant disease. The NHW cancer patients were between 1 in 10 and just over 1 in 3 of all

---

[30] The Rosa Morison House Sub-Committee Minutes are an excellent source for the troubles which beset the new House. See the Minutes of Thursday, 17 June, 1915 and Friday, 22 October, 1915, respectively, for details of the runaway patient, ongoing food protests and patient assumptions about their treatment. See H13/EGA/92 (April 1913-January 1921), LMA.

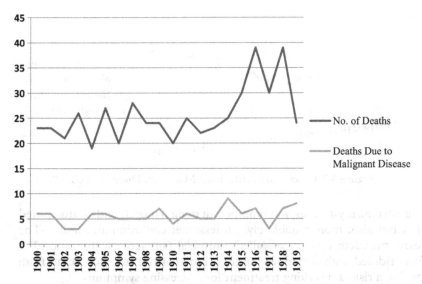

Figure 3.6 Deaths, including Malignant Disease: NHW, 1900–1919.[31]

deaths over this 20-year period. Such statistics, because of the fluctuating numbers, do not suggest that either malignant disease was increasing or that death was inevitable for those patients who visited or who were sent on to the New by their general practitioners. Both concerns were mooted by the medical profession as preventing women from acknowledging their illness early enough. Even in the sixth edition of *Tumours, Innocent and Malignant* (1917), which had a preface acknowledging the 'additions to our knowledge', Bland-Sutton summed up the ongoing pessimism attached to the word 'cancer':

The disease is of very great importance on account of its insidious onset, and, in the earliest stages, painlessness; its progressive and irresistible destructiveness; the manner in which it infects lymph-glands; the extraordinary effects produced in different organs on account of the dissemination of the growth in the form of secondary nodules; the helplessness, misery, and pain it produces when fully advanced; and the inability of medical and surgical art to deal effectively with it, save in the earliest stages. Although this disease was recognised in the dawn of medicine, we not only remain ignorant of its cause, but, in many instances, the diagnosis of the malady is uncertain in the living. This is not due to supineness on the part of investigators, but to the absence of what is called 'specific symptomatology'.[32]

---

[31] Figures collated from *Annual Reports* between 1900 and 1919.
[32] Bland-Sutton, *Tumours*, sixth edition (1917), Preface, p. v; pp. 252–3.

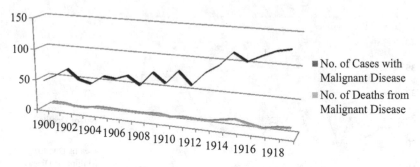

Figure 3.7 Cases and Deaths from Malignant Disease, 1900–1919.[33]

Against the mysterious, but omnipotent malignancy, Bland-Sutton pitted lay, but also, more troublingly, professional confusion and frailty. The early twentieth-century so-called 'universal familiarity with "cancer"'[34] was riddled with misunderstanding, but that did not stop some from taking a risk and seeking treatment for distressing symptoms.

Mortality rates must be paired with the number of patients who sought treatment and were discovered to have a malignant disease in the first place. Although the profession worried about the many moribund patients who finally, but tardily gave in and who could not, therefore, be saved, there were others who, in similar fashion to May Beecham, sought advice as soon as their symptoms appeared. As Figure 3.7 shows, between 1900 and 1919, a patient entering the NHW with any form of cancer had an average chance of 7.7 per cent of not returning home again. The average number of deaths from all patients diagnosed as having malignant disease in the first decade of the twentieth century was 8.7 per cent; this was reduced to 6.7 per cent in the 1910s, with 1917, when only 2.6 per cent of cases died, standing out as the most effective year for patient survival. While this was not, for those leaving, a guarantee of long-term survival, or cure, that their death does not occur in the hospital itself would bode well for the New's reputation as an institution which successfully confronted and attacked one of the most feared contemporary diseases.

The New treated a broad range of cancers in the first two decades of the twentieth century. Figure 3.8 shows the distribution of cases seen by

---

[33] Statistics calculated from *Annual Reports*. There are a few omissions from the tables. They are the number of patients suffering from secondary carcinoma of the pelvis in 1908; those with carcinoma of the vagina in 1915; and the statistics are missing for a secondary deposit in the peritoneum for 1917.
[34] Bashford, 'Cancer, Credulity, and Quackery', 1222.

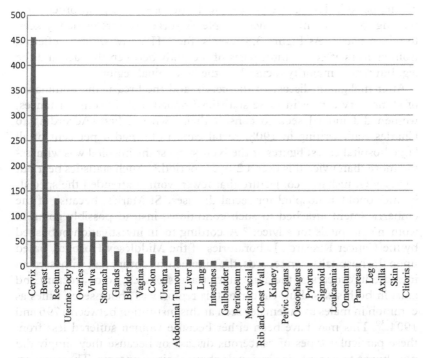

Figure 3.8 Types of Malignant Disease: NHW, 1900–1919.[35]

organ, area or body part between 1900 and 1919. As was to be expected in an institution where the majority of patients were adult women, malignant disease of the female generative organs dominated. Indeed, 30 per cent of all cases were suffering from cervical cancer, 7 per cent from that of the uterine body, and 6 per cent from ovarian tumours. Breast cancer formed the second-highest number of malignant cases seen, with 22 per cent. However, in line with the hospital's general status, there were many patients diagnosed with other forms of malignancy. The numbers suffering from cancers of the alimentary system were particularly numerous. Rectal cancer cases formed 9 per cent of the total number between 1900 and 1919, becoming the third most prevalent cancerous form seen, while malignant disease of the stomach affected 4 per cent of patients. There were no colon cases at all before 1909, but these increased steadily until there were 7 in 1917. Patients diagnosed as having colon cancer formed 2 per cent of all cases, despite only being treated for the second decade

[35] Figures noted under 'malignant disease', collated from *Annual Reports*.

of this period. This corresponded with the rise of surgical procedures relating to the colon, in which the New's surgeons were evidently keen to take a part.[36] As Figure 3.8 reveals, the NHW saw women suffering from cancers affecting most parts of the body between the face and the leg, but with a majority focused on the abdominal region.

After malignant disease of the cervix and the breast, the dominance of alimentary cancer in these statistics implied that, in some instances, women did indeed seek to consult their own sex first. According to Charles Ball, writing in 1908, rectal cancers formed 4 per cent of all large hospital cases; figures at the New suggest the hospital was witnessing more than twice this over a 20-year period.[37] Such statistics bear out Lindsay Granshaw's conjecture that fewer women attended the specialist metropolitan hospital for rectal diseases, St Mark's, because of the embarrassment attached to such conditions, instead possibly going to women's hospitals for advice.[38] According to an investigation published by the Cancer Research Laboratories of the Middlesex Hospital, based upon the hospital's own records, the nineteenth century had witnessed an increase in cancers of the alimentary tract, stomach, colon, rectum and anus in both sexes. But, cancer of this region was about seven times as common in males as in females seen at this institution between 1796 and 1904.[39] This may have been either because women suffered less from these particular types of cancerous disease or because they simply did not choose to consult professionals about their symptoms. The numbers attending the NHW who were eventually diagnosed with cancer of the rectum – 135 over 20 years – may not seem many when compared to the 446 with cancer of the cervix or 336 with malignant disease of the breast, but the fact they chose to come to the New at all suggests more confidence in women doctors than the previous chapter noted was in evidence at the RFH. The unpleasantness of the condition was described by rectal surgeon Harrison Cripps as moving from consciousness of the part, to

[36] See P. Lockhart Mummery, *Diseases of the Colon and their Surgical Treatment* (Bristol: John Wright and Sons; London: Simpkin, Marshall, Hamilton, Kent and Co., 1910), Preface, p. v, and chapter VIII: 'Malignant Disease of the Colon', pp. 249–75. Procedures, Lockhart Mummery comments, were still 'widely different' among surgeons, reflecting a sector in development, rather than characterised by a standardised and uniform approach (p. 273).

[37] Sir Charles B. Ball, *The Rectum* (London: Hodder and Stoughton/Oxford University Press, 1908), pp. 285–6.

[38] Lindsay Granshaw, *St Mark's Hospital* (London: King Edward's Hospital Fund for London, 1985), p. 93.

[39] W.S. Lazarus-Barlow, '"Cancer Ages": A Statistical Study Based on the Cancer Records of the Middlesex Hospital', in *Archives of the Middlesex Hospital V: Fourth Report from the Cancer Research Laboratories* (London: Macmillan and Co, Ltd, 1905), pp. 26–46; p. 45.

a sensation of, if not actual, uneasiness, dull, heavy pain, before physical symptoms manifested themselves in blood-streaked faeces, possibly constipation, alternating with diarrhoea, staining of linen, and increasing emaciation. Secondary symptoms then appeared, affecting digestion, mobility due to swollen legs, and potential spread to the liver. Exhausted by pain and from anal bleeding, without treatment, the patient gradually died. The disease could end fatally in an average of two years if surgical interference was not sought.[40] It may have been this sheer physical discomfort, as well as the hard-to-disguise bowel problems and visible stains, overriding any shame or embarrassment caused by the location of the problem, which sent over 100 women to consult their own sex at the New.

Louisa Aldrich-Blake's pioneering at the NHW of what became known as the 'Aldrich-Blake Method' for excision of the rectum might also explain the large numbers of cases of malignant disease treated when compared with other forms of cancer. Aldrich-Blake had become Surgeon to In-Patients at the hospital in 1902, following Scharlieb's departure for the RFH, and would become Senior Surgeon in 1910.[41] In an issue of the *BMJ* of December 1903, Aldrich-Blake detailed 'Abdomino-Perineal Excision of the Rectum By a New Method', which she had first performed in February of that year at the NHW.[42] 'Simple and efficient', according to its originator, the Aldrich-Blake Method intended to avoid time-wasting by not performing a preliminary colotomy (intended to clear the bowels), unless essential, upon patients, because it would delay proceedings and subject the sufferer to a possible three procedures in total. Excising the disease as soon as possible was crucial to recovery. Previous operations for rectal cancer had been perineal, once the only route to remove malignant disease, but now falling out of fashion in the early twentieth century; sacral, recently pioneered by Swiss surgeon Paul Kraske, to remove growths which extended far up into the rectum; vaginal, utilised when the recto-vaginal septum was affected; and, another late nineteenth-century development, abdominal, which allowed the operator to see immediately the extent of the disease, facilitating a switch to colotomy, if the growth was too widespread, or closure, if the case was inoperable. The latter also permitted radical removal of

---

[40] Harrison Cripps, *On Diseases of the Rectum and Anus*, fourth edition (New York and London: Macmillan, 1914), pp. 333–4.

[41] See *Thirty-First (1902) Annual Report*, p. 6. Lord Riddell's biography, *Dame Louisa Aldrich-Blake* (London: Hodder and Stoughton, 1925), gives an outline of her career, with dates, on pp. 26–7.

[42] Louisa B. Aldrich-Blake, 'Abdomino-Perineal Excision of the Rectum By a New Method', *BMJ*, 2.2242 (19 December 1903), 1586–8.

the lymph glands or any ducts suspected of being infiltrated.[43] Aldrich-Blake's method was therefore a combination of two procedures, bringing together old and new surgical skills. She had devised the operation specifically for one patient, a 54-year-old widow, who had a freely movable, and, therefore, removable, rectal growth. After an abdominal incision, which allowed Aldrich-Blake to see the extent of the disease, the rectum and fatty tissue, containing several enlarged, and thus suspicious, glands, were held forward and now only attached by the superior and two middle haemorrhoidal vessels, which were tied and cut. Due to the shortness of 'Mrs W's' sigmoid, Aldrich-Blake straightened it and carried the lower part to the tip of the coccyx, where a healthy portion of rectum could stretch from the coccyx to the anus. Next, a silk stitch was passed through the peritoneum of the anterior wall of the rectum to guide the operator to the place of division when the bowel should be brought out into the peritoneum. The growth and its diseased attachments were then pushed into the lowest part of the pelvis. Mrs W's abdomen was closed and the patient moved from the Trendelenburg into the lithotrity position. An incision was made in the posterior wall, and, because of the previous movement of the diseased rectum, it was possible to draw it up carefully out of the wound, and then amputate it at the point where the silk suture, previously placed, indicated. Microscopic examination revealed adenocarcinoma, but some of the higher glands removed were free from the disease. The patient made an uninterrupted recovery.

Aldrich-Blake's paper revealed her willingness to adopt, adapt and experiment with different methods of surgical procedure to devise her own operation. Her acknowledgment that she had since managed to save the sphincter of another patient intact, by further refining her technique, pointed to a confidence in tailoring still-novel surgery to the individual patient and their particular condition. As Sally Wilde has noted in an article on prostate operations for a later period, surgery varied from patient to patient, but also surgeon to surgeon; unlike the prescription of standardised drug treatment, surgeons modified, according to experience or level of skill.[44] Aldrich-Blake was sufficiently familiar with rectal surgery to 'devise' her own way of operating; one, indeed, which found its way into Ball's textbook on the rectum in a chapter on surgical 'Cancer Treatment' five years later.[45] As subsequent patients brought their own challenges, Aldrich-Blake, along with many other surgeons of the time, used her previous experience to adopt, adapt and modify to her satisfaction, as well as considering the patient's specific condition. The Senior Surgeon at

[43] See Ball, *The Rectum*, pp. 257–89.   [44] Wilde, 'See One, Do One', 352.
[45] Ball, *The Rectum*, pp. 285–6.

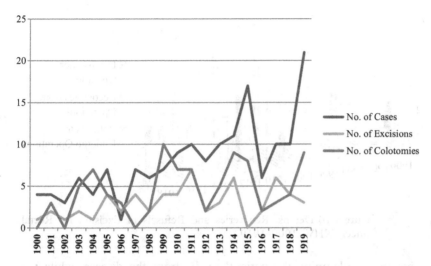

Figure 3.9 Cases of Rectal Cancer, With Surgical Procedures: NHW, 1900–1919.

St Mark's, Frederick Swinford Edwards, described this succinctly by noting that he was not 'entirely wedded' to any one method: 'all cases should be judged on their own merits'.[46] Surgery still had enough of the art and craft about it at this point for surgeons to experiment and hone their skills.

Figures 3.9 and 3.10 show the numbers who sought medical advice for malignant disease of the rectum at the New and the precise way in which they were treated. Not every patient underwent a surgical procedure between 1900 and 1919, but the number of colotomies, coupled with the figures for excision, pointed to the majority receiving some form of relief, if not cure, via surgery. On the whole, colotomies, or the creation of an artificial outlet for faeces, were performed more frequently than excision (Figure 3.9). Given the number of cases of malignant disease, it is likely that colotomies were carried out either as preparation for the excision, a procedure which was not favoured by Aldrich-Blake unless it was strictly necessary, or as a palliative measure for cancers too advanced to be excised. In 1903, William Watson Cheyne, in his 'Observations on the Treatment of Cancer of the Rectum', claimed that there were really only three practical measures for dealing with the disease: to leave it alone and treat medically; to perform colotomy; or to remove the affected portion. The first two options were palliative for Watson

---

[46] Swinford Edwards, 'A Discussion on the Operative Treatment of Cancer of the Rectum', *PRSM*, 4 (1911), 131–2; 132.

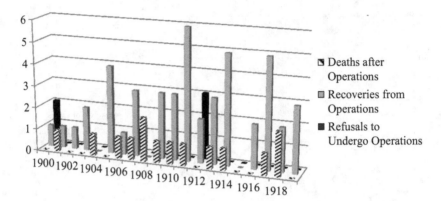

Figure 3.10 Deaths, Recoveries and Refusals in Excision for Rectal Cancer: NHW, 1900–1919.[47]

Cheyne, 'condemning the patient' to die from the disease, while the third attempted to eradicate malignancy.[48] As far as the second option was concerned, Lockhart Mummery pointed out in 1908 that, while deaths from colotomies should be rare when experienced surgeons were operating, they did happen because they were often performed on those for whom it would provide a small amount of relief. For those 'in extremis', with an immovable growth, it could be momentarily life-saving.[49] Colotomies at the NHW over the period between 1900 and 1919 resulted in only four deaths out of a total of 93: one each in 1905, 1910, 1913 and 1915. This represented a 4.3 per cent mortality rate after the operation, with a corresponding 95.7 per cent relief for those patients requiring the procedure.

Given Watson Cheyne's pessimism about the efficacy of the colotomy in providing anything other than a delaying of the inevitable, even if it did offer the patient a temporary measure to combat some of their pain and suffering, it is worth exploring the statistics for excisions performed at the NHW over the same period. Figure 3.10 shows the number operated upon for excision of the rectum out of the total number of patients

---

[47]   The 'Major Operations' figures for 1915 are curtailed in that year's *Annual Report*. There were no operations detailed for rectal procedures at all, but there were 17 patients suffering from the disease noted, as well as 7 unnamed laparotomies for malignant disease and 8 colotomies.
    Figures for 1906 also do not match; there was one patient noted, but two operations, one of which resulted in a death, the other in a recovery.

[48]   W. Watson Cheyne, 'Observations on the Treatment of Cancer of the Rectum', *BMJ*, 1.2215 (13 June 1903), 1360–3; 1360.

[49]   Lockhart Mummery, *Diseases of the Colon*, pp. 280–93; p. 280.

seen. The final year, 1919, offers the anomalous 14.3 per cent, which depresses the average, but, across over the 20 years considered here, excision was the method of choice for, at the lowest, 25 per cent of patients, and the highest 70 per cent. On average, the procedure was carried out upon 36.8 per cent of sufferers from malignant disease of the rectum: 38.6 per cent in the first half of the period, which increased to 41.3 per cent in the 1910s. In 1903, Watson Cheyne had lamented that only around 20 per cent of patients who presented themselves for treatment were suitable for this radical surgical procedure. He noted, more hopefully, that this might be 'somewhat increased' in the near future with ongoing improvements in technique.[50] But a quarter of a century later, Sir William I. De C. Wheeler could still claim exasperatedly that around 70 per cent of patients were found to be suffering from inoperable cancer on admission.[51] If the situation had improved by around only 10 per cent over a 25-year period, the NHW was frequently operating upon more than twice and sometimes three times the number of cases other surgeons were considering. In 1911, for example, excisions were running at a rate of 70 per cent of patients seen; a complete reversal of the inoperable versus operable statistics cited by Wheeler nearly two decades later. Either the female patients at the New were presenting themselves earlier and were therefore more suitable to undergo excisions or the women surgeons at the hospital were taking risks and operating even when the outcome might not be certain or the disease too advanced for success.

The erratic nature of the mortality rates from excision of the rectum at the NHW pointed to this latter proposition. As Figure 3.11 reveals, deaths from this particular operation ranged from none to all. There was little consistency from year to year and vast differences could be seen with only 12 months between cases. So, for example, while 50 per cent of patients who were operated upon in 1901 died, 1900, 1902 and 1903 registered no deaths at all. Similarly, while in 1904, every case died, the year after none did. The statistics stabilised a little after 1909 for nearly a decade, when no more than a quarter of patients died from or following the procedure, but in 1918, the figure rose to 50 per cent again, although it dropped the next year to none. Over the 20 years covered here, the average death rate from excision of the rectum for malignant disease was 24.6 per cent. In 1903, Cheyne had optimistically claimed that while the mortality from cancer of the rectum ranged from 5 to 30 per cent, deaths from excision of a cancerous rectal growth should be no more than 5 to

---

[50] Watson Cheyne, 'Observations', 1361.
[51] Sir William I. De C. Wheeler, 'Discussion on the Early Diagnosis of Carcinoma of the Rectum and Colon', *PRSM*, 21.9 (July 1928), 1543–62; 1543.

10 per cent, due to recent improvements in procedure.[52] However, in 1911, J.W. Smith contemplated his mortality rate of 23½ per cent from a consecutive 34 cases, refusing to offer apologies for his statistics: 'I have operated whenever it was in any way possible to remove the growth and the patient chose to run the very serious risk.' If there was any opportunity to operate it should be advised

however bad it may appear. I have in this way done several cases pronounced inoperable by other surgeons, because in some of the worst and apparently hopeless cases the result has been excellent. I think surgeons who have had a wide experience of the operation would bear me out in this. Of course it means sacrificing statistics, for most of the fatalities have been after operations in such bad cases, but there is no greater hindrance to progress than a too careful eye on statistics.[53]

Given the varying results of serious rectal surgery between 1900 and 1919, those operating at the NHW might have agreed. The chance, however slight, that recovery or at the very least relief from this debilitating condition could be achieved through surgical procedure must have been a good enough reason for those patients willing to undergo operations for cancer of the rectum over these two decades.

Indeed, there were only six refusals to undergo excision of the rectum, and three of those occurred in one year: 1912. Additionally, there were two refusals in 1900 and one in 1907. Of the 161 patients diagnosed with rectal cancer, therefore, only 3.7 per cent would not consent to surgery. Ultimately, refusals formed just 10 per cent of those advised to undergo an operation for their condition. As Figure 3.10 shows, discharging oneself before surgery had taken place had very little to do with mortality rates. In 1912, when 50 per cent of the overall refusals occurred, not one patient died from a rectal excision. Similarly, while there was one death in 1907, there were three recoveries. In 1900, two patients refused the procedure, but the one who did take a chance recovered. The patient perception of the risk attached to the procedure had no concrete link with the number of deaths from that operation. By 1911, as Swinford Edwards made clear, for many surgeons operation was the only possible means of saving the patient: 'All forms of treatment other than operative, whether by radium, X-rays, high frequency currents, trypsin and other digestive ferments, have I think it is generally admitted, proved unavailing, so we can confine our attention to the best

---

[52] Watson Cheyne, 'Observations', 1361.
[53] J.W. Smith 'The Operative Treatment of Carcinoma Recti', *BMJ*, 1.2627 (6 May 1911), 1036–41; 1039.

means of effecting a cure by excision.'[54] Rather than focusing upon alternatives, surgery for rectal cancer, despite its riskiness and high mortality rate, gave the patient the greatest chance of survival. This was evidently how surgeons were recommending the odds to patients because, as Swinford Edwards went on to explain, the practicalities of life after extensive rectal surgery via the abdomino-perineal route, as recommended and performed by Aldrich-Blake, would surely put off many from consenting to the operation.[55] Surgery, however, was even recommended by those purveying one of the non-surgical treatments stated as unsuccessful by Swinford Edwards. The Radium Institute's reports from 1911 to 1914 became steadily bleaker when assessing prognosis following the radium treatment of rectal cancer. By 1914, indeed, for inoperable cases, while the growth might shrink enough to allow surgery to be carried out, for others 'the amount of benefit is rarely so marked or so great as in cancer of the uterus.'[56] Such a statement, which revealed both the efficacy of the surgical procedure in this particular malignancy and radium's lack of success when directly compared with more exclusively women's diseases, could have given the female surgeon an advantage when trying to explain the options to a patient affected with cancer of the rectum. As specialist rectal hospital St Mark's discovered, after trying radium treatment out on their patients, surgery gave better hope as far as long-term prognosis was concerned.[57] At the NHW, either patient desperation, surgical confidence, which had communicated itself very effectively to patients, or a combination of the two meant that 90 per cent of those suffering from cancer of the rectum decided surgery was the correct way to relieve their illness, whatever the possible outcome.

Such reassurance that undergoing a radical surgical procedure was the most beneficial option to take was supported enthusiastically by an insistence on the importance of pathological diagnosis as a confirmation of clinical judgement and a strong belief in the follow-up system for cancer patients. Published articles by early twentieth-century female surgeons at the NHW, such as those by Mary Scharlieb, Louisa Garrett Anderson and the pathologist Kate Platt, made reference to the vital contribution pathology made to surgical scrupulousness, including the

[54] See Swinford Edwards' 'The Operative Treatment of Cancer of the Rectum', *PRSM*, 4 (1911), 99–104; 99. These discussions revealed clearly the differences of opinion between rectal surgeons about the best method of operating for the disease, as well as the ways in which each surgeon operated through modification and adaptation of existing procedures. The 'operability' of rectal cancer was also disputed.

[55] Swinford Edwards, 'A Discussion', 132.

[56] A.E. Hayward Pinch, FRCS, 'A Report of the Work Carried out at the Radium Institute, London, in 1914', *BMJ*, 1.2826 (27 February 1915), 367–72; 369–70.

[57] See chapter 8: 'Conclusions' of Murphy, 'A History of Radiotherapy to 1950', p. 6.

diagnosis, proof and treatment of malignant disease. Garrett Anderson and Platt's 1908 analysis of those patients who had suffered from uterine and cervical cancers emphasised the care with which microscopic sections had been examined and re-examined for their study of 264 cases between 1895 and 1907 in order to ensure that any condition described as malignant was in fact so.[58] Too often in the first two decades of the twentieth century surgeons were accused of unnecessarily removing so-called 'growths' without enough thought or consideration for the patient's actual circumstances. The fear surrounding cancer stoked this assumption in the public mind. Between 1904 and 1909, 'a considerable amount of over-diagnosis' was revealed through data gleaned from hospital statistics: 757 cases were wrongly diagnosed and treated as cancer. This could be contrasted with the 100 per cent cure rate promised through ancient and homely 'quack' methods such as caustics, herbs, ointments, plasters, pills, poultices and vegetable remedies, so derided by professionals and so attractive to the poor, as well as the light treatment, radio-active baths, waters and electric currents which, gaining popularity with some in the profession, stood on the boundaries of acceptability.[59] Surgeons, therefore, had much to prove to potential patients. As articles stemming from experience at the NHW illustrated, confidence in diagnosis through sound surgical judgement, supported by scientific confirmation, made surgery as accurate as it could be, and, importantly, tailored to the individual case rather than the disease itself.

As we saw in chapter 1, Scharlieb had extolled the importance of pathology in print since the 1890s. By 1910, in a debate about malignant and innocent ovarian growths, she laid out a regime which all surgeons should follow for as accurate a diagnosis as possible: a system which put the patient at the heart of the treatment. Scharlieb was shocked at the number of her own cases which had proved malignant and, comparing them with other female surgeons, including May Thorne and Ethel Vaughan-Sawyer, she discovered that her statistics were not unusual. The 'startling proportion' in which the growth was malignant, around one-sixth of cases for all three surgeons, led Scharlieb to label as justifiable the following three rules which should be followed with any malignancy. First, 'that every case shall be carefully recorded; second, that in every case the specimen shall be examined by an expert pathologist; [and] third, that surgeons shall, in all instances, do their best to ascertain the

---

[58] Louisa Garrett Anderson and Kate Platt, 'Malignant Disease of the Uterus. A Digest of 265 Cases Treated at the New Hospital for Women', *JOGBE*, XIV.6 (December 1908), 381–92. This article is discussed by Löwy. See, for example, '"Because of their Praiseworthy Modesty"', 372; 376.
[59] Bashford, 'Cancer, Credulity, and Quackery', 1227.

subsequent history of their patients'.[60] Removal of the cancer through surgical procedure was only one part of the process, according to Scharlieb. Additionally, the more assiduously attention was paid to the exact details of each case, the more frequently specimens were examined by expert pathologists, even if they appeared innocent initially, the more easily surgeons would be able to prolong or save lives.[61] Louisa Aldrich-Blake went even further in her belief that follow-ups were essential to surgical success. Garrett Anderson and Platt made reference to a case whereby a woman was operated upon for ventral hernia, three years after a hysterectomy. When opening her up to repair the hernia, Aldrich-Blake removed her iliac glands. While the patient had not suffered any symptoms, Aldrich-Blake took precautions. A microscopic examination revealed cancer cells. While the pathological process confirmed Aldrich-Blake's suspicions, which were based upon experience and clinical assessment, it also justified the more radical procedure, performed in the interests of the patient. For Aldrich-Blake, the case further encouraged her to propose more radical surgical solutions to the usual follow-up process. It was only incidentally that deposits of malignancy had been discovered, but they had been found because of surgery for another complaint. Therefore, suggested Aldrich-Blake, why not ensure that the follow-up was a surgical one, via an exploratory laparotomy, every 18 months or two years after the initial operation? As Garrett Anderson and Platt put it, her reasoning was that '[t]he risk incurred from an exploratory operation is slight, and the advantage to be derived from it might be great'.[62] There was doubt at the outcome expressed in the second part of this proposal, but that may well have been enough for those patients anxious to ensure that their disease did not return.

The culture of surgery for malignant disease at the New in the first two decades of the twentieth century belies previous assessment that female surgeons were turning towards less invasive modes of treatment. If anything, the number of procedures increased, as did the seriousness and difficulty of the surgery performed. Additionally, women were not only operating on exclusively female conditions. The fact that rectal malignancy provided the third most prevalent form of cancer seen at the NHW shows that, in contrast to the previous chapter where women had not specifically chosen their own sex as general practitioners, regardless of the embarrassing or 'female' nature of their complaint, women with problems in this area did indeed seek the advice of their own sex. Moreover, they

---

[60] Mary Scharlieb, 'On the Proportion of Malignant to Innocent Ovarian Growths, Founded on a Series of 150 Cases', *PRSM*, 3 (1910), 85–99; 86.
[61] Ibid., 90.   [62] Garrett Anderson and Platt, 'Malignant Disease', 385.

also showed willingness to undergo uncomfortable surgery, with only 10 per cent refusing operations over a 20-year period for cancer of the rectum. These are figures which compared very favourably to the despair experienced by other surgeons who tried and failed to encourage large numbers of resisting patients to undergo potentially life-saving surgery. The suspicions and superstitions which surrounded cancer undoubtedly led many simply to go home in pain, eventually to die. That so many did the opposite at the New illustrated that if the cause was serious enough, trust could be established between patient and surgeon because, as Sally Wilde has noted, of the possibility of cure.[63] This was achieved in spite of the ongoing public fear of surgery and, especially, the efficacy of procedures to remove malignancies. Although discussing benign growths, NHW surgeon Florence Nightingale Boyd commented that she thought 'it unjustifiable that women should be allowed to suffer for years [...] without being afforded the relief that surgery could give'.[64] This was certainly the policy at the New regarding malignancy. The promise of relief, however temporary, for many outweighed the substantial risks. Even the high mortality rates for the excision of the rectum, which, as the statistics showed, sometimes ran at 100 per cent, did not prevent the majority from undergoing the procedure. Women surgeons at the NHW were prepared to take those risks, but so, importantly, were their patients.

The Patient Response to Cancer Diagnosis and Treatment: RFH, 1903–1919

The RFH's wealth of case notes allow the historian to examine more closely those patients who were diagnosed with malignant disease at this institution, the ways in which they were treated, their reactions to their condition, and the trajectory of their illness over time, which crucially takes into consideration the question of cures or ongoing procedures for recurrence. Such detailed accounts also permit an insight into precisely how and where treatment was administered to patients, as well as the reasons behind a surgeon's decision to operate or not, or, indeed, a patient's choice whether to follow medical or surgical recommendations. The notes contain important debate between patient and surgeon, as well as, in the hospital's well-established system of staff consultation

---

[63] See Wilde, 'Truth, Trust'. Wilde notes that at the Middlesex Hospital, which specialised in the treatment of cancer, many refusals were 'patients with cancer of the breast, uterus, or rectum, for which the death rate, with or without surgery, was particularly high', 313.

[64] Contribution of Florence Nightingale Boyd to the 'Discussion on the Indications for Hysterectomy and the Methods for Performing it', *BMJ*, 2.2286 (22 October 1904), 1069–84; 1084.

over tricky cases, between surgeons. Often, the weighing up of physical evidence meant there were delays in dispensing treatment or performing surgery, but this period of watching, learning and eventually deciding what to do for the best revealed that decisions were not made lightly and risk was assessed both by surgeon and patient. Unlike the NHW's team, the RFH surgeons, Mary Scharlieb and Ethel Vaughan-Sawyer, focused primarily on the diseases of women, situated as they were in the specialist gynaecological department of a general hospital. Therefore, the majority of their cases were abdominal and, most frequently, of the female generative organs. Their case notes can be used to explore the impact of the early twentieth-century concern about cancer on the prospective patient and to assess whether or not the profession's greatest fears about working-class women's reluctance to consult medical advice were borne out in actuality or whether the situation was more complicated than had been assumed. They also reveal many of the ways in which surgeons tried to keep track of their cancer patients, through a variety of methods dedicated to the follow-up of often hard to locate working-class women, for whom moving frequently because of changes in financial or personal circumstances was second nature.[65] This section will also examine what impact newer, less invasive treatment – such as X-ray applications and the use of radium – had upon female surgeons at the RFH and how it affected the ways in which they operated.

As noted in the first section of this chapter, in print Scharlieb expressed alarm at the number of malignant as opposed to benign cases she had encountered. Indeed, as Figure 3.11 shows, cancer formed no less than 5 per cent and often more than 10 per cent of the conditions treated by the two female surgeons. Across the period covered by this chapter, an average of 8.3 per cent of Scharlieb's patients suffered from malignant disease between 1903 and 1909, while Vaughan-Sawyer's average caseload was even higher: between 1904 and 1919, 10.9 per cent were diagnosed with or confirmed to have cancer. In 1915, cancer cases peaked at 15 per cent of all patients seen by Vaughan-Sawyer. While both Scharlieb and Vaughan-Sawyer were designated 'Physicians' for the Diseases of Women by hospital literature, the vast majority of their cases were surgical, from minor dilatation and curetting of the uterus to major, lengthy and risky procedures for carcinoma. Weisz has labelled gynaecology at this point 'a rather wild and woolly specialist group', a 'protean' and 'enormous field of activity'.[66] As Cuthbert Lockyer explained in an

---

[65] See Letter No. 49: Very Hard Times, for example, which discusses the necessity of moving when temporary work finishes, *Maternity*, ed., Llewelyn Davies, pp. 76–7.

[66] Weisz, *Divide and Conquer*, p. 206; p. 205.

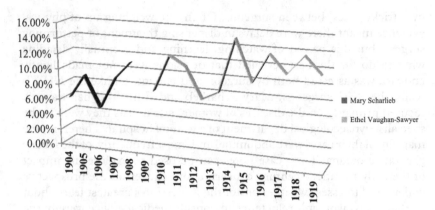

Figure 3.11 Percentage of Cancer Cases to Overall Numbers: RFH, 1904–1919.[67]

article written in 1914, the 'life history' of the specialism proved fascinating. The gynaecologist had started off as a physician, before abdominal surgery had been thought possible, then 'acquired the skill of a surgeon as soon as surgical intervention was required of him for proper fulfilment of his duties'. This 'very adaptable person'[68] had become a surgeon, even if this was not in name. Vaughan-Sawyer was only listed as 'Gynaecologist' and not 'Physician for the Diseases of Women' in 1919, despite carrying out the role for the past decade and a half.[69] While the hospital may have been slow to recognise developing specialties, this particular 'Physician' had been a surgeon from the beginning of the twentieth century.

Malignant disease was, therefore, all too familiar to Scharlieb and Vaughan-Sawyer, who both encountered numerous cancer patients over the years covered by this chapter (see Figures 3.12 and 3.13). It is worth exploring in more detail the kinds of cancers seen by the two women between 1904 and 1919 in order to see which 'Diseases of Women' composed their caseload.[70] The two graphs show similarities, but also a number of key differences between the cases treated by the two women surgeons of the RFH's Gynaecological Department. Firstly, it is clear

---

[67] These statistics are compiled from all cases seen by both surgeons at the RFH, 1904–1919. Between 1904 and 1908, Vaughan-Sawyer's overall caseload was small (73 patients), but over these four years, nearly 11 per cent of her patients had malignant disease.

[68] Cuthbert Lockyer, 'The Future of Radiology', 99. See also Moscucci, *The Science of Woman*, especially pp. 165–206, for changes in the specialism.

[69] *The Ninety-Second Annual Report for 1919* (London: Printed by H.J. Goss and Co., 1920).

[70] Composed from all patient notes of both surgeons between 1904 and 1919, LMA.

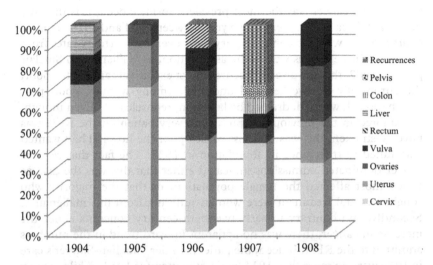

Figure 3.12 Scharlieb's Cancer Cases: RFH, 1904–1908.

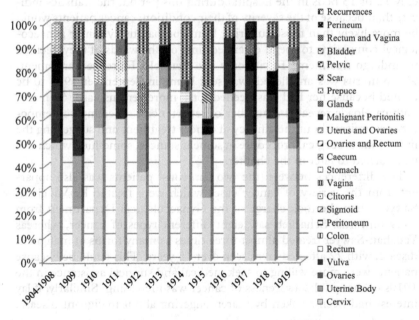

Figure 3.13 Vaughan-Sawyer's Cancer Cases: RFH, 1904–1919.

that cervical cancer was the most prevalent form; indeed, it is the only malignant disease seen every single year between 1904 and 1919. This, of course, tallies with the contemporary fears over the mortality rates from cancer of the cervix, as well as the assumption, as William Japp Sinclair put it in 1902, that the disease 'occurs almost exclusively among the poor, the chronically overworked and underfed, among women, poor, pro- lific, harassed, worried, drained by lactation, reposeless'.[71] Even though, as explored in the previous chapter, not every patient at the RFH was poverty-stricken, this was the class of sick poor the hospital had wanted and aimed to treat since its foundation in 1838. The fact that cervical cancer dominated admissions indicated either that this was the disease which most affected the female population, or that the majority who sought hospital treatment were women suffering from this malignancy. Secondly, and contrary to early twentieth-century concerns about the increase in cancer, there was no apparent upward trend in the numbers admitted to the RFH. Indeed, the patients under Vaughan-Sawyer's care in 1919 were no more than 1911, and not as many as 1913. While she saw three patients in 1912, Scharlieb saw more than twice as many in 1905. Although we do need to bear in mind that both surgeons had access to only 12 or 13 beds in the hospital during this period, the statistics indi- cate that, because of the severity of their condition, cancer patients would be more likely than those suffering from comparatively minor gynaeco- logical complaints to spend extended time on the wards, if they decided to undergo treatment. To cite only one example, Florence Parfrement, whose uterus was anteflexed, was sent home in September 1905 to be treated because her bed was needed for a more serious case.[72] Finally, both caseloads revealed a number of recurrences, reflecting contempo- rary pessimism about the efficacy of cancer treatment and suggesting the limitations of surgical procedure in some instances, something which will be returned to later in the chapter.

The differences between the two surgeons' patients was also appar- ent from the variety of cancer cases which were treated by Vaughan- Sawyer when she took charge of the Gynaecological Department from 1909 onwards. Scharlieb saw eight different types of cancer, whereas Vaughan-Sawyer treated almost three times as many forms of malignant disease, with 22 affected areas seen over 15 years. This could be because patients were more willing to seek medical and surgical assistance in the 1910s or that public awareness of cancer was increasing. Similarly, if lay interest had been awoken by scaremongering about malignant disease,

---

[71] Japp Sinclair, 'Address in Obstetrics', 326.
[72] Florence Parfrement (MS, 1905; Part II).

it could be that general practitioners were more likely to examine their patients and to send them on for specialist advice when cancer was suspected. According to Herbert Spencer, the 'unfortunate state of things' was a combination of patient ignorance regarding suspicious symptoms and the general practitioners' delay in examining those with early signs of malignant disease.[73] Conversely, Vaughan-Sawyer's willingness to take on patients, as well as to operate upon them, even if the case was hopeless, indicated a growing confidence in attempting surgical approaches to cancer. Whereas frequently in the early part of the period covered here, patients were sent home to die without further treatment, the 1910s at the RFH witnessed an increasing desire to do something surgically for those suffering from malignancy. Even if that was a palliative procedure, it became apparent that, in Vaughan-Sawyer's case, as in those of the female surgeons at the NHW, surgery was the answer to the problem of relieving patients, either of their disease, if it was curable, or a short increase in their lives, if it was not.

To explore this latter point, it is necessary to examine the operability figures of the RFH surgeons. This requires assessing whether or not the patient underwent surgery for their condition against the overall number of patients seen. Operability was a particular bone of contention among gynaecological surgeons in the early twentieth century for a number of reasons. Primarily, the concern was that some were offering miraculous success rates due to their careful selection, which was not always acknowledged in print, of patients likely to survive the operation and beyond. Therefore, they either turned away those who could have been saved if they had seen a surgeon more willing to risk their reputation or less promising patients were simply excluded from the statistics. Japp Sinclair commented in 1902 that at the Christie Cancer Hospital in Manchester 'operable cases were seldom seen', they stood at 22 per cent over a decade in the Southern Hospital, and 18 per cent in the Glasgow Western Infirmary, but developments in Germany had indicated that over half of patients could be operated upon and potentially saved.[74] Two years later, Bland-Sutton suggested that his own hospital experience showed that only 5 per cent of 100 consecutive patients suffering from cancer of the cervix were 'favourable subjects for the purposes of operation'.[75] He recommended his 'too exclusive', selection as a defence against the potential discrediting of hysterectomy for malignant disease by the sentimental, superstitious and erroneous. Others, including

---

[73] Spencer, 'A Discussion on Measures', 433.
[74] Japp Sinclair, 'Address in Obstetrics', 327.
[75] Bland-Sutton, 'Discussion on the Indications for Hysterectomy', 1069.

Middlesex Hospital surgeons Comyns Berkeley and Victor Bonney, believed the opposite, claiming in 1913 that: '[i]n estimating an operability rate it is absolutely necessary that it should include every case attending the in and out patient departments, that is, that the patients should not have undergone any previous select'.[76] As Berkeley had noted in 1909:

> We are all agreed that if only early cases are chosen the percentage of cures will be much greater and that of operability much less. Still it is quite evident that most operators have not limited themselves in this way, with the result that many women have been cured whose chances from a clinical examination might have been thought to be hopeless.[77]

For Berkeley, every woman, unless she was incapable of withstanding the operation, should be given a chance, even if the case appeared hopeless upon initial examination. Surgery could provide the best means for prolonging the lives even of those women whose condition was advanced. By taking the risk and increasing the operability rate, cures could be effected.

Surgery for malignant disease in the RFH's Gynaecological Department showed a similar increase to that of the NHW. From not a single operable case in 1904, Scharlieb operated on two-thirds of her patients by 1908, the last full year before her retirement from the RFH (see Figure 3.14). In contrast, Vaughan-Sawyer's cases showed more consistency from the start, as she operated upon 87.5 per cent of her patients between 1904 and 1908. The fewest number of operation cases could be found in 1912 and 1914, where only 50 per cent underwent surgical treatment; in the former year, however, the other 50 per cent were inoperable cases. Of the total number of cancer patients seen by Vaughan-Sawyer between 1904 and 1919, she operated upon an average of 67.4 per cent of them (see Figure 3.15). Although, in 1906 and 1908, two-thirds of Scharlieb's cancer cases underwent a surgical procedure, her average was less than Vaughan-Sawyer, at 41.2 per cent of the total between 1904 and 1908. For the period as a whole, the average 'operability' for both surgeons was 54.3 per cent of in-patients. Similarly, death rates after operation were very favourable. Scharlieb lost only three patients in the last two years at the RFH, while of Vaughan-Sawyer's malignant cases, only 16 did not recover from their surgery over the 15-year period covered by her extant patient notes. For the former, this was an initial success rate of 88.5 per cent; the latter 86.3 per cent. Of the refusals to undergo operative treatment, two of the three Vaughan-Sawyer patients who discharged themselves in 1910 and in 1914 were operable,

---

[76] Berkeley and Bonney, 'Results of the Radical Operation', 146.
[77] Comyns Berkeley, 'Wertheim's Panhysterectomy for Carcinoma of the Cervix', *JOGBE*, 15.3 (March 1909), 145–68; 149.

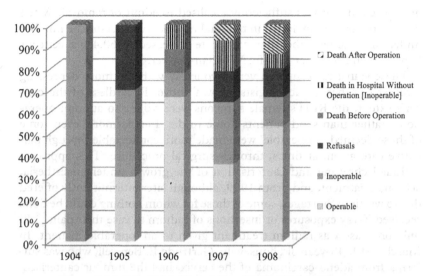

Figure 3.14 Scharlieb's Operability: RFH, 1904–1908.

while one, whose cancer was inoperable, refused all further treatment in 1915. Similarly, of Scharlieb's premature discharges, only one of the seven was offered an operation which might not be successful. The other cases were considered to have consulted surgical advice early enough

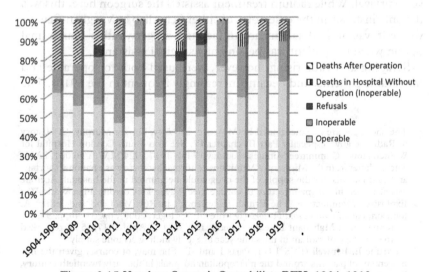

Figure 3.15 Vaughan-Sawyer's Operability: RFH, 1904–1919.

or their condition was sufficiently localised to admit of removal. When these patients were included in the total number seen versus the number undergoing surgery, the operability rate increased to 60.4 per cent for Scharlieb and 69.2 per cent for Vaughan-Sawyer.

These statistics compared very favourably with the more depressing forecast of other gynaecologists, shown above. Regardless of the cancer's extent, the RFH's female surgeons were willing to attempt operations, rather than send patients home to die. Furthermore, even some of those deemed 'inoperable' were made more comfortable through palliative care given, at times, through surgical procedure. This approach included curetting and cauterisation of the growth under anaesthesia, acetone treatment, and, from 1909, although later intermittently offered due to wartime shortages, some of those for whom nothing could be done received X-ray exposures or insertions of radium to ease their pain.[78] In only one case was radium treatment given to an 'operable' patient. In March 1914, 48-year-old housewife, Gertrude E. Benwell, who was suffering from adeno-carcinoma of the cervix, had the tumour cauterised, treated with acetone, and then underwent a series of radium treatments. By the end of April, the growth had shrunk enough for her to be found to have an 'operable' condition. However, while being operated upon, it was discovered that she had a new growth near the orifice of her left ureter, even though her uterus was successfully removed. This nodule had to be left in situ.[79] Mrs Benwell did not return to Vaughan-Sawyer, however, so there was a possibility of a 'cure', at least in terms of a five-year survival. While radium treatment assisted the surgeon here, this was the only instance in the case notes of either Scharlieb or Vaughan-Sawyer where it was utilised as a means to facilitate surgery, rather than a final option when the patient was beyond any surgical assistance.

Scraping and cauterising, however, were used both for operable and inoperable patients, and became increasingly frequent in the 1910s. The

---

[78] The shortages are not mentioned by Moscucci or Löwy, but see Murphy, 'A History of Radiotherapy', especially Part II, chapter IV. See also South London Hospital for Women House Committee Minutes, Tuesday 17 July 1917, H24/SLW/A/06/001, LMA, where a letter from the Ministry of Munitions confirms that there was a national shortage and so no licence for the supply of the drug could be granted to the hospital. Acetone was also used in the manufacture of cordite. See Wayne D. Cocroft, 'First World War Explosives Manufacture: The British Experience', in Roy MacLeod and Jeffrey A. Johnson, eds., *Frontline and Factory* (Dordrecht: Springer, 2006), pp. 31–46; p. 33.

'Radiation in Malignant Disease', *Lancet*, 189.4884 (7 April 1917), 539, remarked on the shortage of radium in the same year as the dwindling acetone supply.

[79] Gertrude E. Benwell (EVS 1914; Parts I and II). She may, of course, given the free movement of patients around the metropolitan hospitals in the early twentieth century, have attended another hospital or died.

removal of obvious parts of growth allowed it to be analysed patholog-
ically, in order to support the surgeon's diagnosis. It also reduced the
levels of pain experienced by the patient, as well as ensuring the extent of
the cancerous area was more perceptible and, therefore, accessible to the
operator. Acetone treatment in the 1910s was enthusiastically embraced
by the Gynaecological Department to cleanse and treat the affected
region after cauterisation. In December 1911, its use for inoperable
cancer was described through Gellhorn's description of his method,
which had originally been published in the *Zentralblatt für Gynaekologie*
of the same year. After scraping as much of the disease away as possible
under anaesthesia, induction was halted, and a speculum inserted into
the vagina and further into the crater remaining after removal of the
growth. Two or three tablespoons of acetone were then poured into the
speculum. After ten minutes, the clotted blood was washed away and
new acetone was introduced: this was left for twenty minutes. Then
the patient was removed from an exaggerated lithotrity position and
any remaining acetone was left to drain away through the speculum. A
gauze plug was inserted and treatment continued at intervals. Gellhorn
claimed that the patient's health and condition could be generally
improved, as well as in many cases where it was possible to prolong life.
It was painless, he noted, and could even be carried out by a general
practitioner.[80] What patients felt about treatments such as acetone and
radium applications, including their ability to relieve suffering, will be
explored later in this chapter. Gellhorn's suggestion about handing
back responsibilities to the patient's own doctor was also interesting,
especially in the light of many gynaecologists' dismay at the generalist's
ignorance about cancer and its treatment. By returning the inoperable
patient to their local practitioner, lessons might be learned. The doctor,
who had perhaps not diagnosed the condition in the first place, or
had not acted quickly enough in seeking specialist advice, would be
compelled to witness their patient's decline. As they would be able only
to care palliatively for them, the stark reality of what could be a slow and
painful death might prompt greater alertness to signs and symptoms, as
well as the necessity of thorough patient examination in the future.

By the 1910s, far from abandoning surgical procedures, Vaughan-
Sawyer was embracing the more radical Wertheim's operation for cancer
of the cervix, along with her contemporaries at other metropolitan
female-run hospitals such as the NHW and the SLHW. Wertheim's

[80] James Young, 'Reviews of Current Literature: Treatment of Inoperable Cancer of Uterus
with Acetone', reporting Gellhorn's article in *Zentralblatt für Gynaekologie*, 35 (1911),
BJOG, 20.6 (December, 1911), 311.

method divided British and European gynaecologists, as both Moscucci and Löwy have explored. The latter has labelled the procedure 'daring' and 'desperate'.[81] In 1911, Amand Routh, president of the Obstetric Section of the Royal Society of Medicine, expressed doubt about the wisdom of such 'heroic operations'. Routh criticised the extremity of contemporary gynaecological surgery, looking forward to a time when treatment could be other than operative and condemning his colleagues recommending surgery because it was the 'easiest way' to deal with a patient.[82] He went on to criticise the use of Wertheim's procedure when the case was very advanced or very recent and feared that the mortality rates did not justify the risk taken both by surgeon and by patient. Briefly, as described by the man himself to a fascinated British audience at the 1905 BMA Annual Meeting held in Leicester, Wertheim had developed his approach seven years previously. While the uterus had been removed formerly through the vaginal route, Wertheim favoured the abdominal option, which allowed the performance of a hysterectomy and the additional removal of surrounding and potentially infected cellular tissue and lymphatic glands. He had adopted and adapted the procedures of others, but with the addition of a vaginal clamp, which would come to bear his name, in order to isolate the cancerous cervix.[83] His justification was that such a radical extirpation decreased the risk of recurrence, allowing 60 to 70 per cent of cases to be 'cured' five years after operation. Most importantly, it permitted those who 'were otherwise irretrievably doomed', having sought advice too late, to be relieved, however dangerous the procedure might be.[84] For detractors, the mortality rate was excessive; even if women survived the operation, death from shock was far too familiar to those who had tried and failed to save their patients. The procedure, at first taking over two hours and only reducing in length with practise, was physically demanding for the operator and required great skill in careful dissection around the bladder and ureters. While Wertheim felt he was offering renewed hope to those 'shut out from life', turned away by other surgeons as incurable, others saw fashionable, but 'homicidal vivisections', cruel experimentation upon dying women.[85]

[81] Löwy, *A Woman's Disease*, p. 33.
[82] Amand Routh, 'The Past Work of the Obstetrical Society of London and some of the Obstetrical and Gynaecological Problems Still Awaiting Solution', *BJOG*, 20.4 (October, 1911), 151–82; 180–181.
[83] Ernst Wertheim, 'A Discussion on the Diagnosis and Treatment of Cancer of the Uterus', *BMJ*, 2.2334 (23 September 1905), 689–704; 689–95. See also Berkeley, 'Wertheim's Panhysterectomy', who considered the impact of the procedure upon British gynaecology. His explanation of what constituted a 'Wertheim' is on 145.
[84] Wertheim, 'A Discussion', 691.
[85] Ibid., and Japp Sinclair, 'Address in Obstetrics', 325.

As both Moscucci and Löwy have charted fully the history of Wertheim's method of operating for cancer of the cervix, I will not do so further here. My interest lies in the adoption of this technique by women surgeons such as Vaughan-Sawyer precisely at the time when Moscucci and Löwy have noted the transition to less invasive procedures and when contemporaries such as Routh were recommending that gynaecologists consider becoming less surgical in their approach to their patients. At the BMA meeting in which Wertheim explained his procedure, Scharlieb commented that abdominal hysterectomy for cancer was not usual in Britain, but she made a point of noting that she had been very much in the minority when advocating this procedure in Oxford just one year earlier. The vaginal route was easier and quicker, but the abdominal was also safe and it prevented any possibility of the recurrence of the disease, as the whole was removed.[86] Of 17 cases of abdominal hysterectomy for cancer, she reported, four were free from recurrence after between two and four years; four had suffered a recurrence (one from cerebral disease), one had died on the day of operation, while the other eight had not been heard of since.[87] Scharlieb had achieved a 23.4 per cent freedom from recurrence as far as those from whom she had heard were concerned, but when the others were added, who had again been diagnosed with cancer, the survival rate beyond ten months was just over 47 per cent. This was clearly the sort of prolongation of life which detractors of the newer methods of abdominal extirpation claimed was torture and supporters viewed as relief. Indeed, as Garrett Anderson and Platt made clear in 1908, women surgeons at the NHW had been carrying out hysterectomies via the abdominal route since 1901, pioneering a method which became routine at this institution a year later. When they compared the results for vaginal hysterectomy with that of the abdominal method, the statistics were enlightening. Twenty-nine patients had the former operation, with only one survival seven years after operation; two had survived for two years, the rest had a recurrence and died soon after, or had not been found. Abdominal hysterectomies provided better results: 26 patients were living and healthy between 18 months and four years after their operation; a further 11 had remained free from cancer for a year and six within three and a half years, while 15 could not be contacted.[88] Vaginal hysterectomy had an extremely low success rate of 3.5 per cent, while 44.8 per cent of abdominal patients had survived for

---

[86] Contribution of Mary Scharlieb to 'Discussions on the Indications for Hysterectomy and the Methods for Performing it', *BMJ*, 2.2286 (22 October 1904), 1084.

[87] Contribution of Mary Scharlieb to 'A Discussion on the Diagnosis and Treatment of Cancer of the Uterus', 698.

[88] Garrett Anderson and Platt, 'Malignant Disease of the Uterus', 385–6.

more than 18 months without recurrence. When recurrence figures were added, 74.1 per cent of the total number had been given an extra year of freedom from the disease. Although nearly 30 per cent of the 'cure' was temporary, the survival rate was far better than either the vaginal option or the depressing statistics of those who would not adopt the riskier methods nor operate on the more advanced cases. To return to the 1904 BMA meeting, where both Boyd of the NHW and Scharlieb of the RFH advocated abdominal hysterectomy for cancer, their optimism was countered by another delegate, Murdoch Cameron, Physician for the Diseases of Women at Glasgow's Western Infirmary, who simply noted that in his experience the great majority of cancer cases had advanced too far for operation.[89] Unlike many of their more pessimistic contemporaries, the RFH's women surgeons were willing to try out and adopt the latest methods, even when others would give up their patients as lost.

Ideally, of course, operability should be based upon the fundamental question: what can be gained through surgery for this patient? By focusing on the benefit, even if it was but a brief respite from malignancy, any procedure could be justified, both to the patient and to the surgeon themselves. British adopters of the Wertheim method recommended the procedure in precisely this way. In 1913, Berkeley and Bonney wrote an article which focused on the 'life-prolonging effects' of radical operations for cancer of the cervix.[90] They explained how they had adapted Wertheim's procedure in order to remove systematically all the glands in the parametric tissue, obturator fossa and the iliac vessels, regardless of whether or not they were enlarged. While this extension added not only to the risk from immediate shock but also the possibility of a more complicated convalescence, their experimentation with technique was both to improve results and allow them to operate on the most advanced cases, who would be considered inoperable by those who only removed the primary growth itself. Berkeley and Bonney's risk-taking, therefore, benefitted surgical advancement as well as the patient herself. By defending the patient's interests, the adopters and adapters of the Wertheim technique could claim that, whatever the cost, they were simply trying to save a greater number in the long run. Even the 'inoperable' could be given a more dignified, less painful death. Without the removal of tissues infected by malignancy, many women would suffer terribly, as the 'great agony' caused by the spread of the disease led to an end characterised by headache, nausea and vomiting. The cruelty, according to supporters of

---

[89] Contribution of Murdoch Cameron to 'Discussions on the Indications for Hysterectomy', 1084.
[90] Berkeley and Bonney, 'Results of the Radical Operation', 145–8.

the radical solution to cancer of the cervix, was actually not to operate in this way. As Berkeley made clear, their procedure freed the patient from the 'foul discharge' of the disease, and, in the majority of cases, the end was more 'peaceful'. 'In some of our own cases', he noted with pride, we 'have had letters from relatives particularly mentioning the absence of pain and distress right up to the end'.[91] Malignant disease of the cervix was horrendous enough for the patient without prolonging her agony by refusing to carry out a more dangerous, difficult procedure for fear of denting one's statistics. For Berkeley, no one 'worthy of the name of surgeon'[92] should be unwilling to help afflicted women.

Female surgeons were similarly inclined to assist their own sex through the performance of radical procedures such as Wertheim's for malignant disease. From early defences of abdominal methods by Boyd and Scharlieb in 1904, to the published statistics of Garrett Anderson and Platt and Vaughan-Sawyer's 'meticulously careful' and 'particularly successful' adoption of Wertheim's at the RFH, British women turned again and again to radical surgery to cure their patients.[93] The 1910s were supposed to have seen a turn away from invasive procedures for cancer, and yet 1918 was the first year where the NHW distinguished Wertheim's from abdominal hysterectomy, and 25 of them were performed.[94] There were 44 patients in the hospital that year for cancer of the cervix; 14 of them were 'unrelieved', so nearly every 'operable' patient underwent a Wertheim. The South London Hospital for Women, which only opened its permanent in-patient department in 1916, went from carrying out 2 Wertheim operations that year from the 5 cervical cancer cases it took in, to 6 in 1917 and 1918, from 13 and 14 patients respectively. By contrast, the SLHW surgeons only performed one vaginal hysterectomy each year between 1917 and 1918.[95] None of the patients undergoing the Wertheim procedure died at either hospital during these years. Although, as we have seen, Wertheim first introduced his method formally to Britain in 1905, British female surgeons at the NHW and the RFH had keenly embraced the abdominal route since the beginning of the century and they continued to take the riskier, more difficult option when Wertheim's procedure began to dominate their surgical treatment of cancer of the cervix.

---

[91] Berkeley, 'Wertheim's Panhysterectomy', 152.   [92] Ibid.
[93] 'Obituary: Ethel Vaughan-Sawyer, MD', 504.
[94] *Forty-Seventh (1918) Annual Report of the Elizabeth Garrett Anderson Hospital* (London: The Women's Printing Society, 1919), p. 21.
[95] Statistics taken from *Fourth, Fifth and Sixth Annual Reports of the South London Hospital for Women and Children* (London: Printed by The Women's Printing Society, 1917–1919).

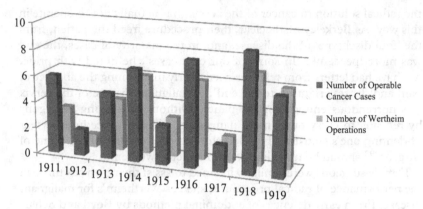

Figure 3.16 Number of Operable Cancer Cases and Wertheim Procedures by Vaughan-Sawyer: RFH, 1911–1919.[96]

At the RFH, Vaughan-Sawyer began carrying out Wertheim's operation at the end of 1910, after having performed abdominal hysterectomies for cancer of the cervix since at least 1904.[97] Forty-five-year-old Nellie Brown, a widowed housekeeper, was the first patient actively noted as undergoing a 'Wertheim'.[98] Over the nine years covered by the extant patient records, Vaughan-Sawyer went from performing Wertheim's on 50 per cent of her operable cancer patients between 1911 and 1912, to 80 per cent in 1913 and 85.7 per cent in 1914. From this point, as Figure 3.16 reveals, Vaughan-Sawyer carried out the procedure on every patient in the years 1915, 1917 and 1919. Overall, between 1911 and 1919, an average of 79.8 per cent of Vaughan-Sawyer's patients with operable cancer of the cervix underwent a Wertheim or a modified form of the operation based on their individual condition. In the last five years of extant notes, this average rose to 90.6 per cent. During the 1910s, therefore, Vaughan-Sawyer, along with her colleagues at the NHW and the SLHW, was not simply performing these 'heroic' operations. They had actually become the procedure of choice for almost all patients with varying stages of cancer of the cervix. In similar fashion to Wertheim himself, as well as Bonney and Berkeley, Vaughan-Sawyer wanted

---

[96] Two of the 1913 cases are interesting: one, Emma Knight (EVS: 1913; Part I), underwent a Wertheim for cancer of the fundus uteri and the other, Hagar Walker (EVS: 1913; Part II), underwent a hysterectomy two years previously (see: EVS: 1911; Part I).

[97] It is very likely that, given Mary Scharlieb's promotion of the abdominal route publicly and at the NHW, they had both been carrying out this procedure since they were employed by the RFH.

[98] EVS (1911; Part I).

her patients to be given a chance of survival. When considering what treatment to give 66-year-old factory worker Emma Knight in 1913, Vaughan-Sawyer strongly recommended Wertheim's because it would mean that her condition was much less likely to recur. Mrs Knight would be given a 'chance' through the more radical operation. In spite of bronchitis and emphysema, conditions which might prevent successful anaesthetisation or even recovery from induction, Vaughan-Sawyer decided to wait 25 days before operating, to allow her patient to regain her health. The pleasure in the success of the patient's recovery was evident in her notes, where remarks about Mrs Knight's 'splendid pelvis' post-operation and the rare confidence in the 'cure' added to the result of the case, showed how the risk taken was replaced by relief in the outcome.[99] As this was Emma Knight's only recorded RFH stay, then it was possible that she was indeed cured by the decision to operate in a more invasive – and, because of her age and condition, doubly risky – manner.

This is not to deny that Vaughan-Sawyer's propensity to gamble always paid off. While Emma Knight benefitted from the more extensive surgery, others did not. Elizabeth Tranter, a 59-year-old widow from Hoxton, also suffered from bronchitis and was a similar age and condition to Emma Knight.[100] Mrs Tranter's health required a longer rest and treatment period, and it was five weeks before she became a more suitable subject for operation. As a very stout, but healthy-looking woman, she was a less appropriate type for a Wertheim than the 'wiry' Emma Knight. A very fat abdomen, indeed, was enough to put off some surgeons from operating in this manner. In choosing cases, Berkeley reminded his colleagues, the very fat, or those who suffered from cardiac, pulmonary or renal diseases were 'very bad subjects' and 'should be left alone', although he did not agree with leaving those over 60 simply because of their age.[101] Other gynaecologists, such as Hastings Tweedy, felt that '[e]xtreme fatness' was a 'hindrance', but should not be viewed as an 'absolute contra-indication' when considering Wertheim's.[102] Vaughan-Sawyer was evidently of the same mind when she made the decision to operate on Elizabeth Tranter. Although warned by her physician colleague Arthur Phear, with whom she consulted over Mrs Tranter's respiratory state, that her patient was not a good subject for operation because of her bronchitis, Vaughan-Sawyer wavered. Initially, she cancelled the procedure, fearing that, as well as the patient's poor physical condition, the growth had possibly

[99] Emma Knight (EVS: 1913; Part I).   [100] Elizabeth Tranter (EVS: 1913; Part I).
[101] Berkeley, 'Wertheim's Panhysterectomy', 166.
[102] E. Hastings Tweedy, 'Method of Radical Extirpation of the Cancerous Uterus Based on a Series of 49 Cases', *JOGBE*, 19.4 (April 1911), 401–9; 406.

extended too far and a recurrence would result. The likely side-effect of a permanent vesical fistula after operation was also feared, condemning the patient to a miserable future, even if the cancer was removed. However, a further delay meant that Vaughan-Sawyer had time to change her mind. A week later, Elizabeth Tranter's respiratory problems were better, and her flesh was firmer and so the procedure went ahead, successfully. There was a double triumph when Mrs Tranter was opened up. The disease had not spread as much as feared and, throughout, the patient remained in an excellent condition. However, four days after the procedure, Elizabeth Tranter died very suddenly from heart failure. This was another side-effect of Wertheim's, due to the length and seriousness of the operation, which exercised detractors because it caused the largest post-operative mortality.[103] Unlike Emma Knight's case, this was one where risks taken did not improve the final outcome.

Yet there was one more thing besides the improvements in Mrs Tranter's medical condition which compelled Vaughan-Sawyer to operate: Elizabeth Tranter had been 'very anxious' to have the procedure. In the light of contemporary medical and lay concerns about women's unwillingness to be operated upon, Mrs Tranter's situation revealed a very different picture of those who had been diagnosed with cancer. As we have already seen, there were refusals to undergo surgery in the period between 1904 and 1919, but the numbers were extremely small in comparison with those who were willing to trust their surgeon's capabilities and judgement. Indeed, as Figure 3.15 showed, only three of Vaughan-Sawyer's patients in the first two decades of the twentieth century refused an operation for cancer. This was just 1.7 per cent of the total number seen and diagnosed with malignant disease. If women were condemned as reluctant to consult in time, then it is hard to see, in this instance, how they could be castigated for not trying to help themselves, even if the outcome might be uncertain when difficult and dangerous surgery was the only answer. As noted in the previous chapter, and as feared by specialists, too often general practitioners were not examining their female patients when they came to them with suspicious symptoms indicating the possibility of malignancy. This broke the link in the referral chain between patient, doctor and gynaecologist, leading to many skipping the middle option and coming straight to the hospital when attempts to seek medical help had failed to produce any answers or effective treatment. Vaughan-Sawyer, in particular, was very keen to encourage her patients to keep her directly informed about their progress. This continuing care extended both to those diagnosed with cancer and those who had been

[103] See Berkeley, 'Wertheim's Panhysterectomy', 159.

warned about the possibility of malignant disease. Berkeley lamented how impossible it was to trace hospital patients in Britain in comparison to the Continent where authorities, such as the police, kept more accurate records.[104] The RFH female surgeons, however, encouraged letter-writing as well as attendance at the hospital's Out-Patients in order to follow their cases. Minnie Fuller's notes did not end with her surgical treatment for chorio-epithelioma, which developed after the miscarriage of a vesicular mole. She was to write to Vaughan-Sawyer fortnightly and to see her doctor very frequently. Unfortunately, Mrs Fuller's letters ceased after a couple of months, when a local reoccurrence, coupled with signs of a cerebral embolus, killed her.[105] Fifty-three-year-old Elizabeth Cuthbert was diagnosed with a malignant ovarian cyst and carcinoma of the rectum in 1910. While the tumour was removed, along with her ovary, the rectal cancer was discovered after the procedure, and was not operated upon at the RFH. After her death, local Norfolk practitioner, Dr Butterworth, wrote to Vaughan-Sawyer, in a letter dated 4 September 1910:

At first she improved considerably in her general condition. She had much less loss although in spite of douching it remained horribly offensive. The growth in the rectum made slower progress than did the ovarian one. Improved so far as to come down stairs and even walk into garden, but complained of feeling heaviness in hypogastrium. Pain relieved by aspirin for some weeks. By middle of July, condition had become much worse; could hardly get out of bed. Large mass of growth in left inguinal region, which felt almost as large as foetal head. At this time she had transient oedema of various limbs; right hand first part to become swollen; tongue remained clean, but had lost all appetite. Abdomen became very distended at about the time and there was some free fluid. Liver enlarged and no doubt full of secondary growths. Pain was most troublesome symptom and was only relieved by large doses of opium. Constipation began to be troublesome at end of July. At beginning of August she was very weak and growth in abdomen felt enormous; died Aug 17th.[106]

This correspondence allowed a rare insight into the condition of a patient with malignant disease for whom only some surgical treatment could be carried out, due to the spread of the condition. Mrs Cuthbert's slow, painful death, after a brief period of respite, as well as the meticulous detailing of her decline by a general practitioner, revealed the desperation many medical professionals felt when faced with inoperable cancer. The prolonging of a patient's life through surgery was a hotly debated topic, but Dr Butterworth's letter, prompted by Vaughan-Sawyer's follow-up system, gave a chance to witness vicariously the last few months of a terminal case.

[104] Berkeley, 'Wertheim's Panhysterectomy', 150.
[105] Minnie Fuller (EVS: 1909; Part I).   [106] Elizabeth Cuthbert (EVS: 1910; Part I).

Additionally, instructing future possible sufferers to return at regular intervals was the most innovative form of patient monitoring in the early twentieth century. Vaughan-Sawyer warned a number of her cases that they had a very strong chance of developing cancer and encouraged vigilance. Ada Humphreys, for example, was tested for malignancy because of two years' constant bloody discharge, combined with an evident family history of cancer. Mrs Humphreys had been attending Vaughan-Sawyer's Out-Patients since the beginning of 1909, and had been treated medically for prolapse and cervicitis, with pessaries and tonics. A year later, Vaughan-Sawyer feared malignancy and a wedge from her cervix was removed for pathological analysis, which returned with negative results. Yet the symptoms worsened, and Mrs Humphreys was admitted. Although her condition was not cancerous, Vaughan-Sawyer concluded that it was 'favourable soil for the growth of malignant cells' and acted accordingly by performing a panhysterectomy, as a preventative measure.[107] After seven children, two miscarriages, many years of pain and suffering and the possibility of developing cancer, Mrs Humphreys was happy for the operation to go ahead.

Alice Briggs was in a similar situation to Ada Humphreys, having suffered from intermenstrual loss for a few years. Additionally, as curettings looked suspicious under the microscope. Vaughan-Sawyer asked her to come up to the hospital frequently for 'careful watching'.[108] Mrs Briggs returned to be observed, so that when her condition worsened again, Vaughan-Sawyer admitted her and performed a panhysterectomy. Similarly, Amy Cook was admitted initially for endometritis, after suffering from continual loss for the past nine months since the birth of a child in June 1910. While pathological examinations did not reveal cancerous cells, further sections were cut to make sure; the latter 'inclining' towards the future development of malignancy. Unsurprisingly, Vaughan-Sawyer wished the patient 'to be watched'.[109] Mrs Cook diligently attended Out-Patients for observation and she deteriorated again in the late summer of 1911, she was admitted for panhysterectomy. While there were no malignancies found in the cases of Ada Humphreys, Alice Briggs and Amy Cook, the suspicious pathological findings allowed Vaughan-Sawyer to act preventively.[110] None of these patients were seen again. Neither were Annie Besnay, Elizabeth White nor Martha Webb, all of whom were warned to come to Out-Patients regularly or to seek medical advice

[107] Ada Humphreys (EVS: 1910; Part II).
[108] Alice Briggs (EVS: 1910; Part II) and (EVS: 1911; Part II).
[109] Amy Cook (EVS: 1911; Part I) and (EVS: 1911; Part II).
[110] On prevention later in the twentieth century, see David Cantor, 'Cancer Control and Prevention in the Twentieth Century', BHM, 81.1 (Spring 2007), 1–38.

the instant they experienced symptoms similar to those which brought them to the RFH in the first place. Although discussing a later period, John Pickstone has described interwar preventive measures as essentially catching the disease early and providing treatment in the hope of avoiding death.[111] At the RFH, however, Vaughan-Sawyer was attempting in the 1910s to prevent cancer before the disease had a chance to manifest itself in some of her patients. This could be seen as a drastic and unnecessary measure in women of active childbearing age, which resembled the 'homicidal vivisections' of Wertheim's procedure. Vaughan-Sawyer, however, was evidently as keen to prevent malignant disease by acting pre-emptively, as she was to 'cure' her patients through radical surgery.

This is not to deny, however, that some cases seen by Scharlieb and Vaughan-Sawyer ignored professional advice. The fact that there were any refusals in life-threatening situations to undergo surgical procedures which might allow the patient to live a little longer or to exist painlessly showed that not all could bring themselves to seek treatment surgically, whatever the cost. As we saw in the previous chapter, this could be due to fear of an anaesthetic, the operation itself, or lack of family support for such a step. Some also discharged themselves because there was no hope or the chances of success were slim. Scharlieb and Vaughan-Sawyer appear to have been honest with their patients about the possibility of a 'cure'. Mary A. Newland, whose husband refused to allow surgery for cancer, was 'not pressed' after the decline of treatment, as Scharlieb felt it was doubtful whether the growth was really operable and the probability of a cure was not great.[112] While the surgeon would take the risk, the patient would not, and Scharlieb respected her wishes. In 1910, Mary A. Maynard was told clearly that her case was inoperable and that the growth had better be left, unless it troubled her, as it could not all be safely removed.[113] By contrast, Ruth Barden's initial refusal to allow a doctor to examine her vaginally and her two-month delay before she consulted female advice at the Bermondsey Medical Mission ensured that, when the latter swiftly dispatched her to the RFH for operative treatment, her cancer of the cervix had spread extensively and become quite inoperable. Mrs Barden discharged herself the day after admission when informed that nothing could be done for her.[114] Unlike those patients described in the previous paragraph, Mary Rose did not follow medical advice. After a severe attack of abdominal pain in August 1908, Mrs Rose went to Clapham Maternity Hospital, where she was

[111] Pickstone, 'Contested Cumulations', 174.
[112] Mary A. Newland (MS: 1908; Part II).   [113] Mary A. Maynard (EVS: 1910; Part I).
[114] Ruth Barden (MS: 1908; Part I).

encouraged to attend the RFH's Gynaecological Out-Patients. There, she was diagnosed with suspected fibroids, but was told to keep attend-ing this clinic so an eye could be kept on her condition. She failed to do so. When Mrs Rose finally returned to Out-Patients in April 1909, her situation was severe enough for admission. She was discovered to have ovarian cancer, which had spread to her pelvis, described as 'choked with growth', and liver.[115] Others were apparently luckier. Thirty-year-old Emily King consulted Vaughan-Sawyer in the nick of time for what turned out to be an epithelioma of the vulva. It had been causing her pain since 1917, forced her to give up her job as a machinist, and was now in an advanced state. Vaughan-Sawyer recommended immediate operative interference because in a few months the growth would have spread to her urethra and femoral sheath and 'all cure would be hopeless'.[116] Mrs King, unsurprisingly, consented to the procedure. However, during the surgery, Vaughan-Sawyer remarked upon the florid nature of the urethra and feared recurrence. She was, unfortunately, proved correct, when Emily King returned to have a new nodule removed from precisely this area in the summer of 1918. Given that she was then sent to the Radium Institute, and what that meant effectively, it could be presumed that Mrs King's late consultation rendered her case eventually inoperable. It was only when her condition became intolerable, not even allowing her to sit down comfortably, that Emily King sought advice. By then, it was too late and despite surgery, treatment became solely palliative.

In similar fashion to Emily King, those condemned as 'inoperable' in the second decade of the twentieth century were often recommended alternatives to surgery as a last resort or momentary respite before death. Rarely, as already noted, were therapeutic measures such as X-ray or radium treatment given for the 'curable' patient in the RFH's Gynaecological Department. Löwy has remarked that while surgery for malignant disease was still dangerous, therapeutic measures offered more attractive options, which were less risky and, even though dogged by some side-effects such as potential infection of the cancerous lesion by pathogenic bacteria, the advantages outweighed those of radical operations.[117] However, it is fruitful, in the final section of this chapter, to explore how women experienced such treatment, especially when being sent to places such as the Radium Institute in these experimental years meant that death was simply being postponed. As reported by the director, A.E. Hayward Pinch, many of the patients at the Institute

---

[115] Mary Rose (EVS: 1909; Part I).
[116] Emily King (EVS: 1918; Part I) and (EVS: 1918; Part II).
[117] Löwy, *A Woman's Disease*, p. 57.

had 'exhausted all the known resources of medicine and surgery, their condition being almost helpless'.[118] It is telling that, in the first year of work recorded at the Institute, 88 patients abandoned their treatment; Pinch explained that this was due to the inconvenience or the expense of travelling to London.[119] While this decreased over the next two years, from 50 to 11,[120] it is worth examining why a supposedly less invasive, more 'humane' treatment put off some of those it was intended to help, to the extent that they stopped their attendance at hospital or at the Radium Institute. For some, indeed, early radiotherapies were little different to quack cures. In her history of this alternative approach to treatment, Murphy places radiotherapy before the Great War 'on the fringes of quackery and orthodoxy',[121] and, unlike surgery, suspicion of this approach was common both to patients and practitioners. Frederick Treves described the use of the X-ray in surgery as a sorry history of hopes dashed.[122] Two years later, indeed, E.F. Bashford, the General Superintendent of Research and Director of the Laboratory of the Imperial Cancer Research Fund, placed 'Radio-activity' alongside 'Nonsense' and 'Faith-healing' in the 'Quack's Armamentary'.[123] Little had changed just before the war, when Cuthbert Lockyer's assertion that radiology should be the future for the gynaecologist was met with deafening silence.[124] Yet, if the medical profession itself was sceptical, how did the patient react to the proposition that they undergo a course of radiotherapy to prolong their lives?

The earliest patient to receive X-ray treatment in the Gynaecological Department was 65-year-old Mary A. Thompson, who became a surgical Consultation Case after being diagnosed with carcinoma of the vagina, which had spread to the wall of the rectum. An operation was not advised in this case, although it could have been 'just' anatomically possible. Vaughan-Sawyer was keen to operate, but, upon consultation with colleagues Scharlieb, Florence Willey and Thomas Legg, and in consideration of the patient's age and poor general condition, X-ray treatment

---

[118] A.E. Hayward Pinch, 'A Report of the Work Carried out at The Radium Institute From August 14th, 1911, to December 31st, 1912', *BMJ*, 1.2717 (25 January 1913), 149–63; 149.

[119] Pinch, 'A Report of the Work', 150.

[120] See Pinch, 'A Report of the Work Carried Out at the Radium Institute, London, in 1913', *BMJ*, 1.2786 (23 May 1914), 1107–11; 1107; and 'A Report of the Work . . . in 1914', 367.

[121] Murphy, 'A History of Radiotherapy', p. 10.

[122] Frederick Treves, 'A Lecture on Radium in Surgery. Delivered at the London Hospital, January 26th, 1909', *BMJ*, 1.2510 (6 February 1909), 317–19; 317.

[123] Bashford, 'Cancer, Credulity, and Quackery', 1225; 1228.

[124] Lockyer, 'The Future of Radiology'.

was 'tried' instead in order to keep the growth down. X-ray applications improved Mrs Thompson's general condition markedly, the pain was a good deal less and the discharge also decreased. Her condition remained inoperable, however.[125] Annie Wheeler, whose womb had been removed for malignancy earlier in the year, came back in November 1912. Miss Wheeler had been suffering from pain in the right groin since August and a large mass of growth on the right side of her pelvis was discovered. She had been treated by a number of different procedures, most of which Bashford and others would have described as quackery, such as radiant heat baths, salt baths, vapour baths, liniments, and, most recently, massage. Despite her exceedingly good condition after the first operation and an entirely uneventful recovery, it was evident a few months later that the cancer had returned and spread to the bladder. After only a month, Miss Wheeler had what she labelled a nervous breakdown, which was followed by pain in her thigh and groin, lasting more or less ever since. When she was readmitted, her condition was considered quite inoperable and X-rays were utilised 'in order to less the pain [sic], and if possible retard the growth'. Despite this proposition, the growth was spreading rapidly, and when she was discharged the pain was better than it was on admission, but actually increased by movement.[126] In these two early cases, X-rays reduced the pain experienced by both women, but they were unable to halt or shrink the tumours to render them operable. Instead, the treatment was simply palliative. Neither woman was seen at the RFH again.

Radium treatment was offered to inoperable patients from 1914, when all other options had failed. The popular press lauded radium as a miracle cure,[127] but none occurred in the gynaecological beds of the RFH. Hagar Walker, a patient since 1906, had undergone a modified Wertheim for carcinoma of the cervix at the end of 1913, but carcinomatous nodules had been discovered in February 1914 and the left sacro-uterine ligament and anterior rectal wall were also found to be infiltrated with growth. After X-ray treatment, which the patient found very painful and weakening, a radium application was tried with a vaginal emanation tube. The pain of this experience was considerable, but it afforded temporary relief and a good night's sleep. Mrs Walker was to come up again for further radium treatment if possible. Despite her frequent attendance at the RFH over the years, she was not seen again.[128] Melia Howlett, who had extensive carcinoma of the rectum, was treated with radium for a year and

---

[125] Mary A. Thompson (EVS: 1909; Part I).   [126] Annie Wheeler (EVS: 1912; Part II).
[127] See Murphy, chapter 8: Conclusions, 'A History of Radiotherapy', p. 20.
[128] Hagar Walker (EVS: 1914; Part I).

three-quarters. In contradistinction to usual procedures, whereby hospitals referred their patients to the Radium Institute, Dr Lynham of the Institute had sent Mrs Howlett to Vaughan-Sawyer. Initially, the patient's doctor had discovered a tumour and advised radium applications to prepare the growth for an operation. Mrs Howlett had consequently been undergoing radium treatment once a month for five days, and for six hours of each day. Then a radium tube was inserted into the rectum. There was very little improvement in her condition and haemorrhage continued. Furthermore, Mrs Howlett had felt much worse in herself, with pain down her right thigh and faintness; a vesico-vaginal fistula had developed and discharge now seeped through both rectum and vagina. Vaughan-Sawyer performed a colotomy upon Mrs Howlett, who began to feel 'very well' because of the surgery. While the growth was still very large and fungating, the switch from radium treatment to surgical procedure made Mrs Howlett far more comfortable than she had felt in a long while.[129] While surgery could not cure her, neither could radium, but the former relieved her situation, whereas the latter exacerbated her pain and suffering. Although this was only a single instance, it is important to note that there was not a one-way trajectory between the Radium Institute and the hospitals. Where one could no longer assist the patient, the other could take over. Radium was not the miracle cure for all, and, where it failed, surgery, as in the case of Melia Howlett, could relieve in ways it could not.

Some experienced pain relief from X-ray applications or radium treatment, but found that it did not work in the long run. Annie Ansell, who attended in 1915 for a Bartholini's cyst, was later discovered to have an epithelioma in her groin. X-ray treatment was tried, but it simply did not 'arrest the course of the disease'; her pain was only relieved by the withdrawal of fluid from the growth. Vaughan-Sawyer recommended that X-rays were stopped and the patient sent to a home or an infirmary, evidently to die.[130] Others were simply too ill to keep going with the processes. Thirty-four-year-old Harriet Croydon, who had a recurrence of malignant disease in the pelvis, had undergone some electrical treatment after her Wertheim's operation in the summer of 1914 and had further X-ray applications in the RFH at the beginning of 1915. These reduced her pain considerably, but, after leaving the hospital and returning every week for repeat procedures, Mrs Croydon was unable to continue to attend the RFH because of the fatigue she experienced travelling from her home in North London.[131] The practicalities of suffering from

[129] Melia Howlett (EVS: 1914; Part I).   [130] Annie Ansell (EVS: 1915; Part I).
[131] Harriet Croydon (EVS: 1914; Part II); (EVS: 1915; Part I).

incurable malignant disease often overtook any desire to continue the hassle of treatment which could only ever prove palliative. In similar fashion to Melia Howlett, it was also recommended by the Radium Institute that Kate Coles' treatment for carcinoma of the fundus be carried out in hospital. Her notes described this procedure in detail: it was neither quick nor without unfortunate side-effects. A radium tube was inserted into the cavity of the uterus and left for 24 hours; this resulted in little pain, but a good deal of bleeding. On 24 June 1915, a second application was made, which caused Mrs Coles some burning pain and an ache in the lower part of the back and abdomen. Two days later, after the tube had been removed, there was more comfort.[132] Neither Harriet Croydon nor Kate Coles attended the hospital again. In May 1914, Elizabeth Fowles did not even have the option of radium applications for a recurrence after Wertheim's procedure a few months before. While such a course was advised, there was no radium obtainable. Neither the Radium Institute nor the Middlesex Hospital could assist the RFH in finding an emanation tube for this patient. Mrs Fowles left the hospital, with only heroin to help her pain and the promise that 'if radium can be obtained she will be treated.' Meanwhile, if she wished it, arrangements would be made to find her a place in a home for the dying. Mrs Fowles' record ended here, and presumably the only option was the last.[133] It was noticeable that after 1915, the suggestion that radium be used in palliative care disappeared and did not return until the summer of 1918. Radiotherapy was not the mode of treatment most recommended by the RFH surgeons for gynaecological cancer patients unless the cases were terminal because surgery was always the first resort, and, even in cases eventually treated with radium, surgery was often attempted first and as much of the growth removed as possible. It is important to remember that the Great War actively prevented radium supplies from being obtained for dying patients.[134] The 1910s might have seen an interest in the properties of radiotherapy, but professional disinterest in what some labelled quack remedies, coupled with the expense and scarcity of radium meant that many, like Elizabeth Fowles, had to forgo this new treatment in favour of powerful painkillers to make the end of life bearable.

---

[132] Kate Coles (EVS: 1915; Part I); (EVS: 1915; Part II).

[133] Elizabeth Fowles (EVS: 1914; Part II). Her previous records are under the name Eliza Fowles (EVS: 1914; Part I).

[134] See Murphy, 'A History of Radiotherapy', chapter 3, about the scarcity of radium supplies before the war and Part II, chapter IV, for the lack of development of radiation treatment at this time.

Conclusion

By exploring in detail the ways in which female surgeons treated malignant disease in the first two decades of the twentieth century, it is possible
to draw the following conclusions. Firstly, and most fundamentally, that,
in spite of previous claims to the contrary, these women specialists, in
the vast majority of cases, resorted to surgery when dealing with cancer.
While other treatments were considered, they were only suggested when
the patient's condition was inoperable. Unlike some of their colleagues,
women surgeons did not scoff at quackeries, but neither did they change
the way they operated when newer possibilities emerged, thanks to the
development of radiotherapy. This form of treatment was not embraced
wholeheartedly by patients either, who suffered the side-effects of applications and even discontinued them. Secondly, women surgeons were
not afraid to try long, hard and difficult surgical procedures in order to
give their patients the best chance of survival, however limited that might
be in reality. As Wertheim had noted the time of the operation could be
reduced considerably with practise. This bypassed the problems which
patients who were designated as unsuitable for surgery might encounter;
which, in turn, allowed more to undergo surgery. By October 1919,
Vaughan-Sawyer took just over an hour to perform a Wertheim, whereas
seven years previously the same operation took twice this time.[135] Neither were female surgeons afraid to modify and rework existing methods.
This satisfied both their own curiosity about the best means to tackle
malignant disease and meant that they were able to tailor their surgery
to each patient, in similar fashion to Aldrich-Blake's development of rectal procedures. Thirdly, a belief in the importance of the pathological
confirmation of disease and a desire to keep track of patients who had
suffered from cancer, as well as those who were likely candidates for
malignancy, showed that surgery had to be supported for the women
surgeons discussed here with scientific confirmation and careful observation. Finally, working-class female patients were attacked as the worst
culprits when it came to taking care of their health. When diagnosed,
however, the majority were more than willing to take risks if an invasive,
potentially life-threatening operation could give them a little longer. For
many patients, early twentieth-century surgery was an 'option worth trying', as Wilde has discussed.[136] Some, such as Mary Keyworth, who was
told by Vaughan-Sawyer in 1910 that her carcinoma of the cervix was

---

[135] See the case of Laura Patchin (EVS: 1919; Part II). Compare this with Ann Brown
(EVS: 1912; Part II).
[136] Wilde, 'Truth, Trust', 327.

operable if she wanted to 'take the risk', decided 'after careful consideration' that they did not want surgery.[137] This did not mean, as this chapter
has revealed, that women surgeons themselves were not prepared to do
everything they could to relieve their patients surgically. For them, the
chance was always worth taking even if there was only a slight possibility
that a life could be saved.

[137]   Mary Keyworth (EVS: 1910; Part I).

4 Inside the Theatre of War

The final two chapters of this book will focus upon the Great War and assess the opportunities it provided for the woman surgeon, both on the home front and, firstly, as near to the various battlefields as women were permitted. It is vital to recognise from the outset that women were aware of the need to take advantage of what warfare could offer them as well as their desire to be as useful as possible to the war effort. No one expected the situation to last beyond the span of the fighting and this was acknowledged at the time.[1] In 1917, the *Girl's Own Paper* warned youthful aspirants to a surgical career not to be 'dazzled by the glamour' of women's co-operation with the allied armies: 'these are temporary conditions, and when peace reigns once more it will not be from the military hospitals that the first demands upon them will be made'.[2] When considering female participation in wartime surgical activities, the excitement of the performance must be measured against the knowledge of its temporality. Additionally, however, the embracing of this moment as an opportunity to enhance wider skills and techniques, the valuable experience gained, must also be acknowledged. The Great War might have provided a chance of a lifetime for women surgeons, but what dominated the thoughts of those involved was that they needed to obtain useful work, rather than worry about its inevitable brevity.

In a recent study of British military medicine between 1914 and 1918, Mark Harrison laments the 'fragmented' nature of medical history focused on this period. While specific, detailed accounts increase in

---

[1] Women's history of this period is full of debate about whether the war advanced or retarded women's prospects in general. For only one recent interpretation, which gives a succinct account of the debate, see David Monger, 'Nothing Special? Propaganda and Women's Roles in Late First World War Britain', *Women's History Review*, 23.4 (2014), 518–42.

[2] A Woman of the World, 'The Queen and Women's Work', *Girl's Own Paper and Woman's Magazine*, 38.9 (March 1917), 457–60; 458, *South London Hospital for Women Press Cuttings 1912–1917*, London Metropolitan Archives, H24/SLW/Y6/1. Future references will be abbreviated to *SLHWPC*.

numbers, works of synthesis are few, ensuring that 'a rounded view of what medicine meant to contemporaries' is missing.[3] Harrison also notes the absence of the mundane from analyses of wartime medicine. Shell-shock or venereal disease has proved more fascinating than the everyday discomforts of trench foot, for example.[4] The heroic actions of a single surgeon in saving the life of a dying patient is far more exciting than the prosaic reality of the team effort required to keep him alive before, during and after the operation itself. In these two chapters, I want to provide a synthesis of women's surgical participation in the Great War in order to examine what performing surgery on soldiers meant to a number of women surgeons and, by extension, their patients. Although I will explore the undoubted thrill experienced by women charting new surgical terri-tories, I agree with Harrison that the quotidian requires attention too.[5] More often than not, the momentary excitement stifled the exhaustion, momentarily. Near the battlefield, the stoic feats of 24-hour operating were few in comparison with the many days of lull, of the treatment of civilians and routine procedures on hernias and appendixes. The watch-ing and waiting alternated with the constant need to generate electricity for vital X-ray equipment, let alone light for the operating theatre. At home, unprecedented new posts in general hospitals increased exponen-tially between 1914 and 1918 for women as more medical men left for the front, but both here and in women-run institutions day-to-day survival necessitated financial support, harder to come by in wartime. Indeed, the division between work at home and at the front does not hold in some instances. Louisa Aldrich-Blake and Agnes Savill, for example, worked both at Royaumont in France and at the RFH and the NHW respec-tively during the war. In considering a variety of wartime case stud-ies, but without losing focus on the vicissitudes of experience, a more

---

[3] Mark Harrison, *The Medical War* (Oxford: Oxford University Press, 2010), p. 13. Ana Carden-Coyne's *The Politics of Wounds* (Oxford: Oxford University Press, 2014) goes a long way to redress the balance, exploring the relationship between doctors and patients. She does not, however, discuss at any length women surgeons.
   This contrasts with Monger's claim that, because of division between historians, it is impossible to discuss 'women's experience' of the Great War.

[4] Harrison, *The Medical War*.

[5] Women's medical work in the Great War has been well explored, but it tends to focus on particular hospitals or organisations. The exception is Leah Leneman's 'Medical Women at War, 1914–1918', *MH*, 38.2 (April 1994), 160–77, which offers a wider perspective. Surgery and suffrage as carried out by Garrett Anderson and Murray has more recently been covered by Geddes in 'Deeds *and* Words', so will not be focused upon here. Eileen Crofton's excellent book about Royaumont is the closest study of all aspects of quotidian life at a hospital run by women: *The Women of Royaumont* (East Linton: Tuckwell Press, 1996).
   For the names and service dates of all personnel involved with the SWH, see the fantastic online resource run by Sue Light at www.scarletfinders.co.uk.

complex picture of the activities of the woman surgeon between 1914 and 1918 can be obtained.

'Surgery Just as Men Do'

Some women surgeons offered assistance to the military as soon as war broke out, but, turned down again and again, their enterprise was largely self-initiated and their services given to their country's allies.[6] The two most prominent organisations established were the Women's Hospital Corps, set up by Flora Murray and Louisa Garrett Anderson in 1914 and backed by the Women's Social and Political Union, and the Scottish Women's Hospitals (SWH), founded by Elsie Inglis, which came into existence a year later with support from the National Union of Women's Suffrage Societies.[7] Garrett Anderson and Inglis had surgical backgrounds, but, as women, were considered unsuitable for frontline service, whether alongside men or on their own. A gamut of reactions to women's proposals, summed up succinctly by Murray, included disapproval, curiosity, amusement and obstinate hostility.[8] Such responses to the female surgeon were, of course, not new, but, after proving themselves in their profession for half-a-century and gradually having gained the acceptance of their colleagues, rejection when their country needed qualified and experienced doctors most was hard to take.[9] Obstinacy

---

[6] The setting up of the women's hospitals has been told many times. For contemporary accounts, see: Barbara McLaren, *Women of the War* (London: Hodder and Stoughton, 1917), especially chapters I and V, and 'Skia' [Vera Collum], 'A Hospital in France', *Blackwood's Magazine*, 204.1237 (November 1918), 613–40.

[7] See Geddes, 'Deeds *and* Words', for the politics of the WHC. For other all-female or mixed teams who set off independently from Britain to assist the war effort, see Leneman, 'Medical Women'. For Inglis, see Lawrence, *Shadow of Swords* (London: Michael Joseph, 1971).

Not every member of the SWH was a suffragist. *Common Cause* noted that Dr Beatrice Russell, member of the Edinburgh Committee, was not part of their campaign for suffrage. See VII.347 (3 December 1915), 450, which claims that her testimony to the 'efficiency' of Royaumont 'is therefore of even greater value than opinions expressed by those who a priori would be expected to uphold the work'.

Russell was a founder member in 1899 of the George Square Nursing Home for Women (later The Hospice) in Edinburgh with Elsie Inglis. See Thomson, 'Women in Medicine', p. 61.

[8] Murray, *Women as Army Surgeons*, p. 126.

[9] Frustration at the obstinacy of the army extends to the historian of medicine. See Ian R. Whitehead, *Doctors in the Great War* (Barnsley: Pen and Sword Military, 2013), on the repeated missed opportunities for harnessing female doctors' expertise. For Steven D. Heys, the Western European ignorance of the Russian surgeon Vera Gedroits' work on the then unusually swift operative treatment of abdominal wounds in the Russo-Japanese War (1904–1905) was similarly inexplicable. See 'Abdominal wounds: Evolution of management and establishment of surgical treatments', in Thomas Scotland and Steven Heys, eds., *War Surgery 1914–1918* (Solihull: Helion and Company, 2013), pp. 178–211; pp. 187–8.

extended both ways, however, and women were undeterred. Garrett Anderson and Murray set up in Paris, impressed the relenting authorities enough to be offered a hospital at Wimereux, and then returned home in 1915 to take charge of what became the Endell Street Military Hospital, run entirely by women. The Scottish Women's Hospitals established units across Europe, treating allied soldiers in France, Serbia, Greece, Corsica, Romania and Russia. An advance casualty clearing station was also run by the Scottish Women at Villers-Cotterets, 40 miles away from Royaumont, until it was overrun by the Germans almost a year after its establishment, in the summer of 1918.[10] When they were presented with what Murray labelled 'an exceptional opportunity in the field of surgery', women surgeons grasped hungrily at the chance afforded them.[11]

In a letter written from Serbia in January 1917, Louise McIlroy, Chief Surgeon of the SWH Girton and Newnham Unit (GNU), lamented the possibility of being forced to share her position with a male Serbian colleague. 'It not only breaks with our trust with the public, who supply us with funds for women only', McIlroy fumed, 'but it takes away from us the one part of our work that has been doubted so much at the beginning, namely the capacity to do Surgery just as men do.'[12] Here, McIlroy illustrated the paradox of the woman surgeon in the Great War. The exclusiveness of the hospitals run only by women, set up initially because of opposition to their serving near the battlefield or with the army, was what made them unique and worthy of financial support. Simultaneously, however, in order to be successful, women needed to draw attention to the fact that they were performing surgery exactly as men did. That, in effect, there was no difference at all in their mode of operating. Ideally, the woman surgeon at the front had to be both female and male in her approach to avoid loss of public support and professional valuation. This tricky balancing act, one which female surgeons had, of course, been carrying out since their entry into the medical profession, was exacerbated by wartime conditions. As such, accounts of superhuman capabilities characterised depictions of surgery by women, which stressed the difficulty of procedures and feats of endurance. Any cracks were to be swiftly covered over. If war was the best school for surgeons, then women were being tested in uncharted surgical territories and could not be found wanting.

[10] For the setting up of Villers-Cotterets, see Crofton, *The Women of Royaumont*, pp. 133–47.

[11] Murray, *Women as Army Surgeons*, p. 170.

[12] Louise McIlroy to Miss May, 18 January 1917, Tin 42: Circulated Letters, 1917–1918, Scottish Women's Hospitals Collection, Glasgow City Archives, Mitchell Library, Glasgow. Future references to this archive will be abbreviated to SWHC.

What was so astounding about the private correspondence of women surgeons who served abroad between 1914 and 1918 was that they did not question their ability to carry out procedures with which they could not have been familiar. Inexperience, according to newly qualified Leila Henry, who became a junior surgeon at Royaumont, was simply not to be acknowledged. Although she had only graduated in 1916 and spent a year at the Sheffield Royal Infirmary, Henry expressed no doubt about her surgical skills, which were honed at an institution situated in a bustling city attacked by Zeppelin raids. Treatment of accidents, common to industrial centres, as well as the more recent German bombing of munitions' targets, gave Henry an insight into injuries caused by the explosions of modern warfare. Despite her youth and what would have been perceived as inexperience, Henry claimed confidently that: 'I felt equally competent to deal with war injuries, given an opportunity'. Initially rejected by the SWH's head office in Edinburgh, Henry retorted that 'youth had nothing to do with it; it was experience that counted!'[13] Although Ruth Verney only witnessed the very end of the war when she left for Salonika in autumn 1918, she was desperate to learn as much as possible, in addition to developing her clinical skills. In a letter to her family, she noted that, along with another young doctor, only a year her senior, 'we feel we must do some work no matter whether it has all been done before or not'.[14] Verney's youthfulness caused a French colleague to wonder if she had begun her studies in the cradle, but Verney did not mind.[15] When looking back upon wartime adventures in the late 1970s, she remembered with fondness her health, strength and unceasing happiness. Everything was 'frightfully interesting', even the treatment of an injured thumb in one of the villages.[16] Adaptation of existing expertise and strong self-belief were what gave women the confidence they could operate as well as men, even if the surroundings and procedures were foreign to them. What they did not know, they could learn as they worked, and they were more than eager to do so.

Isabel Emslie went one step further than Henry and Verney and, in addition to energetic youth and health, added risk to her wartime

---

[13] Leila M. Henry, *Reminiscences of Royaumont 1914–1919*, typed unpublished MS, WW1/WO/054, Liddle Collection, Brotherton Library, Leeds.
Henry was known both as Leila and Lydia, and will be referred to the former here, which is the name she liked to call herself according to Crofton, *The Women of Royaumont*, p. 270.

[14] Ruth Verney to her family, 31 October 1918, WW1/WO/127, LC.

[15] Ibid. Translation my own. All translations from French in this chapter are mine, unless acknowledged otherwise.

[16] Typescript of interview with Ruth Verney in September 1977, Tape 476, WW1/WO/127, LC.

experience. After working with the GNU under McIlroy for three years, in the summer of 1918 she took charge of her own unit in Ostrovo, Serbia. For Emslie, it was either 'lack of foresight' or 'recklessness' which allowed her to live from day to day, accomplishing tasks 'without seeing half the difficulties'.[17] When she stayed on in Serbia after the war ended, operating on civilian cases in Vranja, it was temerity which kept her going. As the only capable surgeon there, Emslie undertook major, specialist operations which would never have 'fallen to [her] lot' at home.[18] Little experience in plastic operations for burns, for example, did not matter. Emslie 'did [her] best and nature gracefully completed my efforts'.[19] The knowledge that war would not last indefinitely haunted the women throughout their time abroad. An awareness that, as Elizabeth Courtauld, surgeon at Royaumont, put it in letters of November and December 1918 that the 'congenial work' of these 'gorgeous times' would soon be over; the parting horrid and the breaking up of everything, though inevitable, distressing.[20] The determination to take advantage of the opportunities was evident; no one wanted to waste a moment. Neither were those who were intending not to utilise their surgical skills in the future as welcome as those were dedicated to the specialty. When Frances Ivens, the Chief Surgeon at Royaumont, sent a request in the early stages of the hospital's existence for a new member of staff, she was very clear about the person she wanted:

We need another good junior surgeon to take the place of Miss Ross in a month. I should like someone who is working for the US [*sic*] or FRCS, having had an H.S. post, if possible, but recently qualified. It is a waste to take on general practitioners who will not make use of the surgical techniques they acquire.[21]

While military surgery was unlikely to sustain most surgeons' careers, Ivens wanted to ensure that those volunteering were there for professional enhancement. Surgery carried out during wartime could only be beneficial to anyone serious about learning and progressing as surgeons when they returned home.

This was precisely how the few who left Royaumont under dark clouds reflected upon the institution's operations. Doris Stevenson, who went to the hospital as an orderly in May 1918, lasted three weeks at her post. Already experienced in nursing, having served six miles from the front since November 1916, Stevenson was horrified by conditions at

---

[17] Hutton, *Memories*, p. 161.   [18] Ibid., p. 177.   [19] Ibid., p. 178.

[20] Elizabeth Courtauld to Ruth, 14 November 1918 and 13 December 1918, WWI/WO/023, LC.

[21] Dr Ivens to Dr Inglis, 11 April 1915, Tin 12: Letters to and from Dr Ivens (CMO) and Miss Ramsay Smith (Secretary): 1914–1918, SWHC.

Royaumont. Among a long list of complaints about the standards of hygiene and chaotic organisation, Stevenson voiced her belief that '[t]his hospital appears to be a school for women doctors at the expense of the sisters and us organised, undisciplined orderlies of good will and intention'.[22] In a later letter, Stevenson claimed that the staff existed in a rarefied exalted state, which bore no resemblance to reality: 'the whole spirit of Royaumont is ludicrous to the few of its members who have seen something of the world, the spirit is positively Prussian in its puffed-upness'.[23] Frances Ivens' retort was blunt, addressing directly the accusation that the surgeons benefited at the expense of the sisters and orderlies: 'such a statement [was] merely malicious and devoid of fact'. She added that the doctors worked 'as hard if not harder than others, and both day and night'.[24] In gathering witnesses to testify against Stevenson's attack, Ivens included a letter from Agnes Anderson who stated, simply, that how the hospital was regarded by the doctors was no concern of the orderlies.[25] While this did not condone the accusations levelled against the surgical staff, neither did it deny them. If Royaumont resembled a school for the development of women's surgical skills, Anderson remained noticeably tight-lipped on the subject, while actively and vociferously defending other criticisms of the way in which the institution operated.

Another woman who left Royaumont dissatisfied with what she saw made pointed accusations about the surgery itself. In October 1915, Dr Margaret Rutherford resigned her post in protest at the recklessness of surgical procedure at the hospital. Since Royaumont's opening at the beginning of the year, cases had been light, but recently, Rutherford remarked, more serious injuries had been sent. Of particular concern for Rutherford were the cerebral injuries; the trephining of two patients, for example, had produced 'grave results'. Three days before her resignation, another case had been received, where surgical treatment was necessary. Rutherford feared a repetition of previous outcomes and advised Ivens, 'for her own sake and that of the Hospital', to seek a second opinion about the advisability of going ahead. Ivens removed Rutherford publicly from the theatre and, despite reassurance that the suggestion had been

22 Miss Stevenson to Dr Russell, Royaumont, 29 May 1918, Tin 42: Circulated Letters 1918 a (January–June), SWHC. She later added attending on 'natives' as one of her concerns over the ways in which the hospital was run. See letters from Doris Stevenson to Miss Ivens, 8 June 1918, and to Dr Russell, 12 June 1918, Tin 42.
23 Miss Stevenson to Dr Russell, Women's Emergency Canteen, Gare du Nord, Paris, 12 June 1918, Tin 42.
24 Dr Ivens to Mrs Russell, 26 June 1918, Tin 42.
25 Miss Agnes Anderson to Mrs Russell, 25 June 1918, Tin 42.

friendly rather than critical, Rutherford felt she could only resign rather than suffer from her chief's lingering resentment at this reaction.[26] Doubt about surgical capabilities in wartime situations was clearly not restricted to male colleagues. This letter was serious enough to ensure that Beatrice Russell, as honorary secretary of the Personnel Committee in Edinburgh, made a swift visit to France, 'as a medical woman can see with expert's eyes what is being done', noted Miss Loudon, Royaumont's adminis-trator.[27] As the women wanted to be seen in the best possible light by the public at home, who were funding their enterprise, it was important that reports placed in suffrage publication *Common Cause* were positive about surgery carried out at Royaumont. Even deaths were concealed. As Loudon noted, only half-jokingly, a few days after Rutherford's resig-nation: 'Another rather dismal report for we have had two deaths (please don't send this information to the *Common Cause*).'[28] This desperation to keep even a small number of fatalities from the public was translated into a report in the periodical which simply noted the visit of Russell and Miss Kemp and told the story of 'A Typical Breton Patient', shoemaker Jean Carron.[29] A week later, Russell's report appeared, although the focus was on the day-to-day running of Royaumont. While the work was 'the real soul of the Hospital' 'one cannot speak in detail in a nonmedical journal'. Confidence and satisfaction dominated this account, however, in what was designated an 'entirely surgical' institution.[30]

This fear of letting the public see inside the operating theatre dogged the SWH. What the women wanted their supporters to see were heroic, superhuman efforts, which saved the lives of their patients; the 'oper-ating, operating, operating' carried out by candlelight during constant threat of attack.[31] Surgeons could 'devise no system of shifts', unlike the rest of the teams, because even if they did have the luck to spend four or five hours in bed, 'they were constantly being called up to serious cases and to emergency operations'.[32] They certainly did not want the circulation of tales about breakdowns, sheer exhaustion and

[26] Margaret E. Rutherford to Mrs Russell, Baillon, Asnière-sur-Oise, 23 October 1915, Tin 6: Letters for which no folios could be traced.
[27] Miss Loudon to Miss Marris, [undated, but very late October or early November 1915 from internal evidence], Tin 12: Copies of Letters Received at Headquarters from July 1915 to October 1916.
[28] Miss Loudon to Miss Mair, 24 October 1915, Tin 12.
[29] V.C.C.C., 'N.U.W.S.S. Scottish Women's Hospitals: Royaumont', *Common Cause*, VII.345 (19 November 1915), 419. The author is Vera Collum, X-ray assistant.
[30] Beatrice Russell, 'N.U.W.S.S. Scottish Women's Hospitals: Some Impressions of Royaumont', *Common Cause*, VII.346 (26 November 1915), 441–2; 441.
[31] Extract from a letter by Miss Florence Anderson, Royaumont, 1 June 1918, Tin 42: Circulated Letters: November 1917–April 1918 (a), SWHC.
[32] 'Skia' [Vera Collum], 'The First Week of the First Great Push. From a Hospital Behind the French Front', *Blackwood's Magazine*, 201.1217 (March 1917), 339–50; 341.

occupational injuries. Ivens' focus in her *BMJ* article on 'The Part Played by British Medical Women in the War' was surgical and scientific achievement, despite personal risk and hardship.[33] This was in stark contrast to some in the official service of the army, who offered franker details of physical and mental collapse. In the *BMJ* of 2 June 1917, two months before Ivens' assessment of women's contribution, Surgeon-General Sir Anthony Bowlby and Colonel Cuthbert Wallace described the current surgical situation in France. They remarked upon the stoicism required for operating day and night at casualty clearing stations near the front and consequent necessity for a relay of personnel. In spite of shift patterns, however, they noted that the work was 'exceedingly trying, and it must be reckoned on that not a few of the staff will be more or less knocked up after three or four weeks of it'.[34] Nearly 60 years after the end of the war, Ruth Verney was asked if she found the work 'too demanding physically'. 'Oh no', she replied. 'I was very healthy. I got jaundice once but it was soon over.'[35] Even in women's private letters, 'knocking up' was viewed with horror. Royaumont was 'not a place for delicate people or those who tire easily', as orderly Agnes Anderson remarked.[36] Minor illness was inevitable, but to be sent home for what the surgeon Elizabeth Courtauld named darkly as 'urgent reasons', even if it meant undreamt-of leave, was dreaded.[37] The terror of missing out was palpable. As radiographer Edith Stoney succinctly concluded: 'I could not have faced the risk of being inefficient. [. . .] We are all out to do the best we can and give the best help we each of us can give – and other things matter very little these days.'[38] Exposure of any weakness to a wider audience was, therefore, tantamount to treason, as one former member of Royaumont was to discover.

Vera Collum, radiology assistant and part-time chronicler of the SWH's exploits for the British press under the pseudonym 'Skia', felt the wrath

---

[33] Mary H. Frances Ivens, 'The Part Played by British Medical Women in the War', *BMJ*, 2.2955 (18 August 1917), 203–8; 203.

In 'Deeds *and* Words', Geddes comments upon the hagiographical style of contemporary reports of the women's work. Letters to and from Royaumont, as we have seen, confirm that this is how the women wanted to be represented to the wider public.

[34] Sir Anthony Bowlby and Colonel Cuthbert Wallace, 'The Development of British Surgery at the Front', *BMJ*, 1.2944 (2 June 1917), 705–21, 707. See also Carden-Coyne, *Wounds*.

[35] Typescript interview with Dr R.E. Verney, September 1977, tape 477, WW1/WO/127, LC.

[36] Miss Agnes Anderson to Mrs Russell, 25 June 1918, Tin 42: Circulated Letters 1918a (January–June), SWHC.

[37] Elizabeth Courtauld to Ruth, Royaumont, 16 July 1918, WW1/WO/023, LC.

[38] Edith Stoney to Dr Erskine, near Malta, 23 October 1915, in Tin 41: Royaumont and Troyes, Miscellaneous Letters, &c, 1915–1916: Second French Unit, Letters, Papers &c, 1916, SWHC.

of her colleagues when her notes were published without permission. As they had successfully concealed any dissent from the *Common Cause* throughout the war, the publication of biographical details, complete with unexpurgated episodes of 'knocking up', created havoc. The offending article appeared at the end of December 1918 and was intended to cheer the Croix de Guerre awarded to the staff of Royaumont and Villers-Cotterets. Instead, gossipy anecdotes drew attention to the breaking down from overwork and overstrain of Augusta Berry, assistant physician and surgeon, Ruth Nicholson, second surgeon, and Miss Martland, surgeon. That it was the surgeons who had 'knocked up' presented a direct link between the operating theatre and the weakness of the female surgeon. Collum was additionally horrified at her own presentation, which had been written in the third person, but had commented on the burns sustained to her hands and neck from persistent X-ray exposure. Again this linked the whole team to physical suffering sustained while carrying out the essential requirements of modern surgery. Such intimate detail caused Collum to shudder: '[t]he allusions to my X ray burns simply made my flesh creep with horror!'[39] The publication of unguarded notes meant for private eyes only 'constituted a breach of good taste'. Collum was now forced to 'smooth down the unfortunate victims'.[40] While her health and strength had not been questioned, Ivens retorted that they 'all feel that it is a pity there is not more supervision of the Press work by a medical member of the Committee who would safeguard our interests from the ethical point of view, and who would see the right papers were supplied with information'.[41] Collum's oversight was all the more surprising given her letter of July 1915 about the necessity of a press campaign to garner more funds for the SWH. Royaumont was doing such good work removing prejudice against women surgeons that it was necessary to '"boom"' it even more carefully in the press. In words that must have come back to haunt her, Collum concluded: 'There is a good deal more method and science in a press campaign than most amateurs realise. Monday's mutton must not be recognisable in Tuesday's stew, especially when the stew and the joint are for different households.'[42] In December 1918, Collum had accidentally permitted communal dining

---

[39] Miss V.C.C. Collum to Miss Cooke, Chelsea, 14 January 1919, Tin 42: Circulated Letters 1919 (a).

[40] Ibid.

[41] Dr Ivens to Miss Ferguson, Royaumont, 14 January 1919, Tin 42: Circulated Letters 1919 (a).

[42] Miss Collum to Miss Craigie, Press Secretary, Royaumont, 18 July 1915, Tin 12: Royaumont: Letters to and from Miss Collum, Miss Allison, Mrs Harley, Mrs Eva McLaren, Mrs Owen, Dr Savill, Miss Tod.

on the meat and bones of the Royaumont staff; her overzealousness in promoting their achievements instead exposed their frailties.

Challenges Posed by Surgery during the Great War

The questioning of surgical ability was not alien to those faced, for the first time, with the horrors of modern warfare. Surgery during the Great War was pursued with caution, doubt and instinct. Experience could be drawn upon, but every injury sustained revealed something new for even seasoned army surgeons.[43] Women were not any different in this respect. Many had, of course, as has been shown throughout this book, considerable understanding of complex abdominal procedures, as well as a desire to take up and perfect risky surgical treatment for malignant diseases. While they had dealt with women and children on the wards, LSMW students had been attending Gate, the RFH's Casualty Department, as part of their training since the association between the two institutions began and would have encountered male victims of industrial accidents, for example.[44] Verney and Henry had gained experience at home in Manchester and Sheffield respectively, dealing with traumatic injuries caused by workplace or wartime incidents.[45] Convalescent soldiers were encountered on the wards by women at home before they departed for service abroad.[46] Cooter's claim that, by the end of the nineteenth century, children's hospitals were predominantly surgical, dealing largely with orthopaedic cases, is pertinent to consider in this context.[47] Many women had experience in children's hospitals and this could have given them greater confidence in approaching the bones and joints of men. In 1912, for example, Garrett Anderson and Murray had established the Women's Hospital for Children in Harrow Road, West London, which held a clinic for London County Council orthopaedic cases on Friday mornings.[48] Elsie Inglis worked at the Edinburgh Hospital and Dispensary for Women and Children and the Hospice, which saw an increase

---

[43] Carden-Coyne makes a similar argument in *Wounds*; see especially chapter 2: 'Surgical Wars'.

[44] For a poetic interpretation of the Gate experience, lamenting the lot of the dresser faced with, among others, 'crushed and septic thumbs' and 'ghastly mutilation', see 'Gate - t.d.s. (A Reminiscence of 1906)', *L(RFH)SMWM*, 38 (October 1907), 805–6.

[45] Interview with Dr R. E. Verney, Tape 476, WW1/WO/127; Henry, *Reminiscences*.

[46] Verney, Tape 476.

[47] Roger Cooter, *Surgery and Society in Peace and War* (Basingstoke: Macmillan, 1993), p. 41.

[48] 'Women's Hospital for Children', *L(RFH)SMWM*, VIII.55 (July 1913), 219.
    Geddes reads women's previous surgical experience differently. See Geddes, 'Deeds *and* Words', p. 86 and 'The Women's Hospital Corps'.

in its surgical work in the decade before the war started.[49] Although the surgery was predominantly gynaecological, Inglis and her colleagues also treated diseases of the bones and joints. It was accepted, both by the public and the profession, that women would care for children, but, as Cooter suggests, this could have given anyone working in such institutions a relatively free rein to experiment with new techniques.[50] This is not to suggest that women were as well prepared for their military surgery as they would have desired, but that they were often little different to male colleagues from general practices, who had perhaps performed only minor surgery in recent years or other men with specialties which were not directly applicable to the results of warfare. That they had carried out any major surgery was an undoubted benefit. Such were the conditions experienced on the Western Front, however, that even the most well-trained professional military surgeon had a great deal to learn.

Articles in the medical press about the progress of surgery during the Great War make interesting reading, allowing an insight into the ways in which surgeons relearned their craft between 1914 and 1918. The newly established *British Journal of Surgery*, for example, was rapidly filled with case studies of every kind of injury.[51] When the Second World War was in its infancy, Ivens reminded colleagues of the need to publish surgical developments for those operating at the front and beyond. In a letter of December 1939 to the *BMJ*, Ivens exclaimed '[m]ay I now too, even after this lapse of time, acknowledge with gratitude the value of the articles on fractures under war conditions by Sir Robert Jones which appeared in your journal in 1916'. 'They were read and reread', she continued, until the pages were ragged!'[52] While surgeons could draw upon experience to assist them, heavily illustrated, multi-part articles advocating best practice were evidently much in demand. Indeed, surgeons learned from the work of others and applied that research to their own circumstances, whether through reading medical journals or actual observation of others' practice. Instinct was only part of the surgical process. At an RAMC

---

[49] The *Annual Reports of the Edinburgh Hospital and Dispensary for Women and Children and the Hospice*, LHB8/7/26, Lothian Health Services Archive, University of Edinburgh.

[50] Cooter, *Surgery and Society*, p. 41.

[51] The journal was established in 1913. At the end of 1914 'Notes on Military and Naval Surgery' appeared in volume 2, issue 8, 701–7; by 1915, the majority of articles were concerned with war surgery. Issue 11, for example, is dominated by the treatment of gunshot wounds.

[52] Letter from Frances Ivens-Knowles to the *BMJ*, 2.4118 (9 December 1939), 1161. The reference is to a heavily illustrated, ten-part series of articles on specific war injuries or conditions, which ran from 1.2887 (29 April 1916), 609–11 to 2.2920 (16 December 1916), 829–34.

meeting in January 1917 to consider the advisability of laying down guidance for the treatment of war wounds, Professor James Swain claimed that 'progress is not made from uniformity', while Sir Berkeley Moynihan offered this assessment on surgical progression: '[t]he whole progress of surgery has depended on the different interpretations that different men have given to the same methods of solving the same problem'.[53] Bowlby and Wallace's 1917 synthesis of 'The Development of British Surgery at the Front' offered a number of ways in which the surgeon at the front learned and relearned how to operate. Really sound opinions could only come when the surgeon had considerable experience of the injury – in this case, the necessity of amputation. Without this knowledge, the advice of those who had been able to form judgement through practise was the best bet before a decision was made. Although they pointed to general rules of operation, Bowlby and Wallace also drew attention to the necessity of departing from ideals when the condition of either patient or limb was in doubt. 'Working out the best method of treatment' was another means of proceeding when new problems arose, as in the prevalence of gas gangrene on the Western Front, something to which this chapter will return later. Surgical 'working out' was encouraged by bacteriological analysis in this particular instance. Without complete answers, suggestions could suffice. The authors continued to discuss treatments 'in vogue at the present moment', implying both that they were not previously popular and that they were likely once again to fall out of fashion. Abdominal surgery, for example, had gone from being considered impossible to prevalent. Confidence was attained, in this field, through attempts, failures, and continual risk: 'each man had to learn the best methods for himself'. Individual experimentation was coupled with 'diffusion of more accurate knowledge', obtained via the ways in which the wounded were transported from field to hospital.[54] Similarly, head injuries had been operated upon immediately, as they were in civilian practice, but observation led to the encouragement of a different procedure, which allowed rest before surgery. Discussion and debate, when coupled with close attention to casualties' reaction to treatment, altered how surgeons operated. When faced with the challenges of modern warfare, specialist surgery was forced to give way to general approaches which then,

---

[53] Swain was Consultant Surgeon to the troops in the Southern Command, 1914–1919, and Moynihan his counterpart in the Northern Command, 1914–1918. Quoted in Whitehead, *Doctors in the Great War*, pp. 163–4.

[54] Thomas R. Scotland, 'Evacuation pathway for the wounded', in Scotland and Heys, eds., *War Surgery*, pp. 51–84.

once again, and through practise, became expertise.[55] Surgery during the Great War developed through the experience of experimentation.

By the 1910s, as we saw in the previous chapter, risky surgical procedures were favoured by those attempting to treat grave malignancies. As Bowlby and Wallace illustrated in 1917, the Great War further revealed the value of a willingness to experiment in order to achieve the best results. However, this radical approach was tempered with a conservative bent. This was especially the case as far as amputation was concerned. It did not take long for surgeons at the front to realise that preservation of limbs was vital for soldiers' eventual return to civilian life.[56] Patients resisted surgery when they became aware that they might come round from an anaesthetic minus a useful body part, whether that was because of their terror at loss of livelihood or their religious beliefs. The administrator of Royaumont, Miss Loudon, wrote to the Edinburgh Committee to relay a conversation she had had with a patient whose finger had been saved by Frances Ivens. "'If I had been in a Military Hospital'", he confided, "I should have lost my finger"'. It would make such a difference in the future if they had the 'proper number of fingers'.[57] When writing about Royaumont in *Blackwood's*, Collum referred to a number of patients who recoiled initially in terror at what they believed were 'senseless slashes of the surgeon's knife'.[58] In an age of the radical approach in some areas, however, amputations, and the pre-anaesthetic, pre-aseptic showmanship that was inextricably attached to such procedures, had correspondingly decreased. With time to operate, thanks to the unconscious patient, surgeons, either in military or civilian practice, were removing fewer limbs than their predecessors.[59] If surgical theory and practice had turned towards conservation for procedures such as amputation,[60] the war forced rethinking about the best way to treat mangled body parts. The injuries seen by surgeons from the battlefields were unlike those

---

[55] Weisz explores the development of specialisation in *Divide and Conquer*.

[56] In contrast, Harrison discusses the ways in which abdominal surgery increased due to public pressure above and beyond the economic necessity of mending soldiers simply to put them back on the front lines. See *The Medical War*, p. 106.

[57] Miss Loudon to Miss Mair, Royaumont, 14 June 1915, in Tin 12: Letters to and from Miss Cicely Hamilton and Miss K. Loudon (Secs) 1914–1917. The patient's response is in French.

[58] 'Skia', 'The First Week', 343; the reluctance of Arab patients to lose their shattered limbs is described as being due to their fear of physical imperfection at death, which meant they would not enter the 'gates of Paradise', 345. Collum ascribes fear of the knife to be an innately 'primitive' reaction.

[59] Cooter, *Surgery and Society*, p. 106. For the surgery of pre-anaesthesia, see Stanley, *For Fear of Pain*.

[60] See Gert H. Brieger, 'From conservative to radical surgery in late nineteenth-century America', in Lawrence, ed., *Medical Theory, Surgical Practice*, pp. 216–31.

experienced even just over a decade earlier on the veldt of South Africa. Differences in the terrain soon made themselves clear. Wounds from modern warfare were exacerbated by the richness of the soil in which the injured fell, which, in turn, swiftly contaminated wounds.[61] Gas gangrene was the bane of surgeons, whose successful operations would be rendered null and void by this evil-smelling, ferocious killer. Medical treatment, and especially tight bandages or plaster of Paris, effectively sealed infections. As Ivens noted in 1939, an application of bandages which under ordinary conditions would earn a special commendation killed rather than cured.[62] Surgeons learned that instant operative action was not always the best course to take. While an urgent response was necessary with war wounds, it was not always surgical. Watching the patient closely was sometimes the best way to react. The result of even slight wounds, if infected, could change the course of treatment or the condition of the injured man instantly. Although they were reluctant to admit it,[63] surgeons needed the assistance of nurses and orderlies, as well as the scientific confirmation which could be obtained through pathological and bacteriological findings or X-ray images. What had once been seen, at best, as ancillary to surgery became vital in this new environment in anticipating and proving surgical diagnoses.

Women's Surgical Experiences

With expertise in a variety of abdominal procedures, a number of women had a surgical advantage over some male counterparts. They had also revealed a willingness to experiment with new techniques, which proved necessary to the vicissitudes of wartime injuries. Adaptations were necessary in some cases, however, in order to permit comfort and ease of movement in the theatre while operating. For example, white overalls sent to Royaumont for the theatre were 'more suitable for the other sex'; they were too short and very full around the waist, while the mackintosh aprons were not long enough to cover skirts sufficiently.[64] What women surgeons actually did during the Great War and how they were received by their patients has been obscured by rhetoric, the hagiography that Geddes has discussed, and the lack of available statistics.[65] For example,

---

[61] Scotland and Heys, 'Setting the Scene', in Scotland and Heys, eds., *War Surgery*, pp. 23–50; p. 49.

[62] Letter from Frances Ivens-Knowles, *BMJ*, 2.4118 (9 December 1939), 1161.

[63] Harrison, *The Medical War*, p. 108.

[64] Frances Ivens to Elsie Inglis, 9 March 1915, Tin 12: Letters to and from Dr Ivens (CMO) and Miss Ramsay Smith (Secretary): 1914–1918.

[65] Geddes, 'Deeds *and* Words'.

the problematic Corsican Unit, in 1917, was described as having 'very confusing and badly kept records', and this was not unusual.[66] Women had a different war to some men in that they did not operate at casualty clearing stations but at base hospitals further down the line or, as Garrett Anderson, Murray, or the radiologist Florence Stoney served, in military hospitals at home.[67] This meant that they often received wounded who had been patched up and sent on, ensuring that they had to deal with the results of initial treatment as well as carrying out their own procedures. Royaumont, for example, was 25 miles away from the firing line and ten from Creil, which was the distributing centre for the French wounded.[68] It also meant that they received a number of cases whose injuries were slight, but who went on to develop gas gangrene. They were, therefore, in an ideal position to utilise experimental resources produced by laboratory studies. Royaumont, as we shall see, carried out trials of serum produced by the French to combat gas gangrene and Endell Street was given bismuth-iodoform-paraffin paste (B.I.P.P.) which ensured wounds could be healed quicker without constant, disruptive changing of bandages.[69] Women's hospitals were sites of scientific, as well as surgical experimentation. Consequently, they are ideal for examining the relationship between very different members of a surgical team and assessing the ways in which surgery between 1914 and 1918 was assisted by, relied upon and incorporated developments in radiology and bacteriology. This is not to claim that the contact between surgery and its satellites was without friction in practice, but that debates between them invigorated surgical technique and saved lives and limbs.

In similar fashion to trench warfare, there were rushes and lulls in surgery near the front lines. Most accounts published about women's hospitals focused on the difficulty of the cases and the skilfulness of the treatment given, prompted by the surgeons themselves and the

---

[66] Dr Erskine to Mrs Russell, Ajaccio, 25 March 1917, Tin 42: Circulated Letters, 1918–1922: Copies of Letters (sent from Edinburgh), Troyes and Salonika, 1917.

   John D. Holmes remarks that 'presumably because of the pressure of work', the new plastic surgical procedures were not recorded in similar fashion to other specialties in the profession's journals. See 'Development of Plastic Surgery', in Scotland and Heys, eds., *War Surgery*, pp. 257–80; p. 266.

[67] The work of Florence Stoney, the sister of Edith, will be considered in the following chapter.

[68] Progress Made 1st November, 1914–13th January, 1915, First News Letter, attached to Appeal Leaflet, in Tin 41: S.W.H.: Agenda and minutes of meetings of Hospital Committee for 1915, SWHC.

[69] See Louisa Garrett Anderson and Helen Chambers, 'The Treatment of Septic Wounds with Bismuth-Iodoform-Paraffin Paste', *Lancet*, 189.4879 (3 March 1917), 331–3. Also Helen Chambers and J.N. Goldsmith, 'The Bacteriological and Chemical Action of Bismuth-Iodoform-Paraffin Paste', ibid., 333–335. See also Carden-Coyne, *Wounds*, for problems with B.I.P.P., pp. 122–9.

committees concerned with press matters at home. Mrs Curnock's *Daily Mail* account of a 'Women's War Hospital' in October 1914 followed a day's action at the Hôtel Claridge in Paris, recently established by Garrett Anderson and Murray. The tone was sentimental, stressing the devotion of the 'wonderful women doctors' who operated tirelessly '[a]ll day and all night' to save 'plucky' Tommies, who arrived in a constant stream, filling all eighty beds.[70] Beyond the seriousness of the operations, head and limb cases were mentioned; the two interviewees had 'smashed thighs' and were proud of their 'twin' injuries. By far the most dramatic, heavily publicised encounters were those of the SWH. Two instances provoked especially awed coverage. In Serbia, Elsie Inglis, the Commissioner of the SWH, and her units were the focus of much scrutiny when the enemy overran the country. Inglis' unit and that of Dr Alice Hutchinson remained to tend to their Serbian patients, while the others retreated across the mountains.[71] The *National Weekly* in April 1917 focused on the perilous experiences of escape and imprisonment, while stressing the women's professional disappointment at not being able to go on caring for their charges.[72] Elsie Inglis 'related her adventures' to an eager *Common Cause* on her return via Zurich in the late winter of 1916, noting that they had also treated Germans when their hospital was taken over.[73] By the autumn of 1916, the indefatigable Inglis was off again in order to set up another unit in Russia. Upon her death after returning from the Russo-Romanian front in November 1917, obituaries were filled with accounts of stoicism, freedom from self-seeking, and professional detachment combined with 'born leadership'.[74] Eulogies stressed her universal appeal. She was '"Our Doctor Inglis"',[75] deeply beloved and venerated. For her colleagues, she was an exemplar of high energy and unselfishness, the ultimate stimulation to greater effort.[76]

---

[70] Mrs Curnock, 'In a Women's War Hospital. British Lady Doctors at Work', *Daily Mail*, Friday, 16 October 1914, in *SLHWPC*.

[71] For correspondence about these experiences, see *Between the Lines*, ed., Audrey Fawcett Cahill (Bishop Auckland: The Pentland Press, 1999).

   For a contemporary account, see the entry on Inglis in McLaren, *Women of the War*, pp. 19–23.

[72] 'Scottish Women's Hospitals', *National Weekly*, 14 April 1917, 45, *SLHWPC*.

   For a succinct contemporary account of conditions in Serbia, see also Ivens, 'The Part Played', 205–6.

[73] 'Return of Dr Elsie Inglis and Her Party', *Common Cause*, VII.360 (3 March 1916), 621–2.

[74] 'Elsie Inglis: Obituary', *BMJ*, 2.2970 (1 December 1917), 743. Also, 'The Death of Dr Elsie M. Inglis', *Lancet*, 190.4918 (1 December 1917), 832.

[75] 'Elsie Maud Inglis, M.B., C.M.', *Common Cause*, IX.452 (7 December 1917), 421.

[76] Florence Stoney to Mrs Laurie, Fulham Military Hospital, 30 November 1917, Tin 12: Letters to and from Miss Stoney, Radiographer.

The second prominent exposure of the woman surgeon's selfless courage came in June 1918 at Villers-Cotterets. 'Bombed Hospital Amputations by Candlelight' was the sensational headline in the *Glasgow Herald*. This was succeeded by the personal account of X-ray assistant, Marion Butler, which stressed the privations experienced by the surgeons, who even had to prostrate themselves in a field to escape German planes.[77] Collum also provided a detailed account of the hospital's candlelit operations during German aerial bombardment and the staff's daring escape.[78] In this article, Collum used the ways in which the women operated during the aftermath of the Battle of the Somme and the summer of 1918 as evidence of theory in practice:

So chance – or destiny – flung our little emergency unit of women into the one spot in the whole of France where it could prove of greatest value during that great struggle, and that later struggle – for Paris – in June-July 1918, and where it could also seize the opportunity to translate its experiment into successful enterprise, its improvisation into a perfected organisation, functioning at high tension during two critical periods of stress and strain.[79]

Both periods of surgical frenzy tested resources. Collum adopted a rope metaphor to examine how the women fared during the physical and psychological strain of a rush. After the Somme, they were 'stretched taut', but 'not a strand of the rope was frayed'.[80] During the events of May and June 1918, they were 'tried up to and beyond our strength'; but with a 'frayed' rope, even with some broken strands, 'it held'.[81] At the end of May, Villers-Cotterets had been bombarded aerially night and day, which necessitated a blackout everywhere except the operating theatre. This was run by carefully shaded candlelight and appeared a 'hell and a shambles'. Wounded men were 'carried just as they had fallen'. There were '[n]ine thigh amputations running; men literally shot to pieces; the crashing of bombs and thunder of ever-approaching guns': '[T]he operating hut, with its plank floor and the tables and the instruments on them literally dancing to the explosions; the flickering candles; the anxiety lest the operated cases might haemorrhage and die in the dark.'[82] This frenzy was compounded when staff and wounded made their way back to Royaumont. In 15 days, noted Collum, they had brought in, X-rayed and operated upon 1,000 wounded. Collum herself made 85 X-ray examinations in 24 hours. Two emergency operating theatres opened, ensuring that there were three working all day, two at night. With such pressure, Ivens and her deputy, Ruth Nicholson, slept only three hours

[77] 'Bombed Hospital. Amputations by Candlelight', *Glasgow Herald* (Friday 7 June 1918), Tin 12: Letters to and from Dr Ivens (CMO) and Miss Ramsay Smith (Secretary): 1914–1918.
[78] 'Skia', 'A Hospital'.   [79] Ibid., 615.   [80] Ibid., 621.
[81] Ibid., 633.   [82] Ibid., 627.

a day for a fortnight. X-ray and the rest of the theatre teams worked 18 hours, while resting for six. Thanks to their superhuman efforts, only 40 of the 1000 wounded men died.[83]

Personal correspondence, manuscripts and reports confirmed the dramatic nature of the summer offensive. The matron, Gertrude H. Lindsay, remarked on the surgical staff's incredible commitment; they 'worked magnificently', carrying on without any awareness of the change between day and night, not one member 'showed any nervousness'.[84] '[S]leep was out of the question, and one never felt it advisable to undress', concluded Elizabeth Courtauld. They worked all night, 'hard at it and working under difficulties. Terrible cases came in': 'Between 10.30 and 3.30 or 4am we had to amputate 6 thighs and 1 leg, mostly by the light of bits of candle, held by the orderlies'. Courtauld gave anaesthetic 'more or less in the dark at my end of the patient'.[85] After her return from Salonika, Edith Stoney went to France and joined the Villers-Cotterets team. In June, she wrote to the Committee about the frantic packing, unpacking and repacking of valuable X-ray equipment, when orders were given more than once to evacuate: no mean feat, given the circumstances. Staff had to ensure patients, but also dressings, bandages, drugs, splints, and, of course, X-ray apparatus, made the journey back to Royaumont. A false alarm about evacuation meant the replacement of electric wiring and the reinstallation of necessary equipment for the many injured who were pouring into the hospital. Florence Anderson, once orderly and now masseuse and radiographer's assistant, exclaimed that the dismantling and then reconstruction of the X-ray installation was a 'tour de force', which ran successfully all night.[86] Less romantically than Collum implied in her *Blackwood's* article, Stoney noted that, as well as candles, she was responsible for the lighting of a 50-candlepower electric lamp, which was carefully shaded by being stuck in a cocoa tin. As they had already evacuated the electrician, Stoney had to assist in working the engine for

---

[83] Ibid., 632.

[84] G.H. Lindsay (Matron), 'In reply to Miss Stevenson's statements with regard to the evacuation of Villers-Cotterets', dated 24 June 1918, and appended to Ivens' letter below.

In addition to her other complaints, and even though she was not present at the clearing station, Stevenson claimed that wounded men were left at Villers-Cotterets. Ivens considered this comment 'sufficiently damaging for me to place in the hands of the Medical Defence Union. It is absolutely untrue', Dr Ivens to Mrs Russell, 26 June 1918, Stevenson had remarked that 'stores and luggage could have been easily saved, there was at least a car which came down empty, wounded and luggage were left', Miss Stevenson to Dr Russell, Women's Emergency Canteen, Gare du Nord, Paris, 12 June 1918. All in Tin 42: Circulated Letters 1918a (January–June).

[85] Elizabeth Courtauld to her father, 31 May 1918, Royaumont, WW1/WO/023, LC.

[86] Extract from a letter (recipient unknown), Royaumont, 1 June 1918, Tin 42: Circulated Letters: November 1917–April 1918 (a) (*sic*).

the X-rays. The surgeons operated all night; Stoney went to bed at 4 a.m. Three hours later, operations were still being performed. Upon the final evacuation warning, the staff left, with as much as they could transport. All the while, they remained under heavy bombardment. When they made return visits to Villers-Cotterets, to collect equipment, it was noticed that personal items had been looted, boxes broken into, X-ray plates spoilt and apparatus broken or lost. The loss of their own clothes and effects brought home after the fact the horrors of what they had gone through. Courtauld was frustrated at the loss of her rubber bath, others their books and 'knic-knacs'. The former had even wanted to dig up and burn vegetables grown by the staff to avoid the 'Hun' profiting from them, but only managed to pick a bunch of radishes, which then had to be abandoned.[87] Yet, within 24 hours of recovery, the reclaimed Gaiffe table was running at Royaumont and 600 examinations were made on it by Stoney herself.[88] As the number of casualties was so enormous, the bravery of the X-ray team in returning to Villers-Cotterets to collect what was left paid dividends when they were able to mobilise the reclaimed equipment to assist at Royaumont during its busiest days. To use Collum's analogy, the events of May and June 1918 proved that the rope could be partially unravelled, but that this did not affect its overall strength. The experiment was a success.

Not every week was as exciting. More variegated detail can be obtained from private letters or official documents sent back to Britain. It was apparent that the Corsican Unit of the SWH undertook 'Very few major operations', for example, while the GNU in Salonika was initially bombarded with medical cases, rather than wounded, which led McIlroy to look forward to an advance and the resulting 'plenty of work to do in surgery again'.[89] Also in Salonika, new recruit Verney complained on Armistice Day that she found 'the work unutterably slack and time on my hands', but with 'champagne and aste spumante for dinner', she exclaimed with glee: 'your daughter is _not_ what she was!'.[90] Royaumont posted weekly reports to the Committee in Edinburgh, for example, although precise statistics were not often included. In April 1915, however, a very detailed assessment of the situation since January was submitted and allows an insight into how the hospital functioned in its first few months. It is quoted in full to illustrate the types of cases received by the institution.

[87] Courtauld to her father, 31 May 1918, LC.
[88] Edith Stoney to Mrs Walker, Royaumont, 30 June 1918, Tin 12: Letters to and from Miss Stoney, Radiographer.
[89] Dr Erskine to Dr Russell, Ajaccio, 25 March 1917, Tin 42; Dr McIlroy to Miss Kemp, Salonique, 3 March 1916, Tin 42.
[90] Verney to her family, 11 November 1918, Letters 1918–1919, WW1/WO/127, LC.

Patients admitted: Jan 13-Feb 13	74	
Feb 13-March 13	77	
Operations performed: Jan 13-Feb 13	11	
Feb 13-March 13	36	
Deaths: Jan 13-Feb 13	1	
Feb 13-March 13	1	
Patients admitted week ending March 20	67	
March 27	45	
Operations performed week ending	17	
March 20		
March 27	25	
Patients in hospital week ending March 20	135	
March 27	158	
X Ray examinations. Jan 13-Feb 13	27	
Feb 13-March 13	44	
week ending March 20	41	
week ending March 27	53	
Photographs taken Jan 13-March 27	119	

Analysis of Cases: Jan 13-March 27

Surgical		Medical	
Shrapnel Wounds	62	Pleurisy, Bronchitis, Pneumonia	36
Bullet Wounds	32	Septic Throats	4
Joint Injuries	17	Rheumatism and Sciatica	21
Fractures	14	Typhoid	5
Contusions	10	Gastritis	5
Septic Wounds	10	Skin Affections	10
Appendicitis	7	Commotio Cerebri	5
Gland Afflictions	6	Nephritis	2
Haemorrhoids	5	Jaundice	3[91]
Grenade Wounds	5		
Burns	3		
Frozen Feet	3		
Typhoid abscess	1		
Haemorrhage Colitis	1		

This rare case analysis was striking because of the number of operations performed. Between January and March 89 procedures were carried out; the figures more than doubled over the three months. In her letter accompanying the report, Ivens exclaimed at the 'enormous increase' of work over the past five weeks, but, in comparison with the type of press coverage women surgeons were receiving, these numbers were small.

[91] Report, received 5 April 1915, attached to a letter from Frances Ivens to Miss Crompton, Tin 12: Letters to and from Dr Ivens (CMO) and Miss Ramsay Smith (Secretary): 1914–1918, SWHC.

Patients were starting to come directly to the hospital from the front because of the facilities provided by the rail network and some were now not passing through the distribution centre at Creil.[92] Yet, while the 200 beds were almost full at times, they were not always occupied by surgical patients.

The mixture of medical and surgical cases was especially interesting, given the focus on women's surgical skills and the designation of the hospitals as centres of pure surgery. Overall, for example, two-thirds (66.3 per cent) of the total number of patients between January 1915 and February 1919 at Royaumont and Villers-Cotterets, both military and civilian, were operated upon, but that left a third who were medical patients.[93] There were 176 surgical cases over the three-month period between January and March 1915, but a corresponding 91 medical cases, ensuring 65.9 per cent of patients, rather than the much higher numbers suggested by supporters, were designated surgical. Of these, at least 19 had conditions not associated with warfare. In amongst evident war wounds caused by bullets, grenades or shrapnel were the more quotidian appendicitis, gland afflictions, colitis, or even more prosaic haemorrhoids. Three had frozen feet, the sort of condition that Harrison remarked attracted little interest from medical historians of the conflict. As the report revealed, exciting and new surgical challenges were not the only ones experienced by the surgeon at the front. In an interview from 1977, Verney remarked succinctly that the GNU in Salonika 'had an awful lot of work which you wouldn't see in England. It was rather interesting in that way and then we had the ordinary well, casual appendix and so on'.[94] Often such all-too-familiar ailments presented themselves for treatment, as well as medical complaints associated with lung problems, aching joints and the frustrating inconveniences associated with the immobility of trench fighting.[95] In fact, it was not until October 1915 that the hospital experienced its first amputations. As Loudon noted, one

[92] Miss Hamilton to Miss Crompton, dated 14 March 1915, received 17 March, Tin 12: Letters to and from Miss Cicely Hamilton and Miss K. Loudon (Secs) 1914–1917. Miss Hamilton also notes that a very large proportion of patients come to the hospital from the region of the Somme. This would, of course, provide the hospital with a considerable rush in July 1916.

[93] Statistics given at the back of Leila Henry's *Reminiscences of Royaumont*, between 13 January 1915 and p.41, WW1/WO/054, LC. There were 7,204 operations and 10,861 patients cared for during the hospital's existence.

[94] Typescript interview with Dr R.E. Verney, September 1977, tape 477, WW1/WO/127, LC.

[95] For a full-colour illustrated early article on the problems for the feet because of the vertical immobility of trench warfare, see R.H. Jocelyn Swan, 'So-called "Frost-bite"', *PRSM*, 8 (1915), 41–6.

day had seen two arm amputations, one right, one left, on different men. These were the 'first', she remarked, as they 'don't count fingers'.[96] One more had been added by 19 October, with several 'on the verge'.[97] This was 'a poor boy of 21 who has had to lose his leg'.[98] The thousandth patient was admitted in August 1915. 'Sergeant Le Begnee' [*sic*] was suffering from appendicitis and appeared not to have come straight from the trenches, even though he had fought at some point in the war.[99] Initially, complained Ivens, Royaumont was not sent many 'big cases'. The work was, therefore, only occasionally 'quite interesting'.[100] Many seriously wounded men were sent elsewhere, as they were expected to take longer to recover than the hospital could support. By 1919, it was concluded that the GNU, which had moved three times since its original establishment in Troyes, had dealt with 6,497 patients: 2,733 of whom were surgical; 3,764 medical. Therefore, 42.1 per cent of the work carried out by the unit was surgery, 57.9 per cent medicine.[101] Endemic diseases, such as malaria and dysentery, dominated in the summer of 1916 when the Unit was in Salonika, and it was only in the spring of 1917 that surgical work became the main focus of the hospital.[102] As the women were to discover, not every case demanded special knowledge; frequently patients were admitted for the most routine of procedures which could be encountered in a civilian hospital at home. Surgical 'interest' was not always piqued by the cases arriving daily.

At times, indeed, institutions near the front must have been confronted with strangely familiar conditions. For Royaumont, it was the expectation of medical and surgical care from local citizens which took them by surprise. During the lulls between attacks, the hospital saw 1,537 civilians for consultations, while general practitioners of nearby villages sent in a further 537 patients for operation. The total number of patients at Royaumont and Villers-Cotterets during the four-year period during which the SHW occupied them was 10,861 and operations were

96 'Weekly Report', Miss Loudon to Miss Mair, 3 October 1915, Tin 12: Scottish Women's Hospitals Royaumont: Copies of Letters Received at Headquarters from July 1915 to October 1916.
97 Excerpts from a letter from Dr Ivens to Mrs Russell, Royaumont, 19 October 1915, ibid.
98 Report from Miss Loudon to Miss Mair, Royaumont, 17 October 1915, ibid.
99 Miss Loudon to Miss Mair, Royaumont, 3 September 1915, received 7 September 1915, ibid.
100 Frances Ivens to Elsie Inglis, 9 March 1915, Tin 12: Letters to and from Dr Ivens (CMO) and Miss Ramsay Smith (Secretary): 1914–1918.
101 Unsigned, 'Report on the Work of the Scottish Women's Hospital (Hôpital Auxiliaire Bénévole 301, Armée d'Orient), Tin 42: Circulated Letters 1919 (a).
102 Ibid.

carried out 7,204 times.[103] French civilians counted for 25 of Royaumont's deaths, which, given that there were only 159 deceased military
personnel between 1915 and 1919 at the hospital, pointed to the severity
of local cases. Courtauld noted that by December 1918, the 'civils' were
being admitted once more and were, consequently, 'flocking in to take
advantage of treatment just before we close'.[104] Civilian care was more
popular in British hospitals, as Courtauld noted in her letter, after the
war had finished, but Royaumont had been involved with the local popu-
lace throughout its existence. When Verney arrived in Belgrade after the
conflict had ended, she worked almost entirely with civilians. As well as
prisoners of war, they were caring for a 'mass' of children sent in by the
Save the Children Fund, and had also contributed to the building of a
well for local water.[105] Although every surgical case in wartime or novel
surroundings was an experience, some patients began to look more than
a little familiar.

The surrounding population evidently took advantage of a well-
equipped hospital in their midst and the women surgeons found themselves operating upon their own sex at Royaumont. In a letter of March
1915 to Inglis, Ivens expressed the 'embarrassment' felt at their outpatient facilities. While they did not operate upon women at Royaumont,
they carried out procedures at the nearby Beaumont Hospital when
cases appeared on their doorstep. At the Beaumont, they had received
two cases and a third, who had a bad malignant condition, could not
be persuaded to leave Royaumont, so they had secreted her in a little
room far away from the men. Another woman, who required operative
treatment, had mysteriously 'appeared' that afternoon.[106] The situation
was so unexpected that Ivens had been compelled to send for throat
and gynaecological instruments: 'It was the last thing which I thought
would be necessary!' She also requested a Paquelin cautery, frequently
utilised for gynaecological malignancies, as they were clearly receiving
a 'lot of' conditions requiring cauterisation. As they had already bor-
rowed and broken one, at present, she added ironically, we have nothing
available but the 'kitchen poker'.[107] The frustration of having to deal
with cases she thought were left behind in Britain was obvious in this

---

[103] The overall statistics, comprising all patients seen between 13 January 1915 and 26
February 1919, are taken from Henry's MS, *Reminiscences*, p.41, WW1/WO/054, LC.
Villers-Cotterets covers only a three-month period, before it was suddenly evacuated.

[104] Courtauld to Ruth, 13 December 1918, WW1/WO/023, LC.

[105] Typescript interview with Verney, September 1977, tape 477, WW1/WO/127, LC.

[106] Frances Ivens to Elsie Inglis, 9 March 1915, Tin 12. The tone of this letter, sent from
one surgeon to another, is naturally very different to those sent to administrators.

[107] Ibid.

surgeon-to-surgeon letter. At this point, additionally, there were many surgeons and not enough to keep them busy. In a convoluted sentence, Ivens sighed: '[we] have really not nearly as much as they could do if the need arose'. A feeling of not being wanted for 'serious' surgery pervaded this letter, as well as the boredom of waiting around for action on the battlefield to intensify. Although this was early on in the hospital's existence and the locals were only mentioned when there was a lull, they evidently utilised Royaumont's facilities and the surgical expertise on offer into the final year of the war. While they were only taken in when they needed operative assistance and sent out as soon as possible, in a letter to Miss Kemp of February 1918, Ivens made reference to 16 women patients that day. Around half of them were suffering from appendicitis; several had malignancies. By this point, however, Ivens' attitude to the female patients had changed significantly. Now she remarked upon their 'extraordinary gratitude' and the staff's corresponding feeling that it was 'very gratifying to be appreciated'.[108] Although local women comprised no more than 5 per cent of the now 300-bed hospital, they formed a consistent hospital population over the time Royaumont was open. So much so that Ivens wondered what the civilians would do without their assistance when they closed at the end of the war. Recognition and thankfulness also came from the authorities of the small towns, whose inhabitants received treatment from the women surgeons.[109] The constant presence of female patients must have ensured that their surgeons could not forget either past or future.

'Appreciation' at being necessary to others outside their institutions was also apparent from correspondence. Female expertise in X-ray work was especially sought after by nearby hospitals, who possessed neither their own specialists nor enough suitable equipment to carry out skilled exposures. Mobile X-ray vans in France had been popularised by Marie Curie[110] and the SWH had been keen to invest in such facilities (Illustration 4.1). Agnes Savill, the radiologist at Royaumont, was an early beneficiary of a fully equipped car, and her knowledge and apparatus was in demand by other institutions in the vicinity. In October 1915, for example, her services were required at a hospital a few miles

---

[108] Frances Ivens to Miss Kemp, Royaumont, 7 February 1918, in Tin 42: Circulated Letters 1918a (January–June).

[109] Typed MS (speech?) entitled 'Impressions of Hospitals at Abbaye de Royaumont, France and Italy', p.13, Tin 12.

[110] On Curie's wartime activities, see Alexander MacDonald, 'X-Rays during the Great War', in Scotland and Heys, eds., *War Surgery*, pp. 134–47; p. 145. The *Lancet* was initially more sceptical about their value. See 'A Mobile Surgical and X-Ray Van', 185.4768 (16 January 1915), 160.

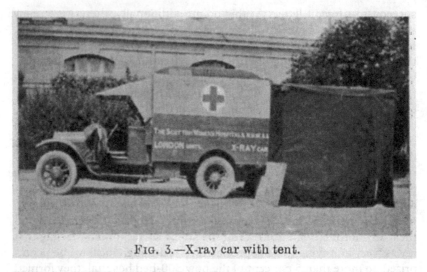

Fɪɢ. 3.—X-ray car with tent.

Illustration 4.1 X-Ray Car with Tent, clearly indicated as belonging to the SWH, *British Medicine in the War 1914–1917* (London: British Medical Association, 1917), Wellcome Library, London.

away, which had only one ambulance and no X-ray equipment. Instead of sending the patients to Royaumont to be X-rayed, which had been the usual occurrence,[111] a mobile unit could go directly to the injured to prevent them from suffering further disruption to their recovery. Sixteen cases were photographed 'on the spot' by Savill. 'Naturally', noted the administrator, Cicely Hamilton, 'the car greatly extends our usefulness in that direction'.[112] *Common Cause* remarked similarly on the value of this 'Travelling' vehicle.[113] Evidently, however, its exceptional nature was overpraised in the same publication. 'We were rather amused', remarked Loudon wryly 'to see the fairy tales in the Common Cause re the X Ray Car'.[114] Indeed, the periodical claimed that the French military

---

[111] See typed MS, 'Impressions of Hospitals', p. 13.

[112] Cicely Hamilton to Miss Marris, [undated, but likely to be October 1915 from internal evidence], Tin 12: Scottish Women's Hospitals Royaumont: Copies of Letters Received at Headquarters from July 1915 to October 1916.

   For footage of the Royaumont X-ray car in action at Villers-Cotterets, see the 1917 film about the SWH online at ssa.nls.uk/film/0035, between 4.22 and 4.54, Scottish Screen Archive, National Library of Scotland.

[113] 'N.U.W.S.S. Scottish Women's Hospitals for Foreign Service: Royaumont', *Common Cause*, VII.351 (24 December 1915), 495.

[114] 'Report', Miss Loudon to Miss Mair, Royaumont, 10 October 1915, Tin 6: Scottish Women's Hospitals Royaumont: Copies of Letters Received at Headquarters From July 1915 to October 1916, SWHC.

authorities had said that 'the car is the finest X-ray car ever used in France' and will enable 'such work to be done much nearer the lines than has hitherto been possible'.[115] It was, by the time Loudon wrote the letter, less hyperbolically going to 'a hospital to see some patients (if one may use the expression)'.[116] Usefulness was less apparent in Greece, however, when the promised car was delayed and then proved ineffective on local terrain. Publicly funded organisations such as the SWH directed their money towards the purchase of such recent technological innovations, which could then be displayed for supporters to admire the utility of their generosity. Such showiness was not popular with Edith Stoney, the radiographer for the GNU in Salonika, who baulked at the tours made in Scotland with the newly purchased X-ray car in the autumn of 1916. The proceeds of a flag day held in Glasgow for the memory of dead nurse Edith Cavell were put towards the purchase and equipment of the car.[117] As it was the first of its kind fitted up in Scotland, great pride in the workmanship and a desire to show it off to the public led to its display. The apparatus was also utilised at Glasgow Royal Infirmary, where sterling work was done on 90 cases a day.[118] This 'local show' astounded Stoney, who suggested no one could admire the car itself, with its polished fittings; the actual photographs based on 'real use' would be the 'best guarantee' of its proper deployment.[119] Keeping it in Scotland was certainly not helping the war effort, she fumed.

Although this purchase eventually proved ineffectual,[120] Stoney was much in demand in Gevgeli and then in Salonika, in similar fashion to Savill in France. 'I have quite a reputation around the other hospitals here for my photos!', she exclaimed with pride to her sister.[121] As she had the only complete tent in the area, others having lost theirs on the journey to Serbia, this allowed her to run X-rays, which had to be strictly rationed for the Unit's own patients. X-ray apparatus was a rarity in Serbia,[122] so Stoney's equipment fascinated. An inspection by the French Medical General from Salonika made 'his best felicitations on [her] photos, and

---

[115] 'N.U.W.S.S. Scottish Women's Hospital: France', *Common Cause*, VII.338 (1 October 1915), 316.

[116] Miss Loudon to Miss Mair, 10 October 1915.

[117] Mrs Laurie to Miss Edith Stoney, 18 March 1916, Tin 12: Letters to and from Miss Stoney, Radiographer from August 1915 to March 1920.

[118] Mrs Laurie to Miss Florence Stoney, 21 September and 30 September 1916, ibid.

[119] Edith A. Stoney to Mrs Laurie, 6 October 1916, ibid.

[120] For a long list of reasons why Stoney was dissatisfied with the car, see a letter addressed from her residence in London to Mrs Laurie, 16 October 1916, ibid.

[121] Edith Stoney to Florence Stoney, Gevgeli, 29 November 1915, Tin 41: Royaumont and Troyes, Miscellaneous Letters, &c, 1915–1916, Second French Unit, Letters, Papers &c, 1916.

[122] Edith Stoney to Dr Erskine, near Malta, 23 October 1915, ibid.

shook [her] warmly by the hand', in anticipation of the good work to come when the Unit reached Greece.[123] When that happened, uncertainty about the course of the war for the Allies in Salonika meant that some hospitals had not felt secure enough to establish their X-ray units. Or, as Stoney put it, 'some cannot put them up, and some do not take very good photos when up'.[124] As a consequence, she had received a number of requests from various quarters for assistance, including a British hospital ship. Stoney had recently examined eight French soldiers from other hospitals, four British soldiers and three British naval officers; two of the British men were doctors. Appreciation by colleagues and patients alike was not reflected in the coverage of Stoney's success at home. Her evident frustration at the lack of publicity afforded the GNU since it had left France was very clear in the May 1916 *Common Cause* article about their experience at Gevgeli. This piece was written by one 'F.A.S.', evidently Edith Stoney's sister Florence. It opened with an admonition that 'very little has appeared' in the press about the voyage of the Unit to the East and stressed that the staff had been 'kept so busy that they have had little time to write'.[125] The focus of the article was on the X-Ray department and the skill of its head. Despite the danger of setting up in a very small room, Edith Stoney's expediency in purchasing a petrol engine in Paris ensured that even in an 'out-of-the-way' Serbian village location the X-ray Department was up and running from the outset. When the hospital was ready, the first rush came for Stoney; in two days, she received four chest cases, two head wounds, two abdominal, 11 leg and three arm injuries. Stoney's accuracy in localising, depth and position, was particularly valued, as her assessment could be utilised by the surgeons to remove bullets precisely from wounds. Such precision was also necessary in judging whether it was wiser or more expedient not to operate. The successful running of X-ray equipment contributed to the hospital's excellent reputation and led to Stoney being in demand with other hospitals who sought out her expertise.

This article also made clear how primitive the living and working conditions were for the SWH Units, especially those in Eastern Europe. It illustrated the very personal contribution members of the whole team made to the smooth running of the operating theatres they established. If her sister had not purchased the engine, reminded Florence Stoney, the hospital would be without an X-ray department, but, even more basically, lacking in electric light. Edith Stoney's Cambridge physics education came in handy more than once during her service with the SWH. While

---

[123] Edith Stoney to Florence Stoney, diary entries, dated 30 November 1915, ibid.
[124] Edith Stoney to Florence Stoney [?], Salonika, 17 February 1916, Tin 42.
[125] F.A.S., 'N.U.W.S.S. Scottish Women's Hospitals: Girton and Newnham Unit at Ghevgeli', *Common Cause*, VIII.371 (19 May 1916), 78.

fundraising at home was directed towards obtaining state-of-the-art technological apparatus, such as the X-ray car, more fundamental resources, such as heat and light, were required by those operating abroad. On the first night at Gevgeli, indeed, Stoney 'lighted the whole hospital' with electricity from her recently procured engine. Now, 'instead of spending the long winter by the dim light of candles, they had the one luxury of good illumination'.[126] Electricity made the light source constant and more reliable, allowing manipulation in the operating theatre to scrutinise particular areas of the body.[127] Stoney's letters were full of the ways in which the women adapted to the difficulties of the surroundings and the circumstances in which they found themselves. The fact that she owned a great deal of her X-ray equipment belied the insistence of the original SWH appeal leaflet on its purchase before leaving of the 'most modern surgical appliances, dressings and drugs'; X-ray apparatus being 'an indispensable adjunct to modern surgery'.[128] Radiology was still a developing, semi-professional surgical 'adjunct'. Its experimental nature was encapsulated by the personal investment in equipment by those wealthy enough to have a try; some owned the apparatus utilised in institutions, for example.[129] It was precisely this ownership of vital resources and personal investment in equipment which led to dissent between Edith Stoney and the Committee at home. Alongside the falling out over the X-ray car, Stoney and the Committee were engaged in a longstanding battle over her engine, which was used to power the radiological equipment. Misunderstandings over its usage led to a stalemate, whereby the Committee thought that Stoney had agreed to sell them the engine and the radiographer had insisted that she had not made this promise.[130] Part

---

[126] Ibid.

[127] For electric light's value to the context of the operating theatre, see Howell, *Technology in the Hospital*, p. 58.

[128] Appeal Leaflet (1914); *Progress Made 1 November, 1914–13 January 1915 First News Letter* (1915), Tin 41: S.W.H.: Agenda and minutes of meetings of Hospital Committee for 1915.

For an account of the Stoney sisters' careers, see Adrian K. Thomas and Arpan K. Banerjee, *The History of Radiology* (Oxford: Oxford University Press, 2013), pp. 50–4 and Jean M. Guy, 'Edith (1869–1938) and Florence (1870–1932) Stoney, two Irish sisters and their contribution to radiology during World War I', *Journal of Medical Biography*, 21.2 (May 2013), 100–7.

[129] Caroline Murphy gives the example of Louisa Martindale, whose personal wealth allowed her to buy radiation therapy equipment, which she then used at her New Sussex Hospital in Brighton, 'A History of Radiotherapy', Part II, chapter IV, pp. 5–6; Part II, chapter 5, p. 26.

[130] This complicated debate lasts for some time, and never really disappears in the correspondence, but Edith Stoney sums up her position most clearly in a letter to Mrs Russell, Salonique, 10 March 1916, Tin 12: Letters to and from Miss Stoney, Radiographer from August 1915 to March 1920. The 'List of X Ray Goods', signed and dated 26 September 1917, by Stoney, was eventually agreed to be sold for £150, 'by special request from Dr McIlroy'.

of the problem was due to the fact that it was 'an absolute necessity' for
the GNU, as a moving surgical corps, to keep all the vital apparatus for
which it had won its good name. But, correspondingly, as engine, coils
and Stoney's artisan assistant were to be left behind in Salonika upon her
resignation, the Committee would effectively remove her usefulness, as
her own apparatus was fundamental both to the furthering of her career
and her efficiency as a specialist war worker.[131] With an X-ray specialist
came equipment and vice versa; one could not exist without the other.
This complex situation, where private property became one foundation
stone of a unit's success, revealed the tension which existed between
individual member and the wider surgical team under desperate conditions. For Stoney, her value could not be separated from the control of
her X-ray apparatus. The Committee, however, were untroubled about
separating technology from operator, and took a different perspective,
choosing to retain the former to keep the unit going.

As Stoney's problems with her own resources illustrated, equipment
led to dispute. The Edinburgh Committee were ever alert to the cost of
what could appear extraneous from a distance.[132] So many letters and
telegrams were requests for more. Four months into Royaumont's activities, Ivens enclosed a list 'which had nothing to do with equipment',
but was added solely because of 'wear and tear'. Without surgical necessities arriving, such as gauze, dressings, linen, wool, and needles, work
was at a standstill. It was cheaper to order material from British sources,
as French prices were increasing swiftly, and every day 'runs away with
a large quantity of material'.[133] In October 1915, Ivens responded to
Beatrice Russell's letter about the cost of gloves. As Ivens noted, gloves
were 'patched' and nurses were 'as economical as possible in their use'.

Chief Surgeon of the Unit, Louise McIlroy, was baffled by Edith Stoney. For her
version of events, see Dr McIlroy to Mrs Russell, 28 January 1917, Tin 42: Circulated
Letters, January 1917.

[131] Edith Stoney to Mrs Laurie, 5 April 1916, Salonique, Tin 12: Scottish Women's Hospitals. Troyes. Letters to and from Mrs Harley (Administrator) and Lists of Personnel,
&c 1915 (sic).

[132] For only one warning about the French prices of surgical equipment rising, see Miss
Loudon to Miss Swanston, 25 September 1915, Tin 12: Scottish Women's Hospitals
Royaumont: Copies of Letters Received at Headquarters from July 1915 to October
1916.

[133] Frances Ivens to Miss Crompton, dated 1 April 1915, received 5 April, Tin 12: Letters
to and from Dr Ivens (CMO) and Miss Ramsay Smith (Secretary): 1914–1918.
See also Miss Loudon to Mrs Laurie, Royaumont, 25 October 1915, which includes
a newspaper article from 18 October on the 'Doubled Prices' of 'Housekeeping in
France' as an illustration of the 'many and serious' challenges faced by the French
housewife, Tin 12: Copies of Letters Received at Headquarters. From July 1915 to
October 1916.

Despite their best intentions, however, tetanus had been found in at least five patients: 'the frightful risk of communicating these appalling germs either from one patient to another or to nurses and orderlies is always with us'.[134] The surgeons required rubber gloves and dismissed any attempts by the Committee to order cotton. Thick and impermeable material was fundamental to prevent sepsis.[135] Despite every aseptic precaution, 'appalling germs' infected both patient and surgeon. 'Even with the greatest care', warned Ivens, 'two doctors have sore fingers this week'.[136] Collum's X-ray burns were not the only injuries she suffered; they were supplemented with a septic finger in August 1915.[137] The heroic aspect of operation upon operation against the terrors of wartime was tempered in reality by the aching, fatigued and, most worryingly, diseased fingers. Shortages of vital equipment and physical suffering led to a united front of institution against administration, practicality over financial concerns.

The holding together of the surgical team was not always in evidence, however. In her *Blackwood's* article of 1918, Collum presented an intriguing image of the democracy operating at Royaumont:

During the first year's service we were practically without rules of any description. We were roughly divided into doctors, nurses, and orderlies, but the lines of demarcation were fluid and hardly existed outside working hours. The doctors made no attempt in the early days to keep up their position as officers, except in the wards and the operating theatre and so on. From the point of view of discipline it may have been a mistake, but it produced a hospital organisation that is surely unique.[138]

Such an idyllic atmosphere of equality in leisure time evidently spilled over into the working life of the institution. Even though Collum demarcated the professional spaces of the operating theatre and the wards from areas of rest and relaxation, the lines between the team members, lay and

---

134 Excerpts from Dr Ivens to Mrs Russell, Royaumont, 19 October 1915, Tin 12: Scottish Women's Hospitals Royaumont: Copies of Letters Received at Headquarters from July 1915 to October 1916.
135 Miss Loudon to Miss Swanston, Royaumont, 25 September 1915, Ibid.
        For further reading on the slow British adoption of surgical gloves from the very late 1890s onwards, see Wangensteen and Wangensteen, *The Rise of Surgery*, pp. 476–84. For a more recent discussion and wider context which considers issues of control, see Schlich, 'Negotiating Technologies'.
136 Excerpts from Dr Ivens to Mrs Russell, Royaumont, 19 October 1915.
137 Dr Agnes Savill to Miss Marris, Royaumont, 15 August 1915. For another account of Collum's burns, where she was 'so badly burned with the old Butt Table's want of adequate protection that she could do no X-Ray work', see Edith Stoney to Mrs Walker, 30 June 1918, Tin 12: Letters to and from Miss Stoney, Radiographer from August 1915 to March 1920.
138 'Skia', 'A Hospital in France', *Blackwood's Magazine* (November 1918), 618–19.

medical, were fluid rather than hierarchical. The overriding impression of Collum's assessment was harmony. Louise McIlroy's unit in Salonika was criticised by its own administrator, Miss Beauchamp, for lax discipline. 'Petty details, such [as] my riding, entertaining British Admirals, giving permission for the staff to have their friends in their recreation tents, were brought up as evidence against me'. However, she fumed, 'the work is just as good as ever'.[139] Enjoyable leisure activities and hard graft were not incompatible for McIlroy. However, SWH correspondence and papers could disagree. Dr Dorothy Cochrane Logan had the unusual distinction of being the only member of medical or surgical staff to be dismissed from Royaumont or, indeed, from any unit of the SWH.[140] From the letters of Frances Ivens and the minutes of the Personnel Committee, it is possible to piece together the reasons for her dismissal. Ironically, given Collum's reading of Royaumont's politics, Logan was removed from the hospital precisely because she refused to accept hierarchical standings.

In an undated letter, received by the Edinburgh Committee on 20 July 1918, Ivens told her side of the tale: 'I did not accept Miss Logan's resignation for I was not aware that she had resigned'. In fact, she continued, 'I dismissed her because she refused to give an anaesthetic when asked to do so'. Such ill-discipline and questioning of orders from the Chief Surgeon relieved Royaumont of someone who 'did not overwork'.[141] Evidently Logan felt differently, as 'poisonous remarks about sweating' had been enough to cause the London Committee to visit their Scottish counterparts. 'Any suggestion of disunion created such a bad impression', concluded Ivens. She was very glad to have Logan out of the hospital.[142] 'Sweating' had very particular connotations in first two decades of the twentieth century, as it had in the nineteenth, but would have been a cruel blow when directed at professional members of a surgical team. Low pay, poor conditions, long hours, and often specifically female, working-class and immigrant oppression were composite factors for the 'sweated' toiler.[143] Indeed, in the words of social investigator Clementina Black,

---

[139] Louise McIlroy to Mrs Russell, Salonika, 15 February 1917, Tin 42 A: Copies of Letters (sent from Edinburgh). Troyes and Salonika, 1917.
See Verney's letters for the evidently mesmeric effect McIlroy had upon her team; Verney was starry-eyed by her CMO and throve in the sociable atmosphere of the unit. '[E]very man here raves about Dr McIlroy's charm – really it is perfectly marvellous!', Verney to her family, Salonika, 27 December 1918, WW1/WO/127, LC.

[140] Although, as the Scarletfinders website notes, Miss Mary Elizabeth Bush, a nurse at Royaumont was dismissed in October 1918. See www.scarletfinders.co.uk/137.html.

[141] Frances Ivens to Mrs Russell, undated, received 20 July 1918, Tin 42: Circulated Letters: November 1917–April 1918 (a).

[142] Ibid.

[143] For a contemporary exploration of sweating, see, for example, Clementina Black, *Sweated Industry and the Minimum Wage* (London: Duckworth & Co., 1907). The Anti-Sweating League had been formed the year before.

sweating was a 'morass exhaling a miasma that poisoned the healthy elements of industry'.[144] Sweating's link with the tailoring trade, one requiring accurate stitching, like surgery, also made Logan's comparison contextually fascinating.[145] For Logan, the regime at Royaumont was akin to nightmarish, exploitative working conditions; for Ivens, her junior was lazy and unruly. Whether Logan refused to give an anaesthetic because she was exhausted and overworked, concerned about doing so, or because she felt that it was beneath her is not clear.[146] The fluidity of relationships at Royaumont, however, was neither as free from hierarchy nor as nonchalantly regarded as Collum would have her readers believe.

Tensions between Louise McIlroy and Edith Stoney also tell another story from that publicised by Collum. The latter saw herself as the saviour of the GNU: 'I saved this corps from utter inefficiency as a surgical corps in Serbia (there was no main electricity at Guevgueli)', she retorted, 'by buying an engine with my own money'.[147] In spite of writing a testimonial for Stoney which stressed her co-operative stance within the team, this was not how McIlroy saw her radiographer in personal correspondence.[148] McIlroy felt that Stoney had lost interest once hostilities had ceased, which had led to the drying up of surgical, and, consequently radiographic, work. Now electrical treatment dominated Stoney's X-ray agenda rather than the localisation of bullets and shrapnel upon which she prided herself. There was no 'friction' in the Unit, however, claimed McIlroy.[149] Stoney offered another assessment of the situation. From the outset, her letters expressed concern over her non-medical background, even though her Cambridge education impressed her colleagues. While assistance was forthcoming from the surgeons, Stoney could not interest them enough to 'work the apparatus with the patients', nor did she feel happy about her 'lack of anatomy', which 'makes me very lame', she noted sadly.[150] Although X-rays showed 'the

---

144 Black, *Sweated Industry*, x.

145 For an exploration of the sweating in the late nineteenth-century tailoring trade, see William Fishman, *East End 1888* (Nottingham: Five Leaves, 1988/2005), particularly pp. 67–106.

146 Logan persisted in her attempts to have salary and maintenance paid by the Committee into 1919. She had evidently kept her dismissal out of the dealings with them and, after receiving Ivens' letter, they would not allow Logan to pursue her claims. See Wednesday, 18 December 1918 and 21 January 1919, Tin 41b: Personnel Committee Minutes, 1918–1920.

147 Miss Edith Stoney to Mrs Russell, Salonique, 10 March 1916, Tin 12: Letters to and from Miss Stoney, Radiographer from August 1915 to March 1920.

148 Louise McIlroy, 'Testimonial for Edith Stoney', dated 8 August 1916, Salonika, ibid.

149 Dr McIlroy to Mrs Russell, 28 January 1917, Tin 42: Circulated Letters, January 1917.

150 Edith Stoney to [Florence Stoney?], Salonika, 17 February 1916, Tin 12: Letters to and from Miss Stoney, Radiographer from August 1915 to March 1920.

real surgical work of the hospital', Stoney evidently felt her lack of medical expertise disabling.[151] Those who were 'not medical', she commented later in 1918, were 'so eaten up these days with the dread of not getting useful enough work' that their desire to help was visceral.[152] She also made exactly the same point as McIlroy about the hierarchy of interest in the GNU, but turned it back on her colleagues. The surgeons themselves, remarked Stoney, inevitably found purely surgical cases more '"interesting"' than the fight against disease, which dominated current work in Salonika.[153] Undoubtedly, however, McIlroy and Stoney respected each other's qualities. The former praised her radiographer's exceptional photographic and localisation skills, her minute and thorough grasp of the physical sciences rendering her far more useful than a medical graduate could have been.[154] 'I have never failed to find pieces of projectiles in wounds which have been photographed by Miss Stoney's stereoscopic process', McIlroy asserted.[155] Stoney, meanwhile, looked admiringly at her Chief's surgical abilities: 'Dr McIlroy is a very beautiful operator – in no case localised by me has she failed to find the bullet from my localising.'[156] It is remarkable how both women praised each other through the prism of their own specialty. Despite their many differences, confidence in their own ways of doing things united Stoney and McIlroy.

Working Together

Whether the X-ray was fundamental to wartime surgery depended on who was asked. For Edith Stoney, it was questionable that a unit could be a surgical one if it did not have X-ray apparatus: 'The front station from Ostrovo Unit has been left without any X rays at all through the worst of the awful Serbian fighting tho' a supposed surgical unit.'[157] The British were slow to adopt the technology, as Bowlby and Wallace noted in their 1917 analysis:

At the beginning of the war x rays were not supplied at the front, but, coincidentally with the development of operating work in the casualty clearing stations, the need of these became apparent. [. . .] [N]ot only have x rays been of great use in

---

[151] Ibid.
[152] Edith Stoney to Mrs Laurie, London, 18 July 1918, Tin 12: Letters to and from Miss Stoney, Radiographer.
[153] Edith Stoney to unknown recipient (probably Mrs Laurie) (undated: 1916/1917?), ibid.
[154] McIlroy, 'Testimonial for Edith Stoney'.   [155] Ibid.
[156] Edith Stoney to Dr Erskine, near Malta, 23 October 1915, Tin 41: SWH: Second French Unit, Letters, Papers &c, 1916.
[157] Edith Stoney to Dr Erskine, London, 30 August 1917, Tin 12: Letters to and from Miss Stoney, Radiographer.

guiding the operator, but in many of the abdominal wounds where the missile has been retained they have been of the greatest service to the surgeon in deciding whether or no operation should be done at all. In many other cases, such as some of the wounds of the head or of the knee-joint, it has been found better not to undertake an operation without a preliminary x-ray examination, so that in the present stage of development of surgery at the front the x-ray plant has become essential for the work of the casualty clearing stations.[158]

Even within this one comment it is possible to see how X-rays were initially considered unnecessary, then necessary, but as an accessory to surgery. Bowlby and Wallace discussed radiology as an associate, an advisor or a guide to the surgeon rather than a replacement for surgical understanding. The surgeon should and indeed did retain control over diagnostic decisions. As Alexander McDonald has remarked, there was considerable variation in the extent to which X-ray equipment was used in France and Belgium.[159] In addition to any scepticism about the value of the technology, Edith Stoney's correspondence also reflected on the difficulties of running apparatus in parts of Europe where even the means to run basic electricity might be scanty. The accounts of the retreat from Villers-Cotterets in the summer of 1918 revealed the practical difficulties involved in the installation of X-ray machinery, as well as the fragility of the easily broken plates and tubes. Disputes over the status of a layperson running equipment and their place in the surgical team could also lead to divisions between radiographic and surgical operators. There were, however, three particular instances where surgery and radiography worked in tandem during the Great War: localising bullets or shrapnel; therapeutic treatment for the wounded; and diagnosing gas gangrene.

The localisation of foreign bodies was vital to surgical success. By accurately pinpointing a bullet or a piece of shrapnel an X-ray could provide the surgeon with a precise location for surgery. As Bowlby and Wallace acknowledged, it might also indicate the advisability or otherwise of operation. If an object was too dangerous to extract, an image of its position could save the patient's life as equally as a surgical procedure would if it was removable. Similarly, those men who survived the war with shrapnel embedded within them, as we shall see in the next chapter, required further surgical care when internal damage resulted.[160] This did occur in wartime, too, either where the patient had not been X-rayed in

---

[158] Bowlby and Wallace, 'The Development of British Surgery at the Front', 708.

[159] McDonald, 'X-Rays during the Great War', in Scotland and Heys, eds., *War Surgery 1914–1918*, pp. 134–47; p. 141.

[160] See Cooter, *Surgery and Society*, for similar problems with limb amputation where nerves and blood vessels had not been adequately sutured or no allowance made for post-operative muscle or skin retraction, p. 110. See also Carden-Coyne, *Wounds*.

the first place or where the surgeon had failed to remove all the debris. Stoney remarked upon four head cases seen in Salonika in 1917. One had been wounded over two months before and had become blind in one eye; the other was temporarily sightless. The blind eye was removed, but the 'good' eye, upon localisation, was found to have metal in the orbit, causing the loss of sight. There were also two cases with metal in their lungs. One was 'awfully thin', but had benefited from accurate localisation of the detritus which had then been removed by McIlroy. The other had an inch of metal in his face and a piece of shell in the lungs, again identified by X-ray.[161] For abdominal cases, localisation was necessary to 'distinguish between the different organs in which the foreign body may lie'.[162] Given initial reluctance during the Great War to operate on abdominal cases, an accurate image could determine whether the patient's condition was hopeless or salvageable. Stoney commented that she had never localised a foreign body which the surgeon had not then gone on to find, so the skill was in great demand under the exigencies of wartime surgery.[163] In her 1917 book *Women of the War*, Barbara McLaren designated such surgical assistance 'invaluable'.[164] Confidence in Stoney's technique was such that during her later post at Royaumont, her value was acknowledged when the 'surgeons ~~refused to operate on~~ wished me to overlook all localisations'.[165] The crossing out here is intriguing in relation to the place of the non-medical radiographer within the surgical team. In contradistinction to Bowlby and Wallace's assessment of the usefulness of the X-ray, surgery did not take place at Royaumont without radiographic confirmation of surgical diagnosis.

The aftercare of patients was complemented, especially at the GNU in Salonika, with therapeutic X-ray treatment. Any scepticism female surgeons had about treating women's malignant disease with rays rather than surgery, as we saw in the last chapter, was not felt when it came to the post-surgical rehabilitation of soldiers. McIlroy was especially passionate about the value of this form of treatment as far as recovery from orthopaedic procedures was concerned. She conveyed her keenness in a letter to the Committee at home. McIlroy believed electro-therapeutic and gymnastic work was 'special' and would 'try to restore the deformed

---

[161] Edith Stoney, NUWSS Scottish Women's Hospitals for Foreign Service: Report XXVIII, Salonika, 14–21 April 1917, Tin 12: Letters from Miss Stoney, Radiographer.
[162] Edith Stoney to Mrs Laurie, London, 16 October 1916, ibid.
[163] Ibid., 17 October 1916.
[164] 'Miss Edith Stoney and Dr Florence Stoney', McLaren, *Women of the War*, pp. 41–5; p. 44.
[165] Edith Stoney to Mrs Laurie, Paris, 7 October 1918, Tin 12. For 'overlook', read 'oversee'.

to a certain extent to a healthy life, and thus build up a little from the
mass of useless lives'. The 'immediate treatment of the wounded' dominated concerns, but what of those recuperating?[166] A whole hut was later
devoted to massage and mecano-therapy when the hospital was moved
to a larger and better site in the autumn of 1917, alongside the establishment of a department for orthopaedics.[167] Verney remarked in an
interview she gave in the 1970s that the physiotherapy unit at Salonika
was 'a new thing. It was the only one in the whole of Salonika and everyone used to come and see us.'[168] While McIlroy felt that Stoney was a
reluctant convert to therapeutic treatment, the radiographer did a great
deal of work in this area and was keen to learn more. When Stoney left
Salonika, she even wrote to Mrs Laurie at home to express her desire to
'have a couple of months to study electric treatment and physical methods with disabled men'.[169] At Salonika, she had been able to treat stiff
joints which required movement to recover mobility. Weight-lifting was
encouraged and Stoney and her assistants set up pulleys and springs and
'ran the engine for electric massage four to five hours most days'.[170] Ioni-
sation was also utilised for the healing of wounds with, as McLaren noted,
'beneficial results'.[171] Unlike the British or French surgeons who could
send their countrymen home for rest and recuperation,[172] the GNU had
to treat 'war weary and nerve racked', predominantly Serbian, men on
site.[173] Specialist Orthopaedic Centres had been set up at home and in
France, but there was nothing for the Serbians, who preferred very much
to be treated near their homeland.[174] For McIlroy and her team surgical
success could be measured only when patients had been rehabilitated to
the best of their abilities. This could be carried out through whatever
means they had at their disposal, no matter how amateurish the devices
or modern the technology.

[166] Dr McIlroy to Mrs Russell, Salonika, 28 January 1917, Tin 42: Circulated Letters,
January 1917.
[167] 'Report on the Work of the Scottish Women's Hospital (Hôpital Auxiliare Bénévole
301, Armée d'Orient)', Tin 42: Circulated Letters 1919 (a).
[168] Typescript of interview with Ruth Verney in September 1977, Tape 477,
WW1/WO/127, LC.
[169] Edith Stoney to Mrs Laurie [no date; June? 1917 from internal evidence], Salonika,
Tin 12: Letters from Miss Stoney, Radiographer.
[170] Edith Stoney, 'N.U.W.S.S. Scottish Women's Hospitals for Foreign Service. Report
XXVIII, Salonika, 14–21 April 1917, Tin 12.
[171] McLaren, *Women of the War*, p. 44.
[172] See Thomas R. Scotland, 'Developments in Orthopaedic Surgery', in Scotland and
Heys, eds., *War Surgery*, pp. 148–77, especially pp. 166–71 for the establishment of
Orthopaedic Centres. For the importance of team work to successful orthopaedic
rehabilitation, see Harrison, *The Medical War*, p. 101.
[173] Edith Stoney to Dr Erskine, London, 30 August 1917, Tin 12.
[174] Dr McIlroy to Mrs Russell, Salonika, 28 January 1917, Tin 42.

In an article written in 1917, Royaumont's radiologist, Agnes Savill, provided a key reason for the final way in which the wartime surgeon was reliant on ancillary members of the surgical team. 'Undoubtedly the most terrible of all the horrors connected with the war which came under the notice of the surgeon', she began, 'is gas gangrene':

Dramatic in the suddenness of its onset, the rapidity of its progress, and the repulsiveness of its too frequently fatal outcome, it has reaped a cruel harvest of our young and vigorous manhood. Throughout the labs of Europe the bacteriologists are working to unravel this sinister problem. Just as tetanus has practically disappeared, so we may hope that gas gangrene will yield before the knowledge of science.[175]

The fact that surgeons were not always capable of spotting gas gangrene, nor predicting where it might arise, rendered them helpless. While bacteriologists worked behind the scenes to develop ways in which surgeons could begin to attack the infection, X-rays could identify the problem before it killed the patient. Both Savill and Stoney were early pioneers of the use of X-ray photography to identify the presence of gas gangrene. As Mrs Laurie wrote admiringly to the latter about the College of Surgeons War Relics Exhibition: 'I was awfully delighted when in London to hear from your sister that you had sent these stereoscopic slides of yours, and that they were quite the earliest in this war, of gas gangrene.'[176] In her *Blackwood's* article of 1918, Collum gave an insight into the fight against the deadly infection, as the whole team battled to save the lives of the 90 per cent of patients who were delivered to them with gas gangrene. Although dramatic, her prose threw the reader headlong into the smells, sights and sounds of the frenetic wartime operating theatre:

it was a nightmare of glaring lights, of appalling stenches of ether and chloroform, and the violent sparking of tired, rapidly hardening X-ray tubes, of scores of wet negatives that were seized upon by their respective surgeons and taken into the hot theatre before they had even had time to be rinsed in the Dark Room. Beneath and beyond the anxiety of saving men's lives there were [*sic*] the undercurrent anxiety of the theatre staff as to whether the boiling of instruments and gloves could be kept level with the rapidity with which the cases were carried in and put on the table, as to whether the gauze and wool and swabs would last! – and with

---

[175] Agnes Savill, 'X-Ray Appearances in Gas Gangrene', *PRSM*, 10 (1917), 20 October 1916 (Electro-Therapeutic Section), 4–16; 4.

[176] Mrs Laurie to Edith Stoney, 15 September 1917, Tin 12: Letters to and from Miss Stoney, Radiographer. See also an unknown, undated cutting about the 'Record of X.Ray Work by a member of the Scottish Women's Hospital', which explains about the 'War Collections of Medical Specimens' exhibition, which was open to professionals and public alike. The article picks out Miss Stoney's slides and skiagrams from Troyes as of especial interest: 'dated 3rd, October 1915' they were 'probably the earliest record for X.Ray of Gas Gangrene'.

us it was anxiety for the life of our hard-worked, over-heated tubes, anxiety to get the gas gangrene plates developed first to persuade them to dry, to keep the cases of each of the six surgeons separate, to see that they did not walk off with the wrong plates – for we had pictures that were almost identical, duplications of names, and such little complications. And it all had to be done in a tearing hurry, at the end of a day that had already lasted anything from ten to eighteen hours, and no mistakes to be made. I do not think we lost a single case from delay in locating the trouble and operating in all that first terrible week of July [1916]. The losses were due to delay in reaching the hospitals.[177]

In a letter to Beatrice Russell, Savill added of the post-Somme rush that the 'photos had to dry all along the wall in the gallery. You can picture the scene – surgeons demanding their photos and I chained to X-ray room!'[178] Both Collum and Savill captured the race against time and the teamwork required in order to treat patients successfully and thwart the spread of gas gangrene.

Identifying gas gangrene was not an easy task. Often the sickly smell gave away its lurking presence, but, as Ivens explained, it was 'the borderline-cases' where surgeons needed the 'most help, for if the infection is deep-seated and clinical signs are not too obvious, one may be tempted to defer amputation until too late'.[179] An X-ray, therefore, as Savill claimed, had a 'prophetic value'. It could both locate and determine the extent of the infection and, consequently, drive surgical intervention.[180] Savill likened the dependence of the surgeon on the radiologist in cases of infection to the way that a physician relied upon the bacteriologist when diphtheria was suspected. Even more precisely, the radiologist could identify different varieties of anaerobe through the appearance of the gas.[181] In similar fashion to the way in which surgeons had learned and relearned their craft in the light of wartime experience, Savill had observed the work of Dr Pech, the radiologist at Creil, the nearby casualty clearing station. Although Savill lauded the X-ray's ability to reveal to the unsuspecting surgeon the presence of gas gangrene,

---

[177] 'Skia', 'A Hospital in France', 622–3.

[178] Agnes Savill to Mrs Russell, Royaumont, 4 July 1916, Tin 12: Scottish Women's Hospitals Royaumont. Copies of Letters Received at Headquarters from July 1915 to October 1916.

[179] Frances Ivens, 'A Clinical Study of Anaërobic Wound Infection, with an Analysis of 107 Cases of Gas Gangrene', *PRSM*, 10 (1917) Section of Surgery: 13 December 1917, 29–110; 30.

According to Collum, Ivens took off two weeks in order to go to London and read this paper. This was the 'only' time she took off during her service with the SWH, which had run from December 1914 to the demobilisation of the Royaumont Unit in January 1919. See 'N.U.W.S.S. Scottish Women's Hospitals. Decoration of 17 SWH Members of Royaumont and Villers-Cotterets Staff', *Common Cause*, X.507 (27 December 1918), 443–7; 443.

[180] Savill, 'X-Ray Appearances', 16; 5.   [181] Ibid., p. 5.

she warned that it was not infallible. Of the 100 plates which had been taken, 67 per cent were useful. The equipment could let the radiologist down, for example, as plates broke or images were underdeveloped. X-ray technology was still in its infancy, barely two decades old. Certain parts of the body were difficult to photograph, such as the trunk and the hand. The former was too dense; in the latter the amount of bone could conceal the outline of the gas.[182] Yet, as the surgical team at Royaumont and elsewhere learned, while one discipline could ensure misdiagnosis, taken together bacteriology, radiography and surgery could form sufficiently accurate evidence for prompt and life-saving action.

Illustrations 4.2, 4.3 and 4.4, all taken at Royaumont, were just three examples extolling the value of this triple alliance in the fight against gas gangrene. The first example, Illustration 4.2, was a case which did not appear to be severe upon admission. There was little swelling of his forearm, his wound was easily opened and the foreign body removed without a problem. Although Savill did not realise it at the time and discovered only later, the X-ray revealed striation (linear bands) 30 hours before the clinical signs, when the man's forearm was cold, swollen, discoloured and immediately amputated.[183] In this instance, the X-ray predicted the danger before symptoms manifested themselves. Illustration 4.3 was 'Le Soldat G.', a 21-year-old Frenchman who was injured in July by a shell, with a fracture of his left tibia and fibula. He was in a bad condition from admittance, and his left thigh was amputated within three hours; from the head of the tibia, the surgeons removed fractured bone with *capote*, which was an infected piece of clothing the shell carried into the wound.[184] Previous X-ray examination had indicated gas round the embedded shell, which was deep-seated, as well as gas bubbles in the right knee-joint. The bacteriological report confirmed the results. 'G.' was subsequently treated for a week after his operation with a variety of serums to counter the infections; after two injections *Bacillus perfrigens* disappeared from his blood. He was healed by the middle of November.[185] In 'G.''s case, a combination of surgery and serum led to his recovery. Illustration 4.4, 'Le Sergent V.', was wounded in February 1916 by shell, suffering a penetrating wound of the left knee-joint and a perforating wound of the right eyeball, as well as penetration and fracture of the ethmoid. The foreign body was not localised in the eye, while the shell in the knee-joint

---

[182] Ibid., p. 6. For early difficulties in observing certain parts of the body and interpreting findings, see Thomas and Banerjee, *The History of Radiology*, pp. 77–81.

[183] Savill, 'X-Ray Appearances', 16.

[184] Ivens' definition in 'A Clinical Study', 31.

[185] 'Case 31: An Analysis of 107 Cases of Gas Gangrene', ibid., 86. Also discussed in the body of the article, 50–1.

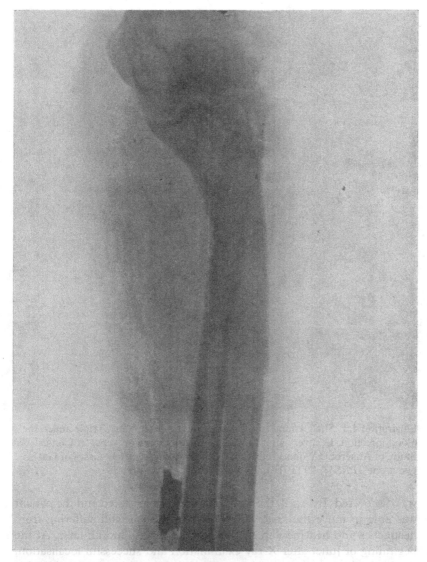

Illustration 4.2 'Coarse striation. Skiagram two days after wounds. (Artery injured and red degenerated muscle). On third day arm blue, cold and swollen. Amputation saved life', Agnes Savill, 'X-Ray Appearances in Gas Gangrene', *PRSM*, 10 (1917), 4–16; 15.

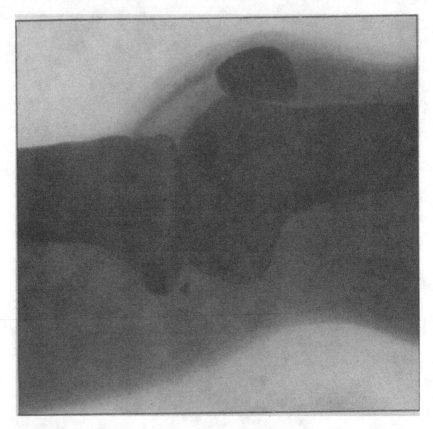

Illustration 4.3 'Shell wound of right knee-joint. Gas in joint. Triple anaerobic blood infection. Recovery after serum treatment', Frances Ivens, 'A Clinical Study of Anaërobic Wound Infection, with an Analysis of 107 Cases of Gas Gangrene', *PRSM*, 10 (1917), 29–110; 70.

was discovered. By April, the wounds were almost healed and the patient was able to move the knee well. However, he was still suffering from headaches and heaviness in the back of his head a month later. At the beginning of June, after X-ray examination and successful localisation, the foreign body was removed through the empty orbit, with considerable haemorrhage from the patient's nose and throat and a discharge of pus from the sinus post-operation. Bacteriological reports from the piece of shell revealed streptococci and *Bacillus perfringens*.[186] The latent nature of the infection in this case showed that it was never advisable to be

---

[186] 'Case L.', ibid., pp. 48–9.

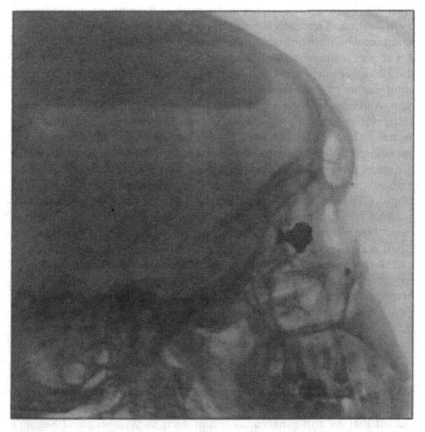

Illustration 4.4 'Latent infection. Shell removed from ethmoid four months after receipt of wound. *Bacillus perfringens* and streptococci present', Ivens, 'A Clinical Study', 76.

complacent in the theatre of war. Although the object was not located for four months, if it had not been, and even though he was effectively recovering, the patient would have died.

The willingness of the female surgeons and their team at Royaumont to put their faith in experimental treatments to combat infection was important to the way in which their work in France was viewed. Royaumont's organisation and direction impressed the Parisian Pasteur Institute's Chef de Laboratoire, Professor Michel Weinberg, who, as the *Common Cause* exclaimed, with its political angle fully to the forefront, 'could not imagine any activity on the part of women that would so effectively further the cause of the women's movement as the work of the Scottish Women's

Hospital'.[187] Weinberg's belief in the work at Royaumont was indicated by his testing of specially developed serum on patients infected with gas gangrene who were brought to the hospital.[188] 'Le Soldat G.' (Illustration 4.3 above) featured in Weinberg and Séguin's 1918 book, where ten of the 126 cases noted are from Royaumont.[189] While 'G' benefited from a combination of treatment, Weinberg and Séguin's serum allowed others, who would certainly have lost limbs from the condition, to receive more conservative surgical procedures. As Leila Henry noted in her memoirs, Weinberg had chosen Royaumont after visiting hundreds of French military hospitals for his experimental research.[190] In 1918, Ivens lamented the slight progress made regarding the preventive treatment of gas gangrene by serum. As she had already established an effective working relationship with the Pasteur Institute and had used their serum with success, Ivens continued to test the value of this treatment on relevant cases. Her results were published in the *BMJ* in October 1918.[191]

Unlike earlier trials, which had often been carried out on patients who had already received some form of initial treatment elsewhere, the majority of soldiers seen between March and September 1918 received their first operation at Royaumont. With the assistance of bacteriological analysis, Ivens observed how many of her cases were suffering from multiple infections with different forms of bacillus, due to the conditions of the battlefield. She expected that mixed or polyvalent serums would provide the best means of a cure and, therefore, utilised three different preparations: a mélange serum of Weinberg; a polyvalent one of Leclainche and Vallée, who had also willingly provided a sufficient quantity for the hospital; and a mixture of the two. The results were impressive. Ivens concluded that an anti-gangrenous serum such as Weinberg and Séguin's could prevent gas gangrene if given before or during surgery. Even in the most serious and advanced cases, when used in sufficient quantity, it could prove of great value as a disintoxicating agent. Leclainche and Vallée's polyvalent serum had a marked influence on those cases who were also suffering with streptococcal infections. By diluting serums with

[187] 'An Appreciation of Royaumont', *Common Cause*, VII.361 (10 March 1916), 633.

[188] For a brief mention of the serum in the British medical press, see 'A Serum for Use in Cases of Gas Gangrene', *Lancet*, 187.4822 (29 January 1916), 257.

[189] M. Weinberg et P. Séguin, *La Gangrène gazeuse* (Paris: Masson et Cie, 1918), pp. 371–2; pp. 384–97.

[190] Henry, *Reminiscences*, p. 29. The impact of such work at the hospital was such that Henry would later write her PhD thesis on the effect of serums on gas gangrene. See Lydia Manley Henry, 'The Treatment of War Wounds by Serum Therapy', PhD thesis, University of Sheffield, 1920.

[191] Frances Ivens, 'The Preventive and Curative Treatment of Gas Gangrene by Mixed Serums', *BMJ*, 2.3016 (19 October 1918), 425–7.

saline, Ivens and her team had discovered that the anaphylactic reaction witnessed in some instances became extremely rare.[192] Although there was very rarely time to analyse microbe reports before surgery due to the necessity of operating on most patients as soon as possible, tailoring the results to the serum to be given was of great advantage. Finally, Ivens recommended that when a secondary operation was required, another fractional dose should be administered as a preliminary. Excision of diseased bone or tissue, coupled with the use of a serum, reduced dramatically the need for amputation. This combination ensured that Royaumont had the lowest amputation and the lowest mortality rate in the area, which, consequently, led the French military to direct the severest cases to Royaumont.[193] Through their willingness to take a risk, the women had proved their openness to experimentation, in addition to enhancing their professional reputation through the success of the surgical team.

'Bons Soins'

This final section will consider how female surgeons were received by their charges. Flora Murray's *Women as Army Surgeons* (1920) was keen to stress how receptive the soldiers were to their novel surroundings. Indeed, she claimed, at the Hôtel Claridge in Paris, 'they trusted the women as they would have trusted men – passing the bullets which had been extracted from their persons from bed to bed and pronouncing the surgeon to be "wonderfully clever"'.[194] Unlike their more suspicious superiors or the incredulous press who came to see whether women really operated alone, the ordinary soldier accepted their lot without complaint. The encounter between the two was, however, open to satire. A *Punch* cartoon from 1915 (Illustration 4.5) imagined a comic outcome when an 'eminent woman surgeon' and suffragist met a familiar patient, a wounded Guardsman who had once been a police constable. According to Murray, such a situation actually occurred at Wimereux when a 'suffragist friend' recognised a patient. '"I remember you", she said. "You arrested me once in Whitehall". "I wouldn't have mentioned it, Miss", he replied with embarrassment. "We'll let byegones be byegones"'.[195] Both versions of the policeman were sheepish and squirming, but both accept the woman in the professional role of the surgeon. No animosity existed in either recounting of the tale.

---

[192] See Ivens, 'A Clinical Study', 63–4, for previous observations concerning anaphylactic reactions.
[193] Henry, *Reminiscences*, p. 29.
[194] Murray, *Women as Army Surgeons*, p. 39.   [195] Ibid., p. 100.

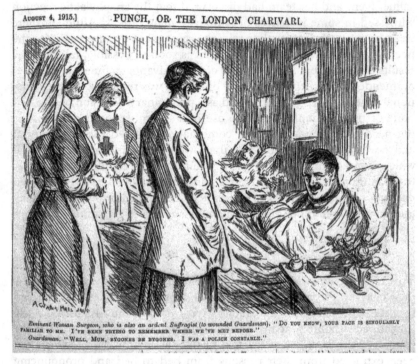

Eminent Woman Surgeon, who is also an ardent Suffragist (to wounded Guardsman). "Do you know, your face is singularly familiar to me. I've been trying to remember where we've met before."
Guardsman. "Well, Mum, bygones be bygones. I was a police constable."

Illustration 4.5 'Woman Surgeon and Suffragette', *Punch* 149 (4 August 1915), 107, Wellcome Library, London.

Curiously, there was, however, a tendency in Murray's account to infantilise the patient and draw disproportionate attention to the motherly aspect of the female surgeon's role. The cases in Paris were described as showing delightful and encouraging enthusiasm for the hospital: 'When they got well and went away, it was like seeing boys go back to school.'[196] They received 'comfort in the presence of women and repose in the case lavished upon them'.[197] While soldiers were duly mothered, male colleagues who focused solely on the interesting aspect of wounds, bypassing the patient himself, came in for strict admonition. Murray recounted the visit of a 'celebrated neurologist', who was an even 'more trying type of visitor' than the 'jocular and semi-familiar' kind which female professionals so disliked: '"I want to see some good head cases. Have you got anything shot through the brain? Any paralysis? No fractures of skull! Nothing good. You don't seem to have much in. Deaf

---

[196] Ibid., p. 40.   [197] Ibid., p. 42.

and dumb! Hm – yes, that's not bad. But I only want to see head cases".'
Murray utilised this visit to stress two things about the very different attitude of the woman surgeon towards her patient. Firstly, the distinguished
visitor treated patients as if 'they were goods on a counter', symptoms
without feelings. And, secondly, by pointing out his appallingly unpro-
fessional bedside-manner, Murray cleverly enhanced the 'human side'
displayed by the women themselves.[198]

This presentation was not confined to the WHC. Collum's *Blackwood's* articles about the activities of the SWH focused upon the close
relationship between woman surgeon and patient. *Common Cause* also
received details about endowed beds, so they could show their readers who was benefiting from their subscription.[199] Royaumont took in
patients from all over France, as well as French North and West Africa.
Collum described the way in which two of their charges reacted to surgery
and Ivens, their surgeon:

One broad-nosed, woolly-headed giant, black as ebony, awakened from the anaesthetic (which drugged these coloured men much less deeply than their white
comrades) on the operating table; he looked round in abject fear, though the
instruments were all in the tray and the orderly had almost finished bandaging
him; then his eyes lighted on the chief surgeon (divested of her gloves and gauze
mask), who, as it happened, had dressed him in the ward and evidently gained
his confidence. A black arm shot out towards her as she made towards the door,
and clutched her hand, which he grasped and laid against his cheek, closing his
eyes contentedly once more as he murmured, 'Moi connais toi'. Another, whose
arm had just been amputated, and who, inadvertently coming round as he was
being borne on the stretcher back to his ward, suddenly leapt from it and made
as if to bolt. The head surgeon came out of the theatre, when he immediately
calmed down, and, letting her take his remaining arm, walked docilely – and
quite capably – upstairs and back to his bed.[200]

If we put aside contemporary racial stereotypes, the patients were devoted
to their surgeon.[201] No longer garbed in her professional uniform, Ivens
was simply a gentle mother-figure to her patients, despite the far from delicate procedures she had just performed. This public image of patients'
innocence was in direct opposition to the bloody, gangrenous stench

---

[198] Ibid., p. 57.

[199] For one example, see Cicely Hamilton, 'Some of Our Patients at Royaumont', *Common
Cause*, VII.348 (10 December 1915), 476, which provided information about five
endowed beds. This included details of the patient's background, his occupation, his
military career and his injury.

[200] 'Skia', 'The First Week', 344.

[201] In contradistinction to this, the orderly Agnes Anderson remarked that 'once a soldier
comes into hospital he is merely a patient and is treated as such regardless of nationality
or colour'. See Miss Agnes Anderson to Mrs Russell, 25 June 1918, Tin 42: Circulated
Letters 1918 a (January–June), SWHC.

of their actual condition, which was concealed from the audience at home. As described when Villers-Cotterets was besieged with seriously wounded in May 1918: 'Black blankets on the beds. On such were men dying, screaming unconscious and delirious.'[202] Women surgeons were dealing not with saints or infants, but with badly injured, confused and frightened men. Elizabeth Courtauld remarked that in April 1918 many of the cases 'are so smelly that to breathe fresh air at intervals is refreshing', even when it was disagreeably cold and snowing.[203] Doris Stevenson, the orderly who had objected to the way in which Royaumont was run, had taken issue with a patient who had 'got up and simply made use of the floor' in the ward, rather than requesting assistance, which an orderly then had to clear up.[204] The ward sister retaliated, stating that the man was 'a head case operated on late the night previous and was not responsible'. He was now 'one of the most helpful and obedient in the Ward'.[205] Men were reduced to children in the messy reality of postoperative conditions, but not in the angelic way they were represented in the press.

Similarly, in a special SWH edition of *Common Cause*, there was little sign of disease and death. Instead, it was the 'divine fingers' of 'the nymphs of Royaumont' which were being extolled by a patient in print.[206] 'Au Fées du Royaumont' by Sergent Auguste Marius Treilles marvelled at the enchanting, fairy-tale atmosphere of the hospital:

> The best-tempered steel of deadly weapons,
> Is transformed in your hands into humanitarian tears,
> And your delicate gentle fingers Miss Nicholson.
> Are thrust into the palpitating body without fear,
> While in a dream Miss Ivens, Miss Heyworth,
> Under the confident spell that your science inspires,
> I see you on waking searching for that smile,
> Comforting balm on the bleeding wounds
> You compassionate women shed uninterrupted.

Treilles' poem was a rare glimpse into the way in which the patient saw the female surgeon. His lines were full of contrasts, which rendered surgery, and by extension the surgeon, simultaneously brutal and delicate, bloody

---

202 Extract from a letter to an unknown recipient from Miss Florence Anderson, Royaumont, 1 June 1918, Tin 42: Circulated Letters: November 1917–April 1918 (a).
203 Courtauld to Ruth, Royaumont, 25 April 1918, WW1/WO/023, LC.
204 Miss Stevenson to Dr Russell, Paris, 12 June 1918, Tin 42: Circulated Letters 1918 a (January–June).
205 Jean Thom (Sister), 'In reference to the statement made by Orderly Stevenson about an Arab using the floor as a lavatory', [undated; June 1918], Tin 42.
206 Sergent Auguste Marius Treilles, 'Au Fées du Royaumont', *Common Cause*, VII.344 (12 November 1915), 397. My translation.

yet kind. Indeed, in spite of the 'gentle' approach, there was only confidence in the procedure, both through the patient's reassurance, but,
most importantly, in the focus and 'thrust' shown by the surgeon herself. The latter operated with professional skill, supported by scientific
understanding. Treilles sought to elevate the French soldier, by stressing
his courage and valour, but he also infantilised the injured as 'our dear
little wounded', over whom the Royaumont staff watched with care all
night and day. Constant devotion, a combination of 'touching zeal' and
'maternal care', concluded Treilles, characterised the hospital and the
way in which it operated. While the women were ethereal beings, they
were also godmothers, looking benevolently over their charges. It was this
mêlée of professionalism and womanliness which clearly impressed both
the female surgeons at Royaumont and the *Common Cause* as supporter
of and mouthpiece for their endeavours.

Junior Surgeon at Royaumont, Leila Henry, kept the letters sent to her
by her patients, which gave a very personal insight into the relationship
between surgeon and soldier.[207] Henry was evidently keen to keep in
touch with those she had treated and from the tone of the letters it was
she who usually instigated the correspondence by evidently asking them
about the progress of their recovery. Taken as a whole, they focused on a
number of related themes. The same words of praise came up again and
again, so that, fascinatingly, if it was not known that Henry was a surgeon
at Royaumont, the letters would give little indication of this fact. Unlike
Treilles, whose published poem extolled the multifaceted women surgeons, without forgetting their professional achievements, the letters sent
to Henry rarely mentioned the success of operations. Instead, they lauded
the care, kindness, devotion, happy memories, spoiling, and food –
usually in contrast to the lack elsewhere. Léon Dramez, for example,
was moved to Chartres along with a number of other former Royaumont
patients, where he lamented the 'very French treatment' he experienced
there.[208] 'Deep respect' also appeared in a number of letters, but it was
not clear if this was for anything other than a usual, formal way to end a
letter. Some correspondents referred to Henry as 'Doctoresse', but only
one as 'Docteur'. Indeed, this man, whose letters survived from a period
of leave Henry took in February and March 1918, was still being treated

---

[207] All the letters are in French, although many are ungrammatical, accents are sparely
used, and the spelling is poor; the handwriting is often difficult to read, due, undoubtedly, to the patient's injuries. Soldiers' names are especially unclearly written in the
form of signatures and the reader has to piece together evidence from the correspondence of other wounded men in order to identify the writer. See collection of soldiers'
letters to Henry, many with extant envelopes, held in WW1/WO/054, LC.

[208] Léon Dramez to Leila Henry, Chartres, 1 January 1919,

by her at the time, whereas the others had been moved and Royaumont closed by the time they wrote to her. H. Wetzel's letter was identical in tone to one received by Louise McIlroy from a grateful patient in 1919. Wetzel was the only correspondent who described how Henry 'saved' him and that it was thanks to her that he was operated upon in time.[209] While McIlroy's correspondent, E. Fontaine, did not explicitly make this point, his implication was the same.[210] Timely surgery had ensured that both would once again be able to embrace their families.

For Fontaine and Wetzel, Henry, McIlroy and their colleagues reunited families, restoring men to their wives and children. As Fontaine added, his wife was confounded by the way in which foreigners served France and her army. For this inexplicable devotion, she prayed daily for the protection of all English and Scottish women.[211] Not one convalescent soldier in extant letters thanked their surgeon for preservation of life and limb for a return to work. Instead the focus was solely private and familial. Gaston Montlouis, a patient of Frances Ivens at Royaumont, wrote to express his gratefulness for the 'assiduous care and devotion which has surrounded him for the five long months [he spent] on his bed of pain'.[212] Now in a rehabilitation centre, where he hoped to spend no more than a month, he looked forward to returning home to his family. Along with many other correspondents, and as 'one of your wounded', he would never forget Royaumont. These phrases appeared numerous times in the letters of former patients and showed how the wounded characterised themselves as part of the wider Royaumont family, with the benevolent matriarch, Ivens, overseeing everything and caring for them all. Indeed, as Paul Huguenin wrote to Henry at the beginning of 1918 before he left to recuperate with his family, France should recognise and reward the SWH for the temporary, but good 'care of its children'.[213] Whether it was having the women around them which made the hospitals resemble home or not, wounded had 'been known to ask to be sent to Royaumont, and one of the young patients asked if he could be evacuated to "another Royaumont"'.[214] When Henry was on leave in early 1918, 'Blanche Ward' was not the same without her; while there was no news to report from the Blanche family according to a letter sent from J.H.

---

[209] H. Wetzel to Leila Henry, Royaumont, 28 February 1918. He also writes on 28 February.

[210] E. Fontaine to Louise McIlroy, Ivry, 27 February 1919, Tin 42: Circulated Letters 1919 (a), SWHC.

[211] Ibid.

[212] Gaston Montlouis to Dr Ivens, Le Mans, 1 January 1919, Tin 42.

[213] Paul Huguenin to Leila Henry, Royaumont, 28 February 1918, WW1/WO/054, LC.

[214] Henry, *Reminiscences*, p. 29, ibid.

Sagnes later in March 1918.[215] Another soldier, back in Algeria, looked fondly on the 'Blanche family', even when returned to his own.[216] Others were comforted by the presence of their ward comrades when they were moved to another hospital. Jules Delavigne, for example, noted that he had arrived at Chartres at 2 a.m., but that he was with Labat, Dramez and several others: all of whom regretted leaving Royaumont.[217] Within the wider Royaumont community, smaller 'families' established themselves, which, in turn, created little enclaves with their own ward surgeon to champion. Even at the end of the war, with the prospect of a return home to anticipate, former patients missed the camaraderie and 'bons soins' of their own particular 'salle'.

Conclusion

Alongside patient gratitude, formal recognition was given to female surgical teams. Louisa Garrett Anderson and Flora Murray were named Commanders of the British Empire; Frances Ivens, Elizabeth Courtauld, Leila Henry, Edith Stoney and Louisa-Aldrich Blake (Illustration 4.6) received the Croix de Guerre; while Louise McIlroy, Isabel Emslie and Edith Stoney received the Order of St Sava.[218] Courtauld compared her position at the end of the war to that of her patients. '[L]ike the rest of the world', she mused, 'I shall never forget these years, but how differently to our poor mutilated men!': 'I come out of them well fed and not a scratch, and having had congenial work to do, no sacrifice at all on my part, all on theirs'.[219] The description of tough, challenging wartime surgery as 'congenial' here was typical of the way in which the female surgical teams discussed in this chapter saw their position in the Great War. It suited them and, despite all protestations to the contrary, they suited it.

On return home from wartime and post-conflict service with the SWH in Salonika and Serbia, Isabel Emslie asked herself: 'Had I been wasting

---

[215] H. Wetzel to Leila Henry, Salle Blanche, Royaumont, 3 March 1918; J.H. Sagnes to Leila Henry, Royaumont, 9 March 1918, WW1/WO/054, LC.

[216] L. Campasse [?] to Leila Henry, Algère, 18 November 1918, WW1/WO/054, LC. Carden-Coyne's *The Politics of Wounds* explores similarly and at greater length the relationships between patients.

[217] Jules Delavigne to Leila Henry, Chartres, 1 January 1919, WW1/WO/054, LC.

[218] See, for example, Murray, *Women as Army Surgeons*, pp. 134–5 and p. 258, for the titles given to the Women's Hospital Corps Team; 'N.U.W.S.S. Scottish Women's Hospitals. Decoration of 17 SWH Members of Royaumont and Villers-Cotterets Staff, on December 13th, With Croix de Guerre, by General Nourisson', *Common Cause*, 27 December 1918, 443–7 and letter from Courtauld to Ruth, Royaumont, 13 December 1918, WW1/WO/023, LC; Dr McIlroy to Miss May, 18 January 1917, Tin 42: Circulated Letters, 1917–1918, SWHC.

[219] Courtauld to Ruth, 14 November 1918, WW1/WO/023, LC.

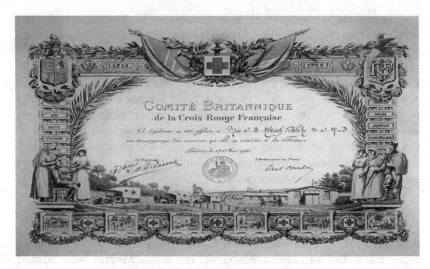

Illustration 4.6 Louisa Brandreth Aldrich-Blake: Comité Britannique de la Croix Rouge Française. Diploma Presented for service to France, 10 May 1920, WMS 5796, Wellcome Library, London.

my time?'[220] The question was essentially rhetorical. Initial doubt gave way to surety. Emslie was convinced that her war responsibilities had been 'experience' and, thus, could never be wasted. As we saw in the introduction to this book, since her student days, she had possessed a 'hankering after the practice of surgery', but this passion had died down and 'was now at rest, having been so amply fulfilled'. Emslie was now 'well satisfied'.[221] In 1939, at the beginning of another conflict, Frances Ivens drew attention to the fact that her research on gas gangrene had been beneficial to her later career. The unmistakable putrid odour had 'since enabled me to recognise the presence of gas infection in a neglected maternity case'.[222] Experience, which saved lives, was certainly not squandered in this case. Women surgeons relished the opportunities that the Great War provided and took advantage of the ways in which new possibilities opened up to them. The pursuit of these chances led them and their teams all over Europe, into dangerous territory and unknown working environments. As SWH Honorary Treasurer, Mrs Laurie, exclaimed to Edith Stoney:

---

[220] Hutton, *Memories*, p. 203.   [221] Ibid.
[222] Frances Ivens-Knowles, 'Treatment of Gas Gangrene', *BMJ*, 2.4116 (25 November 1939), 1058.

as for what all you Members of Staff have endured for the sake of your professional zeal, neither the cold and discomfort of Ghevgali [*sic*] nor the sweltering heat, malaria and dysent[e]ry and all the other horrors of Salonique, seem to have hindered you in doing such wonderfully good work for your patients.[223]

'Professional zeal', identified by both Laurie and the poet-patient Treilles, carried many a surgeon, male or female, through the Great War. So many accounts of women's work between 1914 and 1918 commented on the ways in which women were prevented from continuing with surgical careers when they returned home. But, for many, like Emslie, enough was enough. An opportunity had been grasped with both hands and knowing from the outset that this was not sustainable back in Britain did not depress those involved. The administrator at Royaumont, Miss Loudon, marvelled at Frances Ivens being a 'cormorant for work', returning again and again, tirelessly and hungrily, to the operating table, seeking for more.[224] This surgical greed was satiated during the Great War. When the women surgeons from Royaumont or from Salonika looked back, it was not with regret at opportunities lost. It was with pride in chances taken and surgical work sustained. At a dinner given in her honour in May 1919, Ivens claimed very simply that 'the work she had done had been done because she liked it'.[225] 'The motto for our women's work should be that last word – "efficiency". Don't you agree with me?', Florence Stoney asked Mrs Laurie.[226] During the Great War, women proved that they could operate inside the theatre of war and do so efficiently.

---

[223] Mrs Laurie to Edith Stoney, Edinburgh, 20 November 1917, Tin 12: Letters to and from Miss Stoney, Radiographer.
[224] Miss Loudon to Mrs Laurie, Royaumont, 13 August 1915, Tin 12: Copies of Letters received at Headquarters. From July 1915 to October 1916.
[225] 'The Women Surgeons at Royaumont', *BMJ*, 1.3048 (31 May 1919), 681.
[226] Florence Stoney to Mrs Laurie, Fulham Military Hospital, 8 March 1916, Tin 12: Letters to and from Miss Stoney, Radiographer.

In the March 1917 edition of the *London (Royal Free Hospital) School of Medicine for Women Magazine,* an anonymous poem expressed frustration at being confined to the home front during wartime:

A Lament

I wish I were a doctor bold,
Adoctoring at the front!
But as it is I'm feeling sold,
And want to do a stunt.

My friends who're at the front by now
Are wreathed in happy smiles;
A halo rests on every brow –
You see the shine for miles.

No horrid doubts disturb their rest,
A gentle peace surrounds,
They operate with happy zest,
Or keep the germs in bounds.

My job's their work in circles tame,
A far inferior lot,
And if you think it's all the same,
I firmly say it's not.

Then do you wonder if I scold,
Or yearn to do a stunt?
I wish I were a doctor bold,
Adoctoring at the front![1]

Even if those at home and those serving in Europe performed similar surgery, the surroundings in which they did so were different. For those left behind, work was tame and inferior when compared to that of their bolder sisters. Despite living and working in the theatre of war, gentleness,

---

[1] Anon., 'A Lament', *L(RFH)SMWM,* XII.66 (March 1916), 13.

peacefulness and an angelic calm pervaded the surgery carried out there. Indeed, it was the dazzling shine of frontline achievements which lifted the brave above mere mortals. Such beatific serenity provoked this writer into wishing herself far away from the home front. But her crossness and doubts were combined with something more intriguing. The use of the very recently coined slang term 'stunt' in this context is worth exploring further.[2] Repeated twice here, it encapsulated the yearning of the writer to join her colleagues. That she viewed their actions as 'stunts', however, explained her frustration at the widespread attention they received and the celebratory laurels they garnered. Work at home simply could not compete with such showy and novel escapades.

This final chapter will turn to the woman surgeon on the home front, a more neglected figure, as the writer of 'A Lament' implied, than her counterpart closer to the battlefield. This is not to claim, of course, that she was not as vital to the war effort. While 'A Lament' disparaged the inequality between the two arenas, by so doing the anonymous author effectively focused attention back upon those left in Britain and asked her readers to reassess their worth and value. Was their situation 'lamentable'? Was 'Adoctoring' to civilians less important than treating the military? As male and female doctors rushed to join official and unofficial organisations across Europe to provide medical and surgical care for the wounded, attention had turned by 1915 to the growing dearth of practitioners at home. As Ian Whitehead has calculated, by 1918, over half of Britain's doctors were serving with the forces; civil conscription for practitioners of 55 and under had been introduced the same year in order to combat shortages at the front.[3] The corresponding reduction in the number of medical students was also a cause for concern. Many of those already in university had joined up, leaving their studies to be resumed at an indefinite future date. Additionally, however, those expected to enter medical schools were increasingly turning to the army rather than to scholarship, afraid to miss the action, but also doing their patriotic duty at the front rather than languishing with their books at home. Medicine required at least five years of study and the numbers willing to devote themselves to such an occupation while there was a war

---

[2] The *OED* notes the first use of this term as 1917 and relates it to aerial performance: stunt v.3: http://www.oed.com/view/Entry/192182?rskey=a8eLnM&result=6&isAdvanced= false#eid. See also Julie Coleman, *A History of Cant and Slang Dictionaries. Volume III: 1859–1936* (Oxford: Oxford University Press, 2008), for a grimly humorous definition from an Australian soldiers' magazine, which stresses that while stunts are usually successful, because of the element of surprise, 'a large scale stunt', or a '"push"' does not count success as 'essential', p. 233.

[3] Whitehead, *Doctors in the Great War*, p. 1; p. 83.

going on were falling dramatically. The prospect of there being too few medical practitioners to serve the contemporary civilian population, as well as the possibility of an even more chronic shortage in the future, led to desperate quests for solutions in the medical and lay press to a worsening problem.

There was one sector of the profession, of course, which had not seen a reduction in numbers: medical women. They could not fight, but were they capable of holding the fort while the men were away? It was to them that attention, early on in the conflict, turned. In this chapter, the experience of several women surgeons at all stages of their career on the home front during the Great War will be explored, considering student life, opportunities for newly-qualified women in house-surgeon posts, as well as those experienced in their surgical craft, who were given unprecedented access to disciplines and patients they had never encountered before. Finally, I will consider the realisation during wartime of the South London Hospital for Women and Children. This chapter will examine how women made themselves indispensable to the public, taking advantage of vacancies within medical services in Britain to expand their professional abilities. They were considerably aided by the press in this endeavour; the long-held antagonism towards medical women forgotten in the face of contemporary exigency. Although newspapers and periodicals, both lay and medical, were largely encouraging, as in all walks of life, they were correspondingly keen to stress the temporality of women's professional dominance at home. As the last chapter made clear, it is important to remember that this temporary situation was one into which women in Britain entered with their eyes open. Uncertainties about the length of the war ensured that it was necessary simply to do what one could when one could do it. Hope was there for future change in the ways medical women could operate at home, but it was curtailed by the knowledge that positions were contingent upon the prolongation of the conflict and the absence of male colleagues. Medical women were to act as 'locum tenens for wartime', as the *Times* put it succinctly at the beginning of 1915.[4] Despite this, the press and even some of the more idealistic medical women suffered from collective amnesia during the Great War, unable to imagine a time before women doctors and medical students became vital at home. Opportunities in areas previously considered out of bounds forced many to admit they had no idea why women

---

[4] 'Women Doctors. Enlarged Field of Service. Medical Practice in War Time', *Times*, 22 January 1915, in *London School of Medicine for Women and Royal Free Hospital Press Cuttings, Volume V: Sept 1915–Oct 1920*, H72/SM/Y/02/005, LMA. Future references will be shortened to *LSMWRFHPC*.

had not been allowed more leeway before. More cynical members of the profession knew otherwise. The war might change attitudes in some instances, but over 60 years of struggle would not be erased in a few short months. How these changes and the challenges they brought were experienced by those who encountered them will provide an insight into the ways in which women surgeons could operate during wartime.

Student Life

'The girl who now chooses medicine as her profession is in a much more satisfactory position than the previous students', claimed the *Lady* in 1917: '[s]hould she prefer to study entirely with girls she can still do so, but should she be in favour of co-education the door is open to her'.[5] In a *Lady's Pictorial* article entitled, aptly, 'Out of the Rut', S. Beatrice Pemberton concluded that '[g]irls may rest assured that in choosing' a medical career 'they are choosing the path of the true patriot'.[6] This first section will explore the position of the woman medical student between 1914 and 1918, focusing primarily on the LSMW. War had opened many doors for the aspirant medical woman eager to emerge from the rut of a listless existence. As Louisa Garrett Anderson informed her LSMW student audience in October 1917, expectations for this generation were high. In conclusion to a stirring inaugural, which must have terrified and enthralled the new intake in equal measure, she emphasised their responsibilities: '[w]ork for the school; work for women; work for medicine, and for England'.[7] The choice of speaker that year cannot have been anything but deliberate. Now in charge of a military hospital in Endell Street, the achievements of women surgeons such as Garrett Anderson were lauded in the popular and medical press alike. Such exciting surgical work, whether carried out by the WHC or the SWH, both at home and abroad, proved inspirational for large numbers of young women, excited at the scope promised for meaningful service.

Those already in training, alarmed at the departure of male friends and colleagues, had first-hand experience of the war's effect on medical work and the opportunities they provided for women. Ruth Verney, who had begun her studies in Manchester in 1912, was just about to sit the second MB at Christmas 1914. With disappearance of the male teaching staff to the front, students were taught by demonstrators and

[5] 'New Careers for Women. V. How to Become a Woman Doctor', *Lady*, 22 March 1917, in *LSMWRFHPC*, *Vol. 5*.

[6] S. Beatrice Pemberton, 'Out of the Rut II: Women as Doctors and Dispensers', *Lady's Pictorial*, 3 June 1916, 71, in *LSMWRFHPC*, *Vol. 5*.

[7] 'Inaugural Address', *L(RFH)SMWM*, XII.68 (November 1917), 76–81; 81.

senior students, if they were taught at all. Soon, even the latter had left. When she was interviewed in the 1970s, Verney told the story of a 'Mr White', who was 'very able' and 'the best man' academically: '[q]uite exceptional'. He went 'straight off and he was killed very rapidly [. . .] He was such a brilliant student and one or two others insisted on going but the rest of them were all stopped from going and told they must qualify.'[8] The absence of authority had a stimulating effect on Verney and her friends. They might have had 'very little teaching', but soon began to use their own initiative, by doing their own ward rounds and observing cases which interested them. On the wards, Verney witnessed the sufferings of 'a great many soldiers' who needed to be operated upon and learned much from the haphazard way in which she finished her education. Helena Lowenfeld, on the other hand, was at the end of her studies at the LSMW when the war began. Alongside a number of fellow male senior students, her final qualification was rushed through at the end of 1914. This was because the Army would not grant commissions to those who were not fully qualified; the same attitude, as Whitehead has noted, maintained by the GMC which insisted upon 'the profession's determination that standards be maintained'.[9] When interviewed in the 1970s, Lowenfeld described the 'emergency finals exam' for the MRCS LRCP in late 1914.[10] The action would 'lighten the difficulties' caused by the disappearance of mostly male junior house officers to the RAMC or the ranks by providing new candidates for the posts. Women graduates were, therefore, particularly desirable assets. Of Polish ancestry, but with a German-sounding name, the only suspicions about Lowenfeld's abilities were centred on her spying skills. By taking her British passport with her to the graduation ceremony, the representatives of the Colleges of Surgeons and Physicians were forced to concentrate on Helena Lowenfeld's educational achievements.

If the war encouraged women to qualify in order to fill the gaps provided by absent colleagues, it also brought to the fore a concern which had been dividing medical women since the beginning of the century. Co-education was effectively forced upon male-only medical schools after 1914 because they were desperate to defend their own financial interests by boosting dwindling student numbers. As the *Manchester Guardian* noted cynically in 1920, '[f]ees weighed heavily in the balance against

---

8   Typescript of interview with Ruth Verney in September 1977, Tape 476, WW1/WO/127, LC.
9   Whitehead, *Doctors in the Great War*, p. 94.
10 Helena Wright [née Lowenfeld], written transcript entitled 'Incidents during 1914–18 War' (from interview: tapes 628/639), WW1/WO/148/2, LC. Wright later became a pioneer in the field of family planning and birth control.

prejudice'.[11] A 'war concordat' was signed with St Mary's in 1916, which permitted those studying at the LSMW only to take classes in Paddington.[12] Similar agreements followed in the metropolis at Charing Cross, St George's (1916), Westminster (1917), the London, King's College and University College (1918).[13] Meanwhile, by 1914, many provincial medical schools already admitted women on the same terms as men. Cardiff, St Andrews, Dundee, Aberdeen, all the constituent colleges of the universities in Ireland, Queen's Belfast, Manchester, Leeds, Newcastle, Birmingham, Bristol, Liverpool and Sheffield encouraged women to study medicine. Some stressed their ongoing commitment to educating medical students of both sexes side-by-side. In Glasgow, nearly all the classes were mixed. At Cork, women had a separate dissecting room, indicating that some areas were still considered unsuitable for co-education.[14] Not every female medical student wanted, however, to study alongside her male colleagues nor took advantage of the wartime opportunity to do so. This less frequently acknowledged side of the argument was coupled with the fact that the LSMW, unlike the other medical schools, was bursting at the seams with new students during the war years. They simply could not accommodate all those eager to join the ranks of medical women.

The growing number of women entering medical studies and the corresponding decline in that of their male counterparts was intimately related in the eyes of the medical and lay press. Newspapers began to report a 'national urgency' fewer than six months into the conflict; by January 1915, a shortage of doctors was proclaimed.[15] For the *Daily Chronicle*, the 'stampede of surgeons and medical men to the front and students to the ranks' has left medical women 'in possession'.[16] The LSMW was in a curious position during the war. Firstly, it was receiving an increasing number of applications from girls eager to make medicine their career, spurred on by patriotism, as well as a desire to earn their own money.

---

[11] From a Correspondent, 'Women as Doctors. Problems for the London Medical Schools', *Manchester Guardian*, 5 October 1920, in *LSMWRFHPC, Vol. 5*.

[12] Leopold Spero, 'London Hospital's Tin Hut and What it Means', *Manchester Despatch*, 17 January 1917, in ibid.

[13] James Stewart Gardner, 'The Great Experiment: The Admission of Women Students to St Mary's Hospital Medical School, 1916–1925', *MH*, 42.1 (January 1998), 68–88; 71.

[14] Dr Jane Walker, 'Careers for Girls: VI. The Profession of Medicine', *Educational Times*, 1 October 1914, 464–5; 465, in *LSMWRFHPC, Vol. 5*. For the Irish situation, see Kelly, *Irish Women*, especially chapter 6.

[15] 'Lack of Doctors. Many Required for Immediate Work', *Daily Express*, 22 January 1915, in *LSMWRFHPC, Vol. 5*.

[16] 'War and Women Earners. Employment Lost and Gained. Call for Doctors', *Daily Chronicle* [undated, but evidently January 1915], ibid.

Secondly, however, overcrowding meant that it had either to expand or send students elsewhere. An appeal to the public for money was a risky endeavour when the devastating results of warfare dominated, understandably, requests for charitable donations. The loss of students to other institutions was a delicate topic because of the divide between those who believed co-education was the only way forward for medical women and those who adhered to the entrenched attitude that a single-sex method of study was the most advantageous way for the young to learn their craft. One 1917 article described the problem thus: 'it would not suit the women to be admitted indiscriminately to all hospitals and medical schools as students': 'They would always be in the minority and their interests are far better served by a fortress of their own like the Royal Free.'[17] Students had, therefore, a choice to make. They could take advantage of excitingly novel opportunities elsewhere, which, they were repeatedly informed, would be temporary, or they could pursue the tried-and-tested route through the LSMW, where they would be safely ensconced within a fortress of their own.

It is necessary to examine how students actually viewed these options and the reasons why they made the decisions they did. Octavia Wilberforce, who studied at the LSMW between 1913 and 1920, devoted a chapter of her autobiography to wartime studies. With her friend Pam Kettle, Wilberforce became one of the LSMW students to take up places at St Mary's and described the experience as 'one of the happiest periods' of her life.[18] Despite her education being slowed down by an execrable performance in anatomy, which she had failed several times, Wilberforce finally passed her second medical and entered St Mary's for clinical work. She viewed the invasion of 'such a malebound, prejudiced hospital' as an act which 'mattered enormously' and was advised that she would do well in 'that free air of coeducation', where even the smell of the wards was attractive.[19] Consequently, Wilberforce was thrown in at the 'deep end' as a dresser to the Casualty house surgeon in the autumn of 1917. Although she struggled with anything surgical, and later went on to fail the surgery component of her degree several times, Wilberforce profited from her St Mary's immersion. The poverty of the local area meant that Casualty was indeed a baptism of fire for Wilberforce, but she found the corresponding wealth of insight into patients of 'every class, age and occupation' immeasurably helpful.[20] Such a widening of her education

---

[17] Spero, 'London Hospital's Tin Hut'.
[18] *Octavia Wilberforce* (London: Cassell, 1989), p. 85.   [19] Ibid., p. 82.
[20] Ibid., p. 85. For more on the hospital during this period, see E.A. Heaman, *St Mary's* (Liverpool and Montreal: Liverpool University Press/McGill-Queen's University Press, 2003), pp. 89–168.

encouraged the 'shy' young woman to realise the simplest things about those around her. The St Mary's experience taught Wilberforce 'good manners', such as the need to respond cheerily to porters who wished her a good morning and appreciation of the police force, who brought in her patients. Even though she was surrounded by drunken violence, severe injuries and horrifying sights, mankind 'in the raw' was educational and 'absorbing'.[21] So involved was Wilberforce in her work, indeed, that sheer exhaustion after attendance at emergency operations meant that she slept through the sound of distant guns, sirens and air raids. Although Wilberforce enjoyed her LSMW studies, she was older than most and had found some of her fellow students, those 'herds of girls', alarmingly intense in their schoolgirl crushes.[22] St Mary's provided those who wanted to see life outside 'the fortress' with a perfect opportunity to expand their personal and clinical horizons.

For those who said 'No thanks very much' and were 'really quite contented with the best',[23] staying at the LSMW and walking the wards of the RFH did not mean that they limited their educational choices. A. Lloyd Williams submitted an article entitled 'Impressions of Gate' to the School *Magazine* in 1916, where she described patients as varied as those treated by Wilberforce.[24] Men, women and children thronged the Casualty Department, permitting dressers to experience human life: humour, tragedy and romance alike. The effects of wartime were daily in evidence. Munitions workers, of both sexes, arrived with injuries caused by the hazards of their job, and a man, carrying important papers, had been blinded with a pepper spray in an attempt to steal the secrets within. The pride in the School's success at attracting more and more students was mocked in the annual Topical Play described in the same issue of the *Magazine*, where '500 new and energetic ones being admitted into one ward' led to the mental collapse of the 'revered staff', who were moved to a suitable home of rest.[25] A Prologue to the play reproduced an article about 'Women's Work in War Time', which remarked admiringly upon the increase in the number of women seen at the RFH. Benefits to patients had been 'well nigh incalculable'; surgery, for example, could be performed with 'far greater rapidity when forty assistants are to hand than when there are but three, however capable and experienced those

---

[21] *Wilberforce*, p. 83; p. 85.   [22] Ibid., p. 58; pp. 72–3.

[23] Anon., 'No, thanks very much', *L(RFH)SMWM*, 47 (October 1910), 238. This was written in response to a rumour that the London would open its wards to women students.

[24] A. Lloyd Williams, 'Impressions of Gate', *L(RFH)SMWM*, XI.63 (March 1916), 6–7.

[25] 'The Topical Play. Given at Hospital' and M.E. Burnett and S.I. Walsh, 'Prologue' to the play, reproduced in *L(RFH)SMWM*, XI.63 (March 1916), 13–16.

three may be'.[26] Although poking fun at the School's recent success, the play also stressed the camaraderie between students and between students and staff: strength in numbers, indeed.

Within a month of the war's declaration, the LSMW were urging women to help their country by training to be doctors. In September 1914, Louie Brooks, the Secretary to the School, gave a series of interviews to the press. In the *Daily Graphic*, for example, she was quoted directly: "'Women can render no better national service than qualifying in medicine, where their services can always be turned to national account'".[27] While the urgent demand could not be met by those embarking upon their studies now, their future promise meant that they were performing a national service, 'serving their country',[28] by dedicating themselves to a life of usefulness. By November, the *Morning Post* remarked that there was a decline in the number of students entering medical schools, although numbers were not as low as initially expected. However, older students were departing for the front and the shortage of the fourth and final years was beginning to tell. Guy's had lost nearly 80 senior students; many too had left at St Thomas'. In contrast, however, early propaganda had encouraged a rise in the LSMW's new entrants, 56 in all, bringing the total number of women in training at the School to 212.[29] By December, the LSMW had launched an appeal for extra building space to accommodate its increasing student population. Canny publicity drew upon the School's past value, as well as its sheer necessity in the light of the current conflict and in anticipation of future absences in the profession. Past students, such as Louisa Garrett Anderson, were serving their country and receiving praise for their skilful surgery. Of the 1000 women on the Medical Register, who were now practising all over the world, 60 per cent had been educated at the LSMW.[30] Without their excellent training, and without the LSMW, very few women would be saving lives as medical and surgical practitioners at home and abroad. 'Work of the future' could not be carried out without an expansion of the School either.[31] Famed gynaecological surgeon, Mary Scharlieb, formerly of the RFH, added her voice to the call for a total of £25,000. For Scharlieb, 'practical usefulness' could be obtained no more nobly than

[26] 'Prologue', 15.

[27] 'Women Doctors Wanted. Shortage of Male Practitioners Owing to the War', *Daily Graphic*, 23 September 1914, *LSMWRFHPC, Vol. 5*.

[28] Louie M. Brooks, 'Where Women are Wanted', *Daily Chronicle*, 9 September 1914, ibid.

[29] 'The War and the London Medical Schools', *Morning Post*, 5 November 1914, ibid.

[30] The appeal appeared in newspapers and periodicals across the country. See, for just one example, 'Women and Medicine', *Pall Mall Gazette*, 10 December 1914, ibid.

[31] 'Medical Education for Women', *Daily Graphic*, 10 December 1914, ibid.

through a medical career.[32] With demand for medical women in excess
of the supply, the money requested, argued supporters, was more than
worthwhile.

Despite the belief that war had led to the 'death-blow of an already
moribund prejudice' against medical women, reactions to this appeal
were mixed.[33] While the *Morning Post* had noted that the numbers of
students were not decreasing as fast as had been anticipated, the *Hospital* attacked the LSMW more directly. In March 1915, an editorial
explored the ways in which the School had presented its case and found
it wanting. The periodical acknowledged that in wartime 'foresight and
faith' should not be obscured by 'present national emergency': medical education could serve a 'patriotic purpose'. It went on, however,
to address the 'worthiness' of the School for such beneficence in difficult times. While there was clearly a demand for women doctors and
the increase in students showed that there were ample numbers to meet
the demand, the LSMW was still 'a somewhat detached and sheltered
institution', unstimulated by 'competition and outside criticism'.[34] By
turning the 'fortress' against itself, the *Hospital* struck a nerve. Actual
achievements were undeniable; what the periodical objected to was the
sentimental, tearful tone to the appeal which overwhelmed the practical
and the robust. Promises of 'the good time coming and the better order
which the women doctors will bring' were premature; why not wait and
adjust comparisons 'in the order of time'? This was not the only occasion
the periodical attacked the LSMW's requests for funding. In November
of the same year, another call for support angered the *Hospital* still further and brought to the fore arguments against women doctors which
were thought long buried. War, claimed the periodical, was 'temporary
and exceptional'; the LSMW were asking for money to support those
who could not help the war effort. Students beginning their courses now
would not be qualified for five years, their numbers were limited, so
not worthy of the level of backing requested, and there was a 'widely
entertained view' that many women would forsake the profession for the
'more congenial joys of domesticity'.[35] Such a focus could only excite
public hostility rather than generosity. Despite the antagonism of the
Hospital, the LSMW did achieve its target in only 18 months, through

[32] Mary Scharlieb, 'Women Doctors and the War', *Times*, 8 December 1914, ibid.
[33] 'Medical Education of Women in London', *Queen*, 19 December 1914, ibid.
[34] 'The London School of Medicine for Women', *Hospital*, LVII.1499, 13 March 1915,
523–4; 523, ibid.
[35] 'Women Doctors After the War', *Hospital*, 13 November 1915, in *South London Hospital
for Women Press Cuttings, 1912–1917*, H24/SLW/Y6/1, London Metropolitan Archives.
Future references will be shortened to *SLHWPC*.

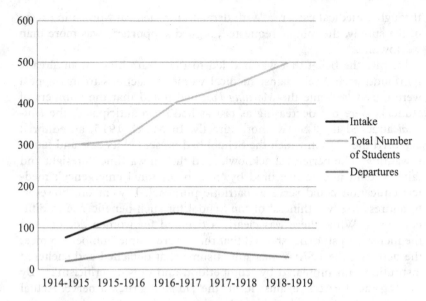

Figure 5.1 Number of Students, New Students, and Departures: LSMW, 1914–1919.

the beneficence of 1,300 donations.[36] The extension was opened by the Queen in October 1916 to widespread jubilation in the lay press. As the *Daily Telegraph* cheered: 'half a century covers the whole of a movement which . . . passionately opposed at the outset, has now converted even its most ardent antagonists, and proved its value with brilliant success since the outbreak of the present war'.[37] The *Hospital*'s admonitions would, however, have an effect on other appeals further into the war, notably, as this chapter will later explore, the way in which the SLHW considered fundraising. A copy of the November piece was pasted, tellingly, into the SLHW's press scrapbook.[38] While, as these articles recognised, the appeal had been successful in garnering public money, the effects of the School's would not be seen for some time to come, nor could the future for women medical students be so clearly predicted.

If the *Hospital* had been privy to the School's entry statistics, it might have extended its scepticism further. Wartime medical study was simply that for large numbers of students. Figure 5.1 measures the intake in

---

[36] 'School Notes', *L(RFH)SMWM*, XI.64 (July 1916), 75.
[37] 'Women Doctors', *Daily Telegraph*, 3 October 1916. This article was also reproduced: 'Leading Article from the "Daily Telegraph". Tuesday, October 3rd, 1916. By Permission', *L(RFH)SMWM*, XI.65 (November 1916), 98–101.
[38] See *SLHWPC*.

Table 5.1 *Percentage of Female Medical Students in Britain Who Began Their Studies Between 1914 and 1918*[39]

	First Year (due to qualify in 1923) (%)	Second Year (due to qualify in 1922) (%)	Third Year (due to qualify in 1921) (%)	Fourth Year (due to qualify in 1920) (%)	Fifth Year (due to qualify in 1919) (%)
London District	41.5	39.4	47.3	25.3	12
England and Wales (inc. London)	35.7	35.2	38.4	27.9	14.9
Scotland	36.1	44.1	36.7	35.8	24.6
Ireland	22.5	18.8	16.5	11.6	9.5
Total	32.6	33.1	31.6	26.6	18

relation to the dropout rate between the 1914–1915 academic year and that of 1918–1919. Reports issued from the RFH described only those who entered the School, while the private School papers record departures.[40]

It is evident that the number of students increased dramatically, from 299 in the 1914–1915 academic year to 499 by the end of 1919. The percentage of new students each year to overall figures reached a peak in 1915–1916, when the former comprised 41.2 per cent of the total. Indeed, the number of those entering the School during wartime did not fall below 24 per cent of students in any single year. Press coverage of the need for future doctors had clearly influenced many. As the *Lancet* indicated, female recruits to the profession were increasing instead of decreasing; on the other hand, it had been recently estimated that 200 to 300 fewer medical men would qualify.[41] By May 1918, the near-parity in the ratio of male-to-female undergraduates in some years, especially in the metropolis, was evident. Table 5.1 shows the percentage of women in comparison to the total number of medical students across the country. Particularly noteworthy was the nearly 50 per cent of women studying in their third year, who would have begun their course in 1915 when the 'shortages' panic was at its height. Until 1918, women accounted for nearly one-third of all medical students; a remarkable statistic given that when the war started there were only 1000 female

[39] Percentages calculated from figures in 'Annotations: The Supply of Medical Students', *Lancet*, 192.4952 (27 July 1918), 113.
[40] Figures calculated from *Eighty-Seventh to Ninety-Second Annual Reports* (1915–1920). Additional information about withdrawals obtained from Student Records of the LSMW, Student Admission Register: 1874–1927, H72/SM/C/01/03/001 and Student Files, H72/SM/C/01/02, LMA.
[41] 'The Medical Education of Women', *Lancet*, 185.4774 (27 February 1915), 451–452.

doctors on the Medical Register. At the beginning of the century, about 5 per cent of medical students were women and not more than 10 per cent before the Great War began.[42] There were 665 in their first year alone in 1918. As the *Lancet* concluded, the shortages were of actual rather than potential medical men and women. The future of health care in Britain was looking more secure by 1918.

When read alongside student records, however, the figures indicate a different picture. It is noticeable that the first three years of medical study contained the most women, while the final two indicated a considerable drop in numbers. This was especially evident across England and Wales where there was a 30 per cent difference between the first and fifth years. Student records for the LSMW exist from 1894, when there were only five withdrawals from the School.[43] Indeed, before 1910, only one year had more students failing to finish their studies: six in 1906–1907. Between 1894 and 1914, an average of around 10 per cent of women left before the end of their course; there was not a single withdrawal in 1897–1898, or in 1905–1906, for example.[44] This rose to 30.4 per cent for the war years alone; a figure which could well be higher, due to a lack of concrete information on the final outcome for 145 students, entering between 1917 and 1919. Of those who left during the period between 1914 and 1919 and for whom there was information, three qualified at a later date, one attended only for 'operative surgery', one re-entered, one withdrew temporarily, one was ominously 'still here', and three died (one of whom 'marries and dies'). Only two went on to qualify elsewhere: one to St Mary's and one who finished her studies at University College London. In the three wartime academic years for which every student had a recorded destination – 1914–1915 up until 1916–1917 – just over half of entrants graduate (53.8 per cent). This can be compared to a 73.4 per cent qualification rate between 1894 and 1914. The much-vaunted and rapidly increasing number of female medical students did not necessarily translate into a similar total of qualified professionals; exactly the sort of hyperbole which the *Hospital* had feared in 1915. Other priorities dominated for nearly half of the women who entered the LSMW during the war years. While the Great War provided unprecedented opportunities for female medical students, not everyone took full

---

[42] Elston, 'Women Doctors', p. 60.
[43] All figures from Student Records of the LSMW, Student Admission Register: 1874–1927, H72/SM/C/01/03/001 and Student Files, H72/SM/C/01/02, LMA.
[44] 1906–1907 and 1911–1912 show an anomalous 33.3 per cent and 40.9 per cent failure rate, respectively, which causes a considerable increase in the average for the two decades between 1894 and 1914. Two of the withdrawals in the latter year later qualified, while in the former one studied abroad and another returned, tellingly, in 1914.

advantage of their chance at a career. For some, it was the start of a life devoted to practise; for others, it was simply something they had done in the war and, ultimately, an occupation to which they would not return.

First Posts

If the writer of 'A Lament' had reread her alma mater's *Magazine* in 1915 she would have been cheered by a recognition of those who chose to stay at home. For St Mary's surgeon Charles Pannett, who wrote from the Hospital Yacht *Liberty*, in December 1914, service was provided 'equally well' by those who were 'carrying on their usual occupations'.[45] Pannett had been encouraged to write the letter because he was embarrassed at the misdirected cheers for everyone who was abroad, even if they, like he, were way behind the front lines. An 'active part in war', as 'A Lament' made clear, was assumed to be far 'more heroic' than the everyday actions of those who were not at the front, even if they were carrying out similar duties. Pannett turned later to women's role in the conflict and his advice was simple: stay at home. By filling posts which men had evacuated, women would assist incalculably. He advised qualified women against leaving for France unless they did so with recognised organisations; otherwise, random acts of charity did not always benefit those they should and became, instead, a 'nuisance' to official bodies. Better to take up the challenges on the home front, where they would be 'most valuable', both to the British public and to their male colleagues serving abroad. If the 'shortage' of medical students was a cause for concern, the loss of the qualified was inevitably leading to panic about the provision of health care in general practice and in hospitals on the home front. The next issue of the *Magazine* crowed that a decision had been made 'to omit from this and future numbers the list of appointments open to medical women. It is quite impossible to keep the list up to date, and at present practically every appointment is open'.[46] For those recently qualified, war brought with it an enormous expansion in their professional, but also their financial, horizons. Those who had graduated in 1914 'all got good positions at once'. Wages were rising swiftly as an incentive. Louie Brooks remarked that the LSMW was being harangued every day for graduate doctors; hospitals were willing to pay 50 per cent more than they had done only a few months before. One former student was registered and appointed to a post on the same day. This position paid

---

[45] 'Correspondence', Letter from Charles A. Pannett to Editor of *L(RFH)SMWM*, X.60 (March 1915), 45.
[46] Editorial, *L(RFH)SMWM*, X.61 (July 1915), 62.

£160 per annum; in addition to the salary, a flat and a maid were included.[47] Such benefits contrasted with the 'disabilities' experienced by women serving with the Army. Although they received the same pay as men, they were not entitled to rations nor billeting allowances, they paid the same income tax as civilians, their contracts were made on a monthly basis only and they were without travel privileges which were afforded even to nurses.[48] Sometimes, it paid to stay at home.

It is important not to forget, as Elston has remarked, that posts at this junior level were always temporary.[49] Inevitably, they would come to an end and the current occupants would move on to their next six-month position. Wartime resident posts should be viewed as useful experience, rather than as jobs from which women were cruelly usurped at the end of the conflict. This was a condition made obvious by the nature of the work itself and the stress, from the earliest days of the war, that women were effectively acting as locum tenens under exceptional conditions. F. Howard Marsh, Professor of Surgery at the University of Cambridge, wrote in the *Cambridge Review* at the beginning of 1915 about women's suitability for resident posts. For Marsh, women were ideal medical students, impressive doctors, and exceptional surgeons. As an examiner, he knew 'women who display every endowment and every qualification necessary for the higher levels of operative Surgery and whose results are as favourable as any obtained by men in similar groups of cases'.[50] Their success could be witnessed every day at the NHW, for example. Despite his belief in women's abilities, Marsh stressed that female substitutes should 'retire in favour' of the returning men if they happened to be holding a position at the end of the war. 'Justice cannot be done', he concluded, 'unless this is a binding compact': '[t]his should be no deterrent. Women who have done good work will readily find other openings.' For the moment, the *Daily Chronicle* noted enthusiastically, hospitals were 'clamouring for' qualified women; it was 'Her Day at Last' concluded the *Birmingham Gazette and Express*.[51] This next section will consider the

---

47 'Women Doctors Wanted. Demands of Hospitals for Resident Physicians', *Evening Telegraph Post*, 15 December 1914, in *LSMWRFHPC*.
48 Jane Walker, 'Medical Women in the Army. Disabilities on Service', *Times*, 4 July 1918, ibid. Walker was writing as President of the Medical Women's Federation, which had been formed in February 1917, and which spent the rest of the war campaigning for the improvement of conditions for female doctors in military service. See Whitehead, *Doctors in the Great War*, pp. 113–14.
49 Elston, 'Women Doctors', pp. 292–3.
50 F. Howard Marsh, 'Scarcity of Doctors', *Cambridge Review*, 24 February 1915, 221–2, in *LSMWRFHPC*.
51 'War and Women Earners. Employment Lost and Gained. Call for Doctors', *Daily Chronicle* [Winter 1915]; 'The Call for Women Doctors', *Birmingham Gazette and Express*, 11 February 1915, ibid.

opportunities with which newly qualified women were presented during the war years, the positions they attained and how they viewed these novel advantages. It is necessary to keep in mind, of course, that short-term contracts were limited by their conditions, as always, but that resident posts could also be curtailed at any point should the conflict come to an end before the period of residence did.

Those who had qualified in 1914, as Helena Lowenfeld had done, found positions opening up instantly. After graduation, she sought a post through advertisements in the medical press. 'Among them', she remarked, when interviewed in the 1970s, 'was a surprise': 'the out-patient department of Hampstead General Hospital' was seeking two resident graduates.[52] They were, as usual, six-month posts, but the 'surprise' was in the location: a general hospital for both sexes. The RFH was unusual in employing male and female staff alongside each other; the war ensured that more situations were available for women to work alongside, as well as instead of, men. Hampstead General (HGH) had been established in 1882 and, unlike the RFH, encouraged paying patients to contribute towards their support. It merged with the North-West London Hospital in 1908, which became the site of its outpatient department, and was recognised as a metropolitan hospital.[53] With Peggy Martland, a friend since their earliest student days, Lowenfeld applied and they were both successful. Their reception was as expected, especially among nurses 'and other workers', who 'received us with some misgivings'. The reason was, Lowenfeld exclaimed, that 'never had there been women house-men before!' Lowenfeld's mixed gendering here gave a good impression of the confusion which must have resulted when she and Martland took up their posts. They were female, but in male roles, as far as the hospital was concerned. HGH proved, however, an excellent environment for the young women to thrive and they had 'a busy, happy six months and learnt a lot'. After six months, the invitation was extended and the two women were moved to the in-patient department: Lowenfeld as house surgeon; Martland as house physician. Lowenfeld described their new conditions as very enjoyable and they 'settled in peacefully'. She had 'a bevy of surgeons to work for' and found it challenging to remember each member of staff's special routines for post-operative patients. The patients themselves were very satisfied with the new house surgeon, about whose 'novelty' they were 'outspoken in their surprise and pleasure'. Although Martland and Lowenfeld had won over

[52] Wright, 'Incidents'.
[53] Ernest Collins, 'The Hampstead General Hospital', *BMJ*, 1.2460 (22 February 1908), 475–6.

their colleagues and their charges, a 'vaguely uncomfortable' atmosphere pervaded the hospital. Lowenfeld's German-sounding surname was to dog her nascent career once more, but this time she was dismissed with a question mark over her 'natural loyalty'. Disgusted at the treatment of her friend, Martland resigned in protest and the experiment at the HGH was over.

It is difficult to know, from Lowenfeld's recollections, whether or not the suspicion of alien activity prompted her dismissal. There was no indication that the (many paying) patients objected and the Board of the hospital expressed 'satisfaction' with her work. According to Lowenfeld, it was 'rumour' which spurred the management's decision; evidently an explanation of her Polish ancestry was not enough to quell this suspicion. Closer examination of the hospital's various committee minutes revealed that the orthopaedic surgeon, Mr Jackson Clarke, drew the attention of the management to the 'undesirability of Miss Lowenfeld's return to the hospital as House Surgeon'. The reason for this, he continued, was that she had recently travelled to Switzerland to meet her father, who was Austrian. There was no recorded debate about this decision and the Secretary was instructed to write to Lowenfeld conveying the information that 'the Committee did not desire her to return to the Hospital'.[54] Lowenfeld evidently consulted solicitors over the manner of her dismissal; HGH later noted that hospital representatives had arranged to meet with Lowenfeld and her advisors.[55] Nothing further was mentioned about the case, so consultation resulted in an end to proceedings. Interestingly, the Medical Committee reacted differently and demanded an explanation from Jackson Clarke as to the 'action he had taken' when he recommended Lowenfeld's sacking. This minute concluded with 'an expression of regret that this action had been taken without previous communication with his colleagues or the Medical Committee'.[56] Whether Jackson Clarke disliked Lowenfeld personally, her parental background troubled him or her movements made him suspicious of her motives, his views were clearly not shared by his colleagues. After taking the plunge and employing Lowenfeld and Martland as house officers, HGH, in dismissing Lowenfeld and losing Martland in sympathy, placed themselves in a precarious position in straitened times.

HGH struggled throughout the rest of the war years to recruit house officers, a situation experienced by any number of hospitals throughout

---

54 House Committee Minute Book. Volume III: 1909–1922, 17 May 1915, Hampstead General Hospital, H71/HG/A/03/01/003, LMA.
55 Ibid., 31 May 1915.
56 Medical Staff Committee Minute Book. Volume I: 1905–1922, Monday 14 June 1915, Hampstead General Hospital, H71/HG/05/01/001, LMA.

the country. Although, given the experience with Martland and Lowenfeld, it was intriguing that the institution continued to employ women in junior roles throughout the war years. Lowenfeld may not have been trusted because of her political loyalties, but the work both she and Martland carried out during their stay first in Casualty, and then, when they were promoted to the treatment of in-patients, told a different story. Two months after Lowenfeld's departure, the Medical Committee remarked that there had been no candidates for a RMO post. As a coda to this statement appeared the following: 'the hospital is seriously inconvenienced by the absence of a resident staff'.[57] While such positions were short-term, this had no bearing upon the absence of candidates in response to advertisements. The end of June saw consideration of a female candidate for a resident post, but she was found unsuitable; by September a male applicant was similarly found unsuited to the role. Temporary measures were put in place and a Japanese man, Dr Nakagawa, took the post of house surgeon for three months.[58] In December, the Medical Committee concluded that it would not be suitable to have two residents who were of a different sex, 'in the interests of the hospital'.[59] This decision was prompted by consideration both for the relationship between house officers and that between those appointed and their patients, but also by something far more fascinating. Within the same minute as the above statement, the Committee reflected that it had simply not found the requisite number of male candidates suitable for either position. This was in spite of the fact that five men had been interviewed and held adequate qualifications.[60] Consequently, women formed both the Medical Committee's first and second choice for each position.

The final year of the war saw a shift in the ways in which HGH valued its women house officers. December 1917 and June 1918 saw the usual six-monthly appointments of female house physicians and house surgeons. The most recent positions of new staff indicated the breadth of choice women were afforded during the war years, in geographical, as well as professional terms, but also the temporality of their positions. For example, Miss Franklin, who was appointed House Surgeon in June 1918, acted previously as House Physician at Bristol Royal Infirmary and held posts as House Surgeon at the NHW and North Staffordshire

---

[57] Ibid., 26 July 1915.
[58] Ibid., 14 June; note about Dr Rachel Cohen as unsuitable in the margin of the minutes and dated 20 June; Dr De Mauric considered unsuitable, 27 September 1915. Dr Nakagawa's temporary position recorded in the minutes of 28 June 1915.
[59] Ibid., 3 December 1915.
[60] Only one, L. Distat Phillips, appeared without an MRCS LRCP; another candidate, A.W. Woo, was evidently of Chinese origin.

Infirmary. Her House Physician colleague, Miss S. Jevons, had been temporary House Surgeon at Charing Cross Hospital, as well as locum tenens at London Temperance Hospital and St Pancras Infirmary.[61] The next round of resident appointments, however, fell a month after the end of the conflict. By December 1918, men formed the top choices of the Medical Committee for both house posts, with women in second place. Melbourne-educated Basil Cohen and J.H.B. Hogg had served respectively with the RAMC and the Belfast Naval Medical Service; the runners-up for the posts were Constance Hart, who had been the Committee's first choice for House Physician only a year previously and was now pushed into second place for the surgical position, and Katherine Waring, who, like Cohen, had served with the RAMC. While there was no explanation as to why the men were chosen over the women in this round of temporary positions, neither their similar experience, as in Waring's case, nor the Committee's personal knowledge of their abilities, counted for anything. Although medical staff at the hospital were willing to consider women throughout the war due to the extremity of circumstances, they thought less favourably upon them when there were suitably qualified male candidates available. The same attitude was evident in the appointment of a gynaecologist in February 1918. Even though they were not able to make a recommendation for a permanent appointment, the Committee were faced with four applicants: three male, one female. After consideration, Eleanor Davies-Colley, the first female FRCS, was deemed the runner-up to Gordon Ley, also FRCS.[62] Evidently, the Committee were happy to contemplate women for the most junior posts at HGH, but, while clearly considering Davies-Colley above two of the male applicants, they placed her behind the other man on the list, even though the position was temporary. In many ways, the more junior the post, the more likely women were to be appointed between 1914 and 1918. Experience might be gained at the lowest level, but hospital management wobbled in their decisiveness when considering female specialists for more senior posts.

In similar fashion to Helena Lowenfeld, Leila Henry, who, as we saw in the last chapter, joined the SHW in 1917, made the most of her situation when she took a post at the Sheffield Royal Infirmary soon after graduating. When the *Queen* periodical wrote about Sheffield University in the winter of 1916, there had not yet been any graduates in medicine. Unlike those who attended the LSMW, for example, Henry was taught

---

[61] Medical Staff Committee Minute Book, 3 June 1918.
[62] Candidates were announced at the meeting on 17 February 1918; Ley was chosen on 20 February.

in much smaller classes where individual tuition was possible; a point to which the *Queen* draws particular attention when discussing the situation of the 14 female medical students. Although Sheffield advocated treating women equally as far as allowing them an education was concerned, they still studied separately for some classes: pathology; obstetrics and gynaecology; and urology.[63] Henry delighted in her studies and embraced all the opportunities open to her, especially in surgery. *Queen* announced that prospects were 'excellent' for clinical studies because students in their final years had access to over 500 beds in the city; those of the Royal Infirmary, the General Hospital and the Jessop Hospital for Women were open to them. In addition to numerous patients, the small cohort and the equality of opportunity as far as appointments for clinical clerkships and dresserships were concerned meant that women had many advantages studying at the university. As *Queen* remarked, female students were able to 'acquire real practical experience, and are not merely hangers-on'.[64] This was extended to the Royal Infirmary in the city, which, at the time the article was published, had three women residents: one assistant house physician and two assistant house surgeons. Sheffield was a fabulous place to work for aspiring surgeons like Henry. As *Queen* concluded, the large works, where frequent serious accidents occurred, meant practical surgical experience was readily available. In autumn 1916, just after Henry had graduated, as one of the first medical women from her university, Sheffield was also hit by a Zeppelin raid.[65] For a year after this, the city was without lighting at night, which contributed to increased incidents in already accident-prone area.[66] This situation, when coupled with munition injuries, meant that Henry was kept thrillingly busy in the Royal Infirmary, in spite of the strenuous trek to her work because she was required to live out, except when she was on night shift in Casualty.[67] It is hardly surprising that she felt herself equal to any other surgeon, despite only being 26. As Henry put it, 'it was experience that counted!',[68] and, thanks to opportunities in her adopted city, there was no shortage of that. Vital training meant that Henry was then capable of transferring her prized surgical skills to wounded military personnel at Royaumont.

---

[63] Crofton, *The Women of Royaumont*, p. 271.
[64] 'Sheffield University and the Medical Education of Women', *Queen*, 12 February 1916, 258, in *LSMWRFHPC*.
[65] For more on how Sheffield was affected by the Great War, see Scott C. Lomax, *The Home Front* (Barnsley: Pen and Sword Military, 2014), especially chapter 16, 'Sheffield's First Air Raid', pp. 172–82.
[66] Ibid., p. 183.   [67] Crofton, *Women of Royaumont*, p. 272.
[68] Henry, *Reminiscences*, p. 5.

When they were still students, Olive Newton and Ruth Verney were thrust into surgical life long before their training had come to an end. The need for house officers was so great that even third-year students, such as Newton, were plucked from medical school to serve their country on the home front. Newton accepted a three-month post in the Casualty Department of Birmingham General Hospital. She found this a 'wonderful experience giving responsibility so early in my career even doing minor surgery'.[69] Just over half-way through her course, Newton was carrying out work more suitable to a qualified house surgeon. She throve on, noticeably, both the opportunity to do surgical work and the responsibility which the role gave her. The absence of suitably registered candidates to fill house posts was not confined to larger hospitals or to institutions which treated both sexes. At the SLHW, run by women surgeons for solely female and child patients, not a single applicant came forward for a temporary assistant surgeon post advertised in November 1915. The Medical Council of the hospital considered, in future, that advertising externally should be coupled with internal requests, to see if any current staff wished to transfer. Advertising in the usual way was, however, decided.[70] Four months later, just before the In-patient Department was due to be officially opened, the Medical Council instructed that assistant positions should be advertised.[71] By May, a preferred candidate was engaged with war work, so a temporary contract was drawn up for another candidate.[72] In July, the two original posts had their titles altered, presumably to encourage those appointed to stay both for financial and professional reasons.[73] Subsequently, the title of assistant was dropped. In the autumn of 1916, the Medical Council voiced concerns, echoed all over the country, that there was an 'extreme difficulty of finding RMOs under present circumstances'.[74] They took steps to advertise and re-advertise for at least two consecutive weeks a month later.[75] When unable to appoint anyone who was suitably qualified, the SLHW turned to medical students. A senior student, Miss Cogan, became acting house surgeon for a month in October 1917 until the chosen candidate was free.[76] In May 1918, a 'partly qualified' fifth-year student, Miss F.M. Spickett, took up a six-month post as house surgeon.[77] Another fifth-year

---

[69] Dr O.M.C. Newton, handwritten 'Recollections (1914–1920)', Recollections M-Y, WW1/DF/148/2, LC.
[70] Recommendations Made by the Advisory Medical Council to the Board of Management: April 1913–May 1934, South London Hospital for Women, 6 December 1915, H24/SLW/A/19/001, LMA.
[71] Ibid., 6 March 1916.   [72] Ibid., 8 May 1916.   [73] Ibid., 13 June 1916.
[74] Ibid., 11 September 1916.   [75] Ibid., 9 October 1916.
[76] Ibid., 5 October 1917.   [77] Ibid., 3 May 1918.

student, Miss K.M. McKeown, became the hospital's house physician a month before the war ended.[78] War work certainly proved more enticing for some young, newly qualified medical women. Miss Peake, for example, who was the preferred candidate in May 1916, had her post held open for her until she was free to take it up an entire year later.[79] Although necessity meant that unqualified students took on roles usually open only to their registered counterparts, hospitals still preferred to turn to the likes of Miss Peake, qualified and with a MD, for more permanent posts. Even among women-run institutions, the hope was for the best rather than simply any applicants; those who were employed temporarily gained practical experience which assisted their eventual career. There were simply not enough women to fill all the available places created by male absence. Those free to choose could work with a wider range of people if, as many did, they sought posts outside the female-only institutions to which they were usually confined. The war, therefore, provided a wealth of different possibilities for those on shorter contracts both to look around for what specifically interested them and to gain more insight into a variety of medical and surgical specialties.

Ruth Verney found her initial experience less palatable than Olive Newton.[80] Even before she had qualified she was 'forced' to go to the Royal Manchester Children's Hospital in Pendlebury as a house surgeon. She found it a 'terrifying', 'dreadful' experience, although did not fully elaborate why this was the case. The only clue she gave was that terror arose 'from facing these grey haired sisters the other side of a child's bed'. Their seniority and her youth and lack of qualification must have ensured that she was made to feel quite unprepared for the work in hand. 'They couldn't get anyone you see', she ruminated when interviewed in the 1970s: 'they had gone'. This rushing of unprepared young women into posts which were unsuited to their training was certainly not the story the press wanted to tell. The heroic aspect of women taking up positions relinquished by their male colleagues dominated accounts of work on the home front. In spite of Verney's fears, she was asked to stay on as house surgeon when fully qualified, whether through necessity, desperation or because she had, despite her misgivings, actually been good at her job. Verney was keen to leave Manchester, and, not enjoying her paediatric work, she moved to the Great Northern Hospital (GNH) in London, where she filled both house physician and house surgeon roles, for the usual six months each. The GNH also took LSMW students as house

---

[78] Ibid., 4 October 1918.
[79] Peake was noted as 'free' from war work in the minutes, ibid., 23 April and 7 May 1917.
[80] Verney, Tape 476.

officers: for example, N. Olivier and E.M. Visick, at the beginning and end of 1918, respectively.[81] While at GNH, female house officers encountered wounded soldiers: 'any amount', according to Verney. GNH formed a section of the Second London General Hospital during the war years and the staff would have been familiar with the wounded sent home from France.[82] Verney remembered an operating-room anecdote from her time at the hospital, which gave a rare glimpse into a space more usually characterised by strict discipline and control.[83] The theatre was on one side of the building, situated around a quadrangle; on the other side, the soldiers were recuperating. Every sound from the other side could be heard while operations were occurring. Miss Beavis, the house surgeon, was asked by her superior to 'hold that tube and she thought he said, what is that tune and she looked up and said, If You Were The Only Boy in the World'. 'It brought the house down in the operating theatre', Verney reminisced: '[t]hat is the sort of side light we used to have'. Evidently, relations between remaining male surgeons and their female house officers at the GNH were more comradely than between youthful, scared residents and judgemental nursing staff in Manchester.

When looking back at 'A Year's War Work' in January 1916, the *Daily Telegraph* claimed that

1915 will take rank as the year of the conquest, final complete, of the medical woman. It is not so much that the War Office asked women physicians and surgeons to assume the care of a military hospital; nor is it on account of their fine work at Malta and in Serbia that their success has been won. Their real triumph is the opening to them of the coveted house-posts at the leading civil hospitals, and these are doors that will never be closed to them again.[84]

Despite women's achievements in surgery at the front and in the formation of Garrett Anderson and Murray's Endell Street institution, the *Telegraph* sought to celebrate the visible presence of female house officers in the wards of hospitals at home as the war's most celebrated advancement to date. The civilian population could read about distant successes, but surely more comforting was the knowledge that women were doing their duty and holding institutional forts in their own country. For young medical women themselves, the sudden professional and financial riches

[81] 'Recent Appointments', *L(RFH)SMWM*, XIII.69 (March 1918), 52; *L(RFH)SMWM*, XIII.71 (December 1918), 157.
[82] 'The War: Home Hospitals and the War', *BMJ*, 2.2815 (12 December 1914), 1041–3; 1042.
[83] Schlich, 'Surgery, Science'.
[84] 'A Year's War Work: Women's New Spheres', *Daily Telegraph*, 1 January 1916, in *LSMWRFHPC*.

afforded by the absence of male colleagues gave unprecedented access to many hospitals all over the country. They were naturally aware of the temporality of their posts, and this gave them a chance to move from institution to institution, garnering experience as they went. If, as in Verney's case, the job proved unpalatable, then many had enough freedom to change disciplines, move to another city and continue to learn while working. 'To be a doctor is to be a permanent and perpetual student', proclaimed Jane Walker in 1914, when describing the profession of medicine as an ideal career for girls.[85] Such an adage proved prescient when considering the wartime experience of young female house officers. Walker concluded that this meant keeping minds alert, hearts young and brains receptive and keen, but she could also have added worthwhile experience gained through a variety of temporary junior posts. The situation on the home front allowed Verney, for example, to pluck up courage to leave a position she hated for one from which she would benefit, or Henry to gain enough surgical confidence to offer her skills to the SWH. Circumstances may have been unprecedented, but senior students and recent female graduates sought opportunities to advance their careers and grasped them while they could, even if the post was only for a few months. Every moment was valuable.

Senior Positions

This chapter has so far considered the ways in which the youngest women took advantage of the opportunities available on the home front during the Great War years. By 1918, however, the age for the call-up of military men had reached 55; a full four years older than their civilian counterparts.[86] The shortage of medical men was not, therefore, simply restricted to the most junior of ranks. As the previous chapter has shown, the novelty of the conditions in which the battles were fought and the complex injuries caused by modern warfare meant surgery at the front was a great leveller. Experience at home counted for little when faced with the unknown. For example, as David Currie has shown, head injuries had been treated in Britain largely by general surgeons and understanding of the devastating damage caused by bullet wounds, coupled with the catastrophic bacterial infections from the fertile battlefield soil, was limited at the start of the conflict.[87] However, the knowledge and expertise of consultant surgeons was eagerly drawn upon; members of the RAMC, like

---

[85] Walker, 'Careers', 465.   [86] Whitehead, *Doctors in the Great War*, p. 83.
[87] David Currie, 'Wounds of the Skull and Brain', in Scotland and Heys, eds., *War Surgery*, pp. 234–56; p. 242.

these civilian counterparts, had not experienced conditions like those in France and Flanders before and co-operation was vital. As Mark Harrison has concluded, power 'came to be vested in civilian consultants who entered the Army on temporary commissions'.[88] This was in spite of antagonism between them in the past. Indeed, by 1918, regulars were outnumbered by civilians 11:1.[89] Absences at the top had to be filled as urgently on the home front as those on the lowest rungs of the career ladder. This next section will explore how two experienced women, the surgeon Louisa Aldrich-Blake and the radiologist Florence Stoney, both of whom served at home and abroad, took on the work of male colleagues at institutions in Britain. Through an examination of patient records in the case of Aldrich-Blake's post at the RFH, I will also explore precisely who was treated by this highly regarded surgeon, willing to take on others' caseloads. In addition to new responsibilities, it is worth considering whether perceived opportunities on the home front led to actual extensions in surgical and ancillary expertise of women such as Aldrich-Blake and Stoney.

When Aldrich-Blake died in 1926 at the age of 60, she had typically been carrying out surgical duties within a month of her death and had been at an administrative meeting only a week before. Aldrich-Blake's prolific 'activity' ran throughout her distinguished career and characterised the tone of her obituary.[90] Her surgical prowess was evident from student days at the LSMW, where she obtained her BS with first-class honours, after having done the same for her MB in medicine and obstetric medicine. After taking her MD, Aldrich-Blake then became the first female surgeon to receive a MS, a distinction she achieved in 1895. Fellow LSMW student, surgical colleague and founder of the SLHW, Maud Chadburn, remarked of her friend's brilliant surgical abilities that 'second best was unknown to her': '[s]he gave full time and thought to every case, whether minor or major. As an operator she was bold, courageous, level-headed, thoughtful; her hands were good to watch at work – her finger-tips obviously carried brains in them.'[91] Although not a quick thinker, she had excellent judgement according to contemporaries; her nature was ideally suited to the complex, lengthy operations developed in the early twentieth century, such as Wertheim's for carcinoma of the cervix and her own procedure for excision of the rectum. As we saw in

---

[88] Harrison, *The Medical War*, p. 99.   [89] Ibid., p. 96.
[90] Information from 'Obituary: Dame Louisa Aldrich-Blake', *BMJ*, 1.3393 (9 January 1926), 69–71. Only one biographical work was published, shortly after her death, by Lord Riddell, President of the RFH from 1924 to 1934: *Dame Louisa Aldrich-Blake*. For more on Riddell's tenure at the RFH, see: Armidon, *An Illustrated History*, p. 49.
[91] 'Appreciations: Miss M.M. Chadburn', appended to 'Obituary', *BMJ*, 70.

chapter 3, she worked primarily at the NHW, having been appointed an assistant surgeon in 1895, full surgeon in 1902 and senior surgeon in 1910. She became Dean of the LSMW in 1914. Aldrich-Blake's surgery during the Great War was far less well-known than her other activities. Riddell, for example, devoted just over a page to the 'manifold duties' of wartime.[92] As her obituarist marvelled, however, it was 'difficult to realise how one individual could have successfully accomplished all the war work which Miss Aldrich-Blake undertook'.[93] Her wartime assistance, at home and in France, was in the form of practical surgery, as well as administrative organisation. In addition to supplying and equipping those keen to set up units near the front, she rounded up women on the Medical Register in order to encourage them to serve abroad in 1916; thanks to her efforts, 80 were sent to Malta, Egypt or Salonika in the autumn of 1916 and then another 50 when the RAMC requested more. Aldrich-Blake utilised her supposed vacations to allow colleagues serving abroad to rest. She worked at Cherbourg over the Christmas and New Year of 1914–1915, and relieved Frances Ivens at Royaumont for two summers in 1915 and 1916. When Ivens wrote back to the SWH Committee after Aldrich-Blake's departure in 1915, she noted her 'most helpful' assistance during a 'very busy fortnight'; she had done 'quite a lot of work' and allowed Ivens, notoriously unwilling to take breaks from her surgical work, to 'get off a good deal'.[94] According to Riddell, despite her brief stays, Aldrich-Blake evidently made an impact on those she treated and became known among the patients at Royaumont as '"Madame la Générale"'.[95] Evidently, her calm confidence and efficiency implied leadership to the injured.

It is not surprising that she was chosen to cover a number of absent surgeons' work at the RFH; a role her obituarist calls 'double duty'.[96] In the 1917 *Annual Report* for the hospital, and despite her seniority and the breadth of her expertise, Aldrich-Blake appeared for the first time as 'Acting Assistant Surgeon'.[97] The *Report* for 1918 omitted her from the list of staff altogether, but she reappeared in the 1919 *Report* with considerable elevation as 'Consulting Surgeon'.[98] During these years, she also acted as visiting surgeon to the WAAC Hospital at Isleworth and consulting surgeon for women patients at the Herbert Hospital in

[92] Riddell, *Louisa Aldrich-Blake*, pp. 51–2; p. 51.   [93] Ibid., 69.
[94] Dr Ivens to Mrs Russell, Royaumont, 16 September 1915, Tin 12: Copies of Letters Received at Headquarters From July 1915 to October 1916, SWHC.
[95] Riddell, *Louisa Aldrich-Blake*, p. 51.   [96] 'Obituary', 69.
[97] *Ninetieth Annual Report for 1917* (Printed by H.J. Goss and Co, Ltd, London, 1918), p. 8.
[98] *Ninety-First for 1918* (1919) and *Ninety-Second for 1919 Annual Reports* (1920), p. 8.

Woolwich, as well as still treating her own private cases.[99] Extant patient records at the RFH reveal that Louisa Aldrich-Blake was carrying out surgery on men and women between 1917 and 1920, when male colleagues began to return. Her reward for the hard work over these years was a consulting role with the 'care of patients'; along with her Deanship of the LSMW, this earned her a seat on the Medical Committee of the hospital.[100] As her RFH colleague Arthur Phear later noted, she was a 'distinguished member' of staff, who achieved 'professional success and worldly distinction'.[101] Aldrich-Blake's solid common sense and good judgement were invaluable when the RFH began to lose its male staff. In its *Annual Report* for 1914, the RFH remarked on the 'many members of the Honorary Medical Staff who have sought and obtained long leave of absence from home duties'.[102] It reassured its subscribers, however, that the work of the hospital would be carried on and the civilian population would not suffer or be placed at any disadvantage by this development. The 'ready and self-denying spirit' which motivated those left behind would ensure that the hospital was able to carry on as usual. Of the surgical staff, the hospital lost Senior Surgeon, generalist, thyroid and cleft-palate expert, Mr Berry, and Assistant Surgeons, Mr Joll, a thyroid specialist, and Mr Pannett straight away, leaving only Surgeons, the generalist and dermatologist, Mr Evans, and the generalist Mr Cunning. Despite absences, the names of all appeared on the list of staff until they were joined in the report for 1916 by the names of those 'Acting' their roles. This emphasised both a desire to ensure continuity throughout the conflict, thus reassuring patients and subscribers, and to make clear that wartime developments were temporary measures.

As the hospital had lost the services of general and specialist surgeons, those covering their caseloads were required to adapt themselves to a variety of different surgical procedures. Between 1917 and 1920 Aldrich-Blake was entrusted with both female and male patients of all ages. From a background in gynaecological and rectal operations, she was expected to carry out more general surgery than she was used to, as well as dealing with industrial accidents, which were regularly brought into the RFH, those wounded during metropolitan air raids, and with soldiers brought back from the front. The hospital, along with many others during the war years, set aside a certain number of beds for military personnel at the request of the War Office. From August 1914, it offered 40 beds, which were continuously occupied by those injured on the battlefield, who

99 'Obituary', 69.   100 *Ninety-Second Annual Report*, p. 15.   101 'Obituary', 71.
102 *Eighty-Seventh Annual Report for 1914* (1915), p. 14.

were transferred from institutions on the Continent back to London. For many, this was a momentary rest before they were sent back to the ranks or reintegrated into industrial life at home.[103] In 1915, the RFH made two wards available for the treatment of war wounded; for this, they were paid 4/- per day for each occupied bed.[104] Temporary buildings were then erected as a Military Section of the institution.[105] By 1919, over a four-year period, it had dealt with 4,128 officers alone.[106] Aldrich-Blake, therefore, gained experience treating military men both fresh from the battlefield when she worked at Cherbourg and Royaumont and after initial surgery when they were transferred to the RFH. In many instances, as Aldrich-Blake and Florence Stoney would discover, and as this section will explore later, they were having to correct earlier injuries overlooked or ignored in favour of more obvious wounds.[107] Due to the patient's ongoing suffering, they were compelled to relocate foreign bodies and then re-operate upon those whose injuries had been too swiftly treated or simply patched up at the front.

Between the autumn of 1917 and spring of 1919, extant case notes indicate that Aldrich-Blake treated 168 male, female and child patients at the RFH. The circumstances of the Great War at home and at the front permitted women to operate on men for the first time in any number. It is fruitful to compare the gender breakdown of Aldrich-Blake's patients over this period to see whether this opportunity was given to her at the RFH. As Figure 5.2 shows, Aldrich-Blake actually treated just over 7 per cent more men than women during the war years, despite her previous expertise as a surgeon for the latter. It was evident that the hospital believed she was able to take on these cases, but also that male patients themselves were happy enough to be operated upon by a woman. The RFH needed assistance in areas other than those in which Aldrich-Blake had specialised, so they utilised her surgical skills to the utmost. This trust allowed Aldrich-Blake to widen her expertise considerably, in terms both of patient gender and in the types of operation she was performing. It may be assumed that, as child patients formed a large number of cases at the RFH, the majority of the males she saw were actually under the age of 14. As with any hospital of its size, and, as Lynsey Cullen has discovered in her sampling of RFH case notes before the war, children under the age of nine made up 24 per cent of patients treated by male physicians and

---

[103] *Eighty-Seventh Annual Report for 1914* (1915), p. 14.
[104] *Eighty-Eighth Annual Report for 1915* (1916), p. 12.
[105] *Ninety-Third Annual Report for 1920* (1921), p. 16.
[106] *Ninety-Second Annual Report for 1919* (1920), p. 14.
[107] For more on patients returned to Britain, see Carden-Coyne, *Wounds*.

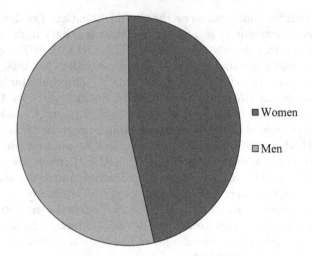

Figure 5.2 Aldrich-Blake's Patients: RFH, Autumn 1917–Spring 1919.[108]

surgeons between 1902 and 1912.[109] In chapter 3, when analysing all Mary Scharlieb and Ethel Vaughan-Sawyer's surgical patients in the Gynaecological Department of the RFH, women in their twenties and thirties dominated their caseloads.. Aldrich-Blake would have similarly treated a majority of similarly aged female patients and for like conditions in her work at the New, as well as some children. It would be expected that, along with the pattern established by her male colleagues at the RFH and other institutions, Aldrich-Blake would have treated smaller numbers of children than adults. An analysis of the age range of her male and female patients reveals that over three-quarters of them were adults over the age of 14. Although she had not operated upon men, except straight from the battlefield in recent years, the majority of patients dealt with by Aldrich-Blake were adult men. Indeed, even of the children, boys dominated, with more than twice as many male as female. In women-run hospitals there were strict edicts about the age of male children. Seven was the limit at the NHW, while at the SLHW, despite campaigning from the Medical Council to raise it to ten, it was fixed firmly by the institution's trustees at six.[110] Aldrich-Blake's patient base

---

[108] Compiled from Miss Louisa Aldrich-Blake's Case Notes, Men and Women, 1917–1920, Parts I and II, H71/RF/B/02/01–02, Royal Free London NHS Foundation Trust, LMA.

[109] Cullen, 'Patient Records', p. 87.

[110] New Hospital for Women House Committee Minutes. Volume V: May 16 1905–Tuesday 24 February 1914, 17 December 1907, H13/EGA/038, LMA; Record of

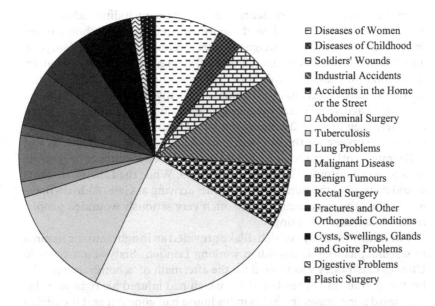

Legend:
- ⊟ Diseases of Women
- ▨ Diseases of Childhood
- ⊟ Soldiers' Wounds
- ▨ Industrial Accidents
- ▨ Accidents in the Home or the Street
- ▢ Abdominal Surgery
- ▢ Tuberculosis
- ▢ Lung Problems
- ■ Malignant Disease
- ■ Benign Tumours
- ■ Rectal Surgery
- ■ Fractures and Other Orthopaedic Conditions
- ■ Cysts, Swellings, Glands and Goitre Problems
- ▨ Digestive Problems
- ■ Plastic Surgery

Figure 5.3 Conditions Suffered by Aldrich Blake's Surgical Patients: RFH, Autumn 1917–Spring 1919.

between 1917 and 1919 at the RFH was considerably different to that of women surgeons' usual demographic. Aldrich-Blake's experience, therefore, broadened the range of cases she would have encountered in peace time, both by gender and by age.

By examining more closely Aldrich-Blake's RFH surgery between 1917 and 1919, a detailed picture can be obtained of the operations she was required to perform. The chart below (Figure 5.3) reveals the general nature of the complaint of all 168 patients treated during this period. Aldrich-Blake's expertise in abdominal surgery was, unsurprisingly, utilised; this category of her patients formed the greatest percentage of overall cases at 23.8 per cent. Most intriguingly, though, the vast majority of these patients were seen by Aldrich-Blake for prosaic hernias and appendicitis. The same routine procedures could be seen with rectal cases, in which, as we saw in chapter 3, Aldrich-Blake excelled. All of the operations she undertook were for haemorrhoids, polyps or abscesses, and only one of the malignant cases was rectal. However,

Recommendations Made by the Advisory Medical Council to the Board of Management: April 1913–May 1934, South London Hospital for Women, Monday 8 February 1915, H24/SLW/A/19/001; Board of Management Minutes, SLHW, Wednesday, 10 March 1915, H24/SLW/A/04/001, LMA.

when the wider area of 'accidents' was added up, including industrial or workplace incidents, as well as those which occurred in the home or on the streets, the same percentage of cases resulted as abdominal surgery. The 'accident' sector dominated when fractures and other orthopaedic conditions were added; of the nine patients who came under this category, two were congenital deformities, and only two more were not the result of an accident. When the numbers of accidental injuries were added together, they formed 26.8 per cent of Aldrich-Blake's caseload. Coupled with surgery for the aftermath of soldiers' wounds, accidental and deliberate injuries came to 31.6 per cent of the total number of patients seen between autumn 1917 and spring 1919. While the LSMW students would be used to the number of accidents arriving at Gate, Aldrich-Blake was leading the treatment of these often very seriously wounded people, rather than simply assisting.

The injuries seen by Aldrich-Blake provided an insight into the hazards of wartime, as well as quotidian working London. Sixty-seven-year-old Charles Champney was treated for the aftermath of 'a bomb dropped by hostile aircraft' in September 1917, which had injured his right foot. He had heard guns firing, the lights in his house had gone out and the ceiling then fell in. Although Champney managed to escape with his daughter and grandson, he only noticed pain in his right foot half an hour after evacuation and saw that his boot was cut open on the outer side. He consulted a very helpful policeman, who cut off his boot and stocking, to discover that Champney had severed part of his little toe.[111] Safety was no longer guaranteed in the home, but neither were the streets nor public transport free from danger. Percy L. Castle, a 48-year-old sorter at the General Post Office, suffered a wound in his left thigh. He had been in a tram on Charing Cross Embankment at midnight when a bomb from enemy aircraft fell near the car. Castle jumped to save himself. Unfortunately, the car floor smashed on impact, an electric fuse ignited and fragments of burning material hit Castle on the left thigh, just below the buttock. He also received injuries to his scalp and left wrist; later there was some conjunctival haemorrhage seen in his left eye.[112] Munition workers of both sexes also formed ten of Aldrich-Blake's patients (seven women; three men). Fifteen-year-old George Hampton was a metal-plate worker in a munitions factory and had been working his treadle when he injured his hand in October 1917.[113] In February 1918, 24-year-old Maud Symes was admitted with ulceration of the arm following a septic wound to her hand. She slipped on a step at work a few months

[111] Charles Champney (LAB 1917: Part I).   [112] Percy L. Castle (LAB, 1917: Part I).
[113] George Hampton (LAB, 1917: Part I).

previously and thought that 'bits of brass' had entered the wound from the floor.[114] Charles Coe's injury caused him problems a long time after his work at a 'Bullet Arsenal' in Woolwich. An explosion in 1915 at the factory resulted in him being hit by a piece of brass. The injuries affected his whole body, from his face all the way down to his leg. More seriously, his right eye was destroyed and he lost the sight in his left eye. Nearly three years later, Coe was still suffering from the effects of his injuries: he had foreign bodies trapped in his eyelid, right temple and under the skin of his left hand, which frequently discharged. Aldrich-Blake removed the first and third, but the second was not found.[115] These were the only three cases where working in a munition factory proved hazardous, although 19-year-old 'munitionette' Ethel Rainbow was found to be infected with secondary syphilis.[116]

If accidents in munitions factories did not provide Aldrich-Blake with too many patients, other industries contributed their fair share. Annie Farrell, who was 63, was in the RFH with a litany of woes. While alighting from a train, she was knocked down by a taxi in December 1917, falling onto her face and bruising it, along with the left hand which had presumably broken her fall. The same taxi then proceeded to run over Miss Farrell while she was prone, hurting her left foot about ankle height. Her foot was set under anaesthetic and a splint was fixed. While an air raid was going on nearly a week later she was carried downstairs at her home without any attention paid by the carrier to her foot. When Miss Farrell came to the RFH the next day, her foot was in a 'bad position'; X-rays later revealed that she had impacted fractures of the tibia and fibula. Aldrich-Blake struggled to reset her foot, but finding very little movement in the seat of fracture, was compelled to use 'strenuous efforts' to achieve a better position. Anyone who felt that women could not be strong enough for such operations would have been amazed by the force this surgeon put into restoring her patient's mobility.[117]

Unlike Annie Farrell's unfortunate accidents, other patients were injured during the working day on the home front. Transport caused problems not only for those utilising its services. Harold Purchase, who was 18 and a packer, jumped from a van and fractured his leg above the

---

[114] Maud Symes (LAB, 1918: Part II).   [115] Charles Coe (LAB: 1918; Part I).

[116] Ethel Rainbow (LAB, 1917: Part I). She was certainly not the only munition worker in these circumstances. See Angela Woollacott, *On Her Their Lives Depend* (Berkeley, CA: University of California Press, 1994), about fears surrounding working-class women's sexual promiscuity when provided with the 'high wages and premature liberty' of munition work, p. 126; also, pp. 134–61.

[117] Annie Farrell (LAB: 1917; Part II). Although this is a case from December 1917, it is out of place in the second box of Aldrich-Blake's records.

ankle.[118] An 18-year-old railway porter, Richard Watson, was required to put a horse into a van. Upon attempting to hit the horse with a whip, he slipped on the wet surface and the van ran over his thigh. He fractured his femur as a result. This was the second time a horse had been the cause of an accident, as the patient had attended Gate in February when one had kicked him.[119] Lift boy, George Munton, who was 16, fell down the shaft by stepping backwards into it when the lift had already gone down. He was bruised and bleeding from the rectum on admission.[120] James Duke, a 44-year-old shunter, was run over by a railway truck, which passed over his right foot and severed it almost completely above the ankle. Unsurprisingly, the patient was in a great deal of pain when he was admitted immediately at 2 a.m. His ankle was removed later.[121] Sydney Farrow, a 46-year-old porter, caught his thumb in a cog wheel, resulting in a compound fracture and a septic injury, which left the thumb black and shrivelled. Aldrich-Blake amputated.[122] Tobacco work was not much safer. In March 1918, Alice Belotti had caught her left foot in a machine, badly breaking and cutting her big toe. Sequestra was removed both in July and August when X-rays revealed that there were several pieces of bone still in the wound, as well as the remains of her terminal phalanx.[123] Bakery was no less dangerous for Stephen Coster, who worked a rolling machine at a biscuit factory and had caught his arm in machinery. It was crushed between two rollers and deeply gashed. The wound required repeated skin grafts and he was in hospital for nearly three months.[124] About 58-year-old French polisher Benjamin Sharp little was added; his pelvis was fractured and he died at 5.10 p.m. on the same day he was admitted in August 1918.[125] That the RFH treated many accidents was evident due to the number of beds set aside for such cases: 17 during the war years out of a total of 200.[126] Only general medical and surgical patients of both sexes were afforded more. Although the war had contributed significantly to the number of maimed and disabled men, accidents, on the street or in the workplace, were causing dangers, as they always had done, to those working on the home front. In similar fashion to her junior counterparts, such as Leila Henry in Sheffield, Aldrich-Blake was able to lead their treatment and restore many to industries vital to keep the country, and war production, moving.

Eight of Aldrich-Blake's surgical patients either were, or had been, soldiers or sailors. As already noted, women surgeons did not only come

---

[118] Harold Purchase (LAB: 1918; Part I).   [119] Richard Watson (LAB: 1917; Part I).
[120] George Munton (LAB: 1918; Part I).   [121] James Duke (LAB: 1918; Part I).
[122] Sydney Farrow (LAB: 1918; Part II).   [123] Alice Bellotti (LAB: 1918; Part II).
[124] Stephen Coster (LAB: 1917; Part I).   [125] Benjamin Sharp (LAB: 1918; Part I).
[126] See, for example, *Ninety-First Annual Report* (1919), p. 51.

across wounded military personnel near the battlefield. Many were still suffering the effects of injuries long after the initial incident had taken place. While surgeons at the front and in base hospitals treated wounds at first hand, those left at home were required to deal with the long-term suffering caused by battlefield injuries. This was not simply obvious problems stemming from amputation, but the more prosaic, such as the effects of trench foot, and the endlessly niggling pieces of shrapnel which tormented those wounded and affected their daily lives. Twelve men were treated at the RFH for trench foot in 1917, for example, while five were suffering from the same complaint a year later. Three men were affected by pain in their amputation stump in 1917, six in 1918, and one in 1919.[127] If we compare the general statistics to Aldrich-Blake's case notes, the patient in 1919 was hers. Clerk Maurice Smith, who was only 20, was admitted in March 1919 with an ulcerated stump. Since his right leg had been amputated a year previously, after a bullet wound in the ankle, Smith had suffered from a persistently ulcerated scar. He had fallen behind enemy lines, been taken prisoner, hospitalised and had his leg removed. Smith was released in September and admitted to Roehampton, where an artificial limb was provided. This aid caused the scar to burst open every time he wore it and it consequently was prevented from healing. While the pressure was not painful, the constant reopening of the wound was obviously causing problems. Aldrich-Blake recommended re-amputation when she saw how gelatinous and unhealthy the remaining parts of Smith's tibia appeared.[128] Men evidently continued to suffer from their injuries even when the cause had been surgically removed. A return to civilian life was neither comfortable nor painless, when old wounds were reopened and further surgical procedures were needed.

It was the after-effects of gunshot wounds, however, which formed the bulk of Aldrich-Blake's military cases. Driver Thomas Cook, a 35-year-old Welshman, was wounded by shrapnel on 18 September 1917, taken to base hospital at Rouen, and X-rayed and operated on a day later for the removal of shrapnel. The same process happened again. Eleven days later, he was brought home and admitted to the RFH. Although Aldrich-Blake operated on his thigh, she was unable to find any remaining shrapnel. The comment that 'patient seems rather depressed; says nerves are much affected still, suffers from sleeplessness' implied that the experience had deeply affected him. Cook appeared to have taken at least two weeks

---

[127] See *Ninetieth*, *Ninety-First*, and *Ninety-Second Annual Reports* for 1917, 1918, and 1919 respectively (1918; 1919; 1920), p. 47; p. 47; p. 47.
[128] Maurice Smith (LAB: 1919; Part II).

to decide upon an operation for the removal of his appendix, for epigastric pain; 'rather worrying' about the procedure, as the notes put it. While his thigh wound continued to discharge, nothing more could be found, and Cook was sent to a convalescent home in December. Two 21-year-old Canadian privates, Russian-born Medensky and McLean, formed Aldrich-Blake's other military patients that autumn. They were admitted the same day with gunshot wounds to the left foot and to the right elbow, respectively. Medensky had been wounded six months before and had been treated at Ypres and Le Havre, but was still unable to walk properly. McLean's injury was more recent – only a fortnight previously. He had moved from a casualty clearing station, to a base hospital and then on to the RFH. Neither appeared to be operated upon, but stayed in the RFH for confirmation of their condition, a small amount of recuperation and healing, and then were moved to convalescent homes. Other men had rejoined civilian life, as we saw with Maurice Smith. Edward Moffatt, who was 40, and now a porter, had been wounded in the head and leg at Ypres in 1916, but was still suffering from the effects of a shrapnel wound in the left buttock. In May 1918 he began to feel pain and throbbing at the site of the buttock injury. Moffatt was X-rayed at the Military Hospital and sent on to Aldrich-Blake. Unlike Cook, Moffatt's shrapnel was located easily, although it had been encapsulated by fibrous tissue. His procedure was a success and he left relieved of pain. James Adams, a 31-year-old painter, came to the RFH in January 1919 complaining of an 'inability to open his mouth'. Two years previously, a shell had burst in his face, injuring his eye. This had been excised and pieces of shrapnel removed. After a good recovery, Adams was cured. Six weeks before his admission, however, he had discovered that his mouth would not open as widely as usual and a swelling appeared on the right side of his head. For the last fortnight, the pain had become increasingly severe and now he was only able to open his mouth one-eighth of an inch and take fluid nourishment. Another swelling had consequently appeared in his right cheek. The difficulty of locating a 'thin flake of metal' made the radiography and surgery of this patient exceptionally hard. Three small foreign bodies were located eventually. Initial surgery proved ineffective and one piece of shrapnel was inaccessible. However, the moving of the shrapnel was momentarily as effective as a cure and meant that Adams could eat solid food and he was discharged at the end of January.[129] In February, Aldrich-Blake located and finally removed the necrosed bone from Adams' face.[130]

---

[129] James Adams (LAB: 1918–1919; Part II).   [130] Ibid. (LAB: 1919; Part II).

The most desperate and frustrating case must have been that of Able Seaman James Smith, who entered the hospital in July 1917, but did not leave until January 1919. He had fractured his left leg, with his tibia and fibula broken at the junction of the middle and lower third. Fragments were separated from each bone and were considerably displaced backwards and outwards. His right leg, a little above and below the middle of the limb, saw each bone broken in two places. Detached fragments were displaced in this leg too. Smith's head wound had been stitched, but he was still suffering from a black eye, so the hospital had received him within a few days of his injury. His tibia was plated by Mr Joll in August 1917 and his right leg was put on a Hodgkin's splint. Alongside surgical treatment, Smith was receiving massage. His bones did not set well, so an extension was performed under anaesthetic in October. Despite apparent improvement, X-rays revealed that the bones were still not healing as hoped and his wounds were discharging. Aldrich-Blake removed Joll's plate in January 1918, as well as a great deal of dead bone and sequestra. By April, Smith was walking on crutches. Aldrich-Blake continued periodically to remove sequestra from his leg wounds; procedures which took an hour or more each time. After a fall in June, Smith was operated upon again and Aldrich-Blake found that the tibia union was only fibrous in his left leg. A month later, when he was attempting to walk, Smith 'felt something snap' in his right leg; X-rays revealed that he had fractured his right tibia at the site of the old injury. In September, there was still no union between the fragments in his left leg, so Aldrich-Blake plated them, in an operation lasting nearly two and a half hours. The leg was now in a good position. Smith's right leg continued discharging, however, into December, and sequestra was extracted at regular intervals. Smith was removed to the Seamen's Hospital at Greenwich in January 1919, where he could be cared for residentially.[131]

Aldrich-Blake's surgical patients provide the historian with a useful insight into what the woman surgeon actually did on the home front when called upon to cover for her male colleagues. While much of her work was undeniably routine and 'unexciting' in surgical terms, she did operate upon a significant majority of men for the first time, as well as carrying out orthopaedic surgery which resulted from the effects of accidents or trauma. Her caseload revealed that those discharged from the military continued to suffer long after receiving wounds. Shellshock has long dominated discussions of medicine during the Great War,[132] and yet

---

[131] James Smith (LAB: 1917–1919; Part II).
[132] Harrison, *The Medical War*, p. 13. Also see Carden Coyne, *Wounds*, for the ongoing physical suffering of military patients.

the physical scars were just as life-changing to those whose injuries would never go away, as we have seen in the cases of, for example, James Smith, James Adams or Maurice Smith. Without the expertise of radiological staff, however, many of these patients would have continued to suffer. It is to a female expert in the field that the last part of this section now turns.

Unlike her sister Edith, Florence Stoney was a qualified doctor and did not suffer from the sense of inferiority which crippled her sibling's confidence at times. Her correspondence, which was largely with Mrs Laurie of the SWH Committee, as well as her sister, allowed more personal reflections than Aldrich-Blake's case notes could into the pressures of war work on the home front. It also compounded the sense, evident in the RFH patient records, of the vital nature of X-ray work for wounded soldiers. Stoney began her war service in Antwerp as head of medical staff and chief of the X-ray department of a unit set up by Mrs St Clair Stobart. When Antwerp fell and the unit escaped to London, she later joined the re-established team who set up at Cherbourg under the French Croix Rouge. Barbara McLaren, in her 1917 account of the Stoneys' work, quoted from Florence Stoney about her experiences abroad. "'Most of our cases were septic fractures'", Stoney remarked, "'badly comminuted as well'": "'The X-rays were much in request to show the exact condition of the part and the position of the fragments'".[133] Easy extraction could result when the pieces were localised. Able to identify, through practice, the dead bone in a comminuted fracture because of its denser shadowy appearance on an X-ray, Stoney contributed to the recovery of the patients by pinpointing pieces for early removal.[134] Stoney and a colleague, Mabel Ramsay, wrote about the hospital's work in a *BMJ* article of June 1915, which described the catastrophic fracture cases, such as those of the cranium, jaw and limbs, they had encountered in the four months between November 1914 and January the following year.[135] This was, as we saw from Aldrich-Blake's record of service, a time when she was also working at Cherbourg. It was not just Stoney's ability to locate shrapnel or dead bone via X-ray which impressed her contemporaries and surgical colleagues. As the *BMJ* commented in 1917, Stoney's images, like those of her sister Edith, were of 'great merit' and stressed their 'workmanship' in detailing the medical history of the war.[136] When

[133] McLaren, *Women of the War*, p. 41.   [134] Ibid., p. 42.

[135] Mabel L. Ramsay and Florence A. Stoney, 'Anglo-French Hospital, No. 2, Chateau Tourlaville, Cherbourg', *BMJ*, 1.2840 (5 June 1915), 966–8. See also Florence A. Stoney, 'The Women's Imperial Service League Hospital', *Archives of the Roentgen Ray*, 19.11 (April 1915), 388–93.

[136] 'The War: The Army Medical Collection of War Specimens at the Royal College of Surgeons of England', *BMJ*, 2.2964 (20 October 1917), 531–4; 532.

the Cherbourg hospital closed in March 1915, it was not surprising that Stoney, who offered her services to the War Office upon her return to Britain, was appointed to the 1000-bed Military Hospital in Fulham. She remained in charge of radiology there until May 1919, when the institution closed. It was at Fulham that she became a key participant in the treatment of so-called 'Soldier's Heart', which was characterised by tachycardia, breathlessness and closely linked, for Stoney, to thyroid hyperactivity.[137] Some manifestations of shellshock or other neurasthenic conditions could be traced back, in Stoney's opinion, to the 'same thing' as hyperthyroidism. Stoney believed that by treating the problem with X-rays and causing the thyroid gland to atrophy with 'vigorous and filtered doses', the patient could be cured without need for surgery.[138]

Yet it was precisely as a fundamental aid to wartime surgery that Stoney's work was most appreciated and needed on the home front. As we have seen with Aldrich-Blake's military patients, unlocalised shrapnel continued to cause problems for the wounded. Case II of the jaw fractures mentioned in Stoney and Ramsay's article described the extensive trajectory of a bullet to the face which fractured the upper and lower maxilla of the patient, who had been fired upon by a German from a tree. A large stellate wound had been created when the bullet had passed through the mouth, and shattered the alveolus posteriorly of the superior maxilla, as well as the entire vertical ramus of the inferior maxilla. The bullet had ricocheted off a button and hit the patient's shoulder; the coracoid was splintered and the bullet embedded in the axilla, where it broke into many pieces. As the patient's carotid artery was exposed and appalling sepsis resulted, the Cherbourg team feared a secondary haemorrhage from the artery. While the face wound healed and parts of the jaw were removed, it was Stoney who was responsible for the location of the extensive shrapnel. '[C]areful localis[ing]' meant that 'most of the pieces' were removed from the 'long track' of injury. Now able to eat well and possessing good movement in the shoulder, the patient was a success story for Cherbourg and emphasised the need for precision in X-ray work.[139] In this article, Ramsay and Stoney stressed that surgery for bullet wounds should not be viewed as a one-off operation; procedures in the plural were necessary 'before finally healing to remove dead

---

[137] See her contribution to the discussion at the Therapeutical and Pharmacological Section of the RSM, published in *PRSM*, 9 (1916), 50–7. For more on the condition, see Joel D. Howell, '"Soldier's Heart": The Redefinition of Heart Disease and Specialty Formation in Early Twentieth-Century Great Britain', *MH*, 29 (January 1985), 34–52.

[138] Stoney, 'Discussion on the Soldier's Heart', *PRSM*, 1916, 54.

[139] Ramsay and Stoney, 'Fractures of the Jaws: Case II', in 'Anglo-French Hospital, No. 2', 966.

sequestra'.[140] Another patient, Case II of the tetanus patients, was shot through both legs, which resulted in extremely septic, foul wounds. The bullet, which had come to rest in the outer side of the head of the fibula, which it had also fractured, was extracted on the second day after admission. This was 'greatly aid[ed]' by Stoney's X-ray and localisation.[141] The 'invaluable' work carried out by Stoney was lauded because of its exactness, which spared the surgeons 'a vast deal of trouble, and also saved useless incisions', benefitting the patients as well. Similarly useless searches did not need to be performed if the bullet or shrapnel was too deeply embedded but difficult to access and not presenting any trouble.[142] Stoney brought her experience at Cherbourg to bear on her work at the Fulham Military Hospital (FMH), where X-ray diagnosis and treatments continued to assist surgical procedures and spare patients unnecessary further trauma.

The nature of surgery's published reliance on heroic radiology concealed a more uneven relationship between the two behind the scenes. Stoney's letters, like those of her sister Edith, revealed the tensions between members of the surgical team; the former, however, wrote at length about health problems faced by the hard-working X-ray operator. When she was awarded an OBE in 1919 for her 'very strenuous' war work, Stoney remarked to Laurie that 'X-ray work is very exacting, though few realise it'.[143] This sense of unappreciated difficulties was compounded by its opposite: the expectation that X-rays could solve anything. Surgeons, Stoney lamented in December 1915, 'always ask more of X rays than they can possibly perform'.[144] Laurie worried in May 1916 that there was 'a great responsibility on [Stoney's] shoulders in Fulham Hospital'.[145] Six months earlier, Stoney had given Laurie some statistics about her time at the institution. She had personally taken over 1800 plates since the end of April that year, as the War Office required every case to be photographed, rather than screened, 'on account of the risk to those working the machines'. This safeguard was undermined, however, by the fact that she had to 'take several plates' in some instances. The hospital did possess a 'lead partition to shield the operators from the rays'.[146] Such a

140 Ibid., 967.
141 'Tetanus: Case II', Ibid., 968. Despite eventual amputation of his right leg the patient died from the effects of tetanus.
142 'Notes', ibid., 268.
143 Florence Stoney to Mrs Laurie, 29 Nottingham Place, 13 March 1919, in Tin 12: Letters to and From Miss Stoney, Radiographer from August 1915 to March 1920, SWHC.
144 Florence Stoney to Mrs Laurie, 2 December 1915.
145 Mrs Laurie to Edith Stoney, 23 May 1916.
146 Florence Stoney to Mrs Laurie, 24 November 1915.

measure meant that Stoney and her co-workers were made safer than her colleagues at the front or in base hospitals, where the usefulness of the X-ray process surmounted concerns about the protection of operator and patient.[147] Fully aware of the problems her own sister was experiencing, she berated the SWH Committee for penny-pinching and putting the health of valuable workers at risk:

if you economise too much in plates – you both don't do as good work and you risk the operator's health – it is really dangerous to do a lot of screen work, such as is necessary if photographic plates cannot be taken – as it is the risk of X-ray work is very considerable for the operators – more with a makeshift room not properly protected – than with a fixed installation.[148]

Protection may have been more adequately arranged in the fixed situation of the well-equipped FMH, but Stoney was evidently physically affected by her time there.

As her obituary made clear, Stoney dealt with more than 15,000 cases at Fulham, many of whom had been 'sent from other hospitals for the localization of bullets and pieces of shrapnel'.[149] Stoney's letters from July 1916 gave a clear indication of pressures faced by her department in the aftermath of a big push. On 6 July, they were receiving 'floods of wounded over from France'. That day alone she had 'X Rayed 25 cases and there are many more waiting to be done tomorrow'.[150] Ten days later, in a few short lines to Mrs Laurie, she noted that '[t]omorrow is a full day. The wounded are coming in so fast from France we are all busy – I have been working all day to try and keep up with the rush.'[151] In August, claustrophobic working conditions were described with grim irony. The 'great number of cases at Fulham from the fighting at the Somme, as well as further north' had darkened the past few months, 'so that these long hot Summer days I have spent in the delightful recesses of my dark room with all the light and air shut out, and with an electric fan going to prevent our melting'.[152] Such cases were still being received at Fulham in the spring of the following year. With pride, Stoney remarked that a recently unsatisfactory case, wounded in August 1916, had arrived at the hospital with a 'bullet behind his heart and his chest all blocked up with effusion', but was about to be liberated of unwanted shrapnel. '[A]pparently', she crowed, 'it has never been localised and dealt with, all these months – he was in a hospital in Portsmouth': 'I expect it will

[147] McDonald, 'X-Rays', in Scotland and Heys, eds., *War Surgery*, p. 137.
[148] Florence Stoney to Mrs Laurie, 24 November 1915.
[149] 'Obituary: Florence A. Stoney, OBE, MD', *BMJ*, 2.3745 (15 October 1932), 734.
[150] Florence Stoney to Mrs Laurie, 20 Reynolds Close, 6 July 1916.
[151] Ibid., 16 July 1916.   [152] Ibid., 4 August 1916.

be taken out in a day or two now'.[153] The omission of her involvement in finally solving the mystery only deepened the importance of the discovery, both for herself and for the patient: a fact of which Stoney was evidently aware. By September 1918, however, she was afraid that her health might not hold up for the end of the war. On the fifth of the month came the dreaded recognition: 'I have knocked up'.[154] Stoney hoped this was a temporary situation and had therefore taken six weeks' 'rest from X-rays': 'it is more exacting that most people realise – and I have had 3 ½ years almost continuously shut up in the dark'. She was back at work in November, reassured that she 'shall hold out now till the end of the war'.[155] Although this was written only three days before the Armistice, Stoney's work at Fulham was not over until the following spring.

As Aldrich-Blake's former military patients illustrated, the war did not end for those who suffered from the physical after-effects of modern warfare. Neither, therefore, did the need for Stoney end on 11 November 1918. Even in March 1919 the work was 'still strenuous' and by this point, the rumoured information that Fulham was to close in May, encouraged a weary whoop of joy: 'I shall be very glad if that is so.'[156] A month later she reiterated her sense that 'few' realised what the 'constant strain of X-ray work in the dark stuff atmosphere and with the X rays about – mean to the workers'.[157] The imagery of light and dark utilised by Stoney is worth further notice. She was desperate to 'be free to get some sunshine again', while she hoped that her sister Edith will one day be 'something like her old bright self again'. Time in the dark with the shadowy pictures left both longing for mental and physical daylight. Both were scarred by their experiences. While the war allowed the Stoney sisters to make themselves useful to the 'great cause of the wounded',[158] their X-ray work robbed them eventually of their health.[159] Florence Stoney would be 'no exception', as the BMJ put it, to the 'usually painful deaths' of the X-ray pioneers, knowing 'quite well what would be the manner of her death'.[160] As McLaren rightly claimed in 1917, Stoney took up her appointment at

[153] Ibid., 29 Nottingham Place, 1 March 1917.
[154] Ibid., Co. Kerry, 5 September 1918. For an exploration of the self-abnegation of early radiologists, see Daniel S. Goldberg, 'Suffering and Death among Early American Roentgenologists: The Power of Remotely Anatomizing the Living Body in Fin de Siècle America', BHM, 85.1 (Spring 2011), 1–28.
[155] Florence Stoney to Mrs Laurie, Fulham Military Hospital, 8 November 1918.
[156] Ibid., 29, Nottingham Place, 13 March 1919.
[157] Ibid., 29, Nottingham Place, 23 April 1919.   [158] Ibid., 2 December 1915.
[159] See obituaries of Florence Stoney in British Journal of Radiology, 5.59 (November 1932), 853–58 and in BMJ, 2.3745 (15 October 1932), 734 and 2.3746 (22 October 1932), 777.
[160] S. Watson Smith, 'The Late Dr Florence Stoney', BMJ, 2.3746 (22 October 1932), 777.

the FMH a fortnight before Endell Street opened. As such she became the 'first woman doctor to work under the War Office in England'.[161] Yet, it was Garrett Anderson and Murray who dominated the press coverage in the spring of 1915; women like Stoney remained 'so often unsung'.[162] They were lauded as providing the 'most glowing and striking tribute' to the work of the woman doctor.[163] And yet without the fundamental assistance of disciplines ancillary to surgery such as radiology, surgeons would have been far more in the dark than they were at home and at the front. Through a consideration of the work of experienced women such as Aldrich-Blake and Stoney it is possible to evaluate the importance of ongoing surgical care at home during the war, whether that be for injured military personnel or for ordinary men, women and children. Surgical procedures were increasingly dependent, especially in the case of delayed reactions to shrapnel or foreign bodies, on the illumination of the X-ray and the skill of the rays' operator. Aldrich-Blake's patient, Edward Moffatt, for example, had been X-rayed at the Military Hospital and sent on to the RFH for operation.[164] Co-operation between surgeons and members of the wider team of medical and scientific professionals ensured those left behind on the home front would continue to receive effective operative treatment in spite of wartime conditions.

Women Surgeons and the Opening of a New Hospital in Wartime

While this chapter has concentrated so far on the expansion of women surgeons' professional work into areas they had not been able to oper-ate in before, it is necessary to explore how their more usual 'sphere' of influence fared during the Great War. Brian Abel-Smith's claim that 'the crisis of war' meant that 'young active males came before women, chil-dren, and old people' can be refuted through an examination of the ways in which the establishment of the South London Hospital for Women and Children focused public attention on the importance of precisely these sections of the population.[165] Epidemiologists and historians of medicine have debated for decades over the causes of the decrease in mortality rate in the second half of the nineteenth century and during the Great War for the civilian population of Britain.[166] I will not argue that a group of

---

161 McLaren, *Women of the War*, p. 42.   162 Ibid.
163 'The Week in London', *Queen*, 27 February 1915, in *LSMWRFHPC*, *Vol. 5*.
164 Edward Moffatt (LAB: 1918; Part I).
165 Brian Abel-Smith, *The Hospitals 1800–1948* (London: Heinemann, 1964), p. 283.
166 See, for example, Thomas McKeown, *The Modern Rise of Population* (London: Edward Arnold, 1976) and Simon Szreter's refutation of his analysis in 'The Importance of

women surgeons deciding to establish a hospital for women and children in 1912, which came to fruition in 1916, led to a decline in the mortality of those social groups. Rather, I want to analyse how this institution was set up and developed precisely to foster and protect these members of the civilian population, during the present exigencies of war and for the future. As we have already seen in this chapter, women doctors and their supporters drew very carefully in wartime publicity upon their vital contribution to the health of the nation and to the well-being of the women and potential children who would people a post-war world. Millicent Garrett Fawcett put this dramatically when she remarked in 1914 that the 'precious lives of men in the prime of life' were being lost every day in France and Belgium: 57,000 alone in the first three months of warfare. Women must, therefore, 'stop the wastage at the outset of life, and secure for the country a larger proportion of healthy "well born" citizens who will be the men and women of the future'.[167] This final section will explore how a group of women behind the establishment of the SLHW were canny in their appeals to the public. They had learnt from criticism of the LSMW's moneymaking tactics and made sure that they tailored requests for support to perceived public necessities. By pushing women and children to the forefront, and, additionally, remarking upon the lack of hospital beds for those who could afford to pay, the women behind the SLHW focused attention away from their own needs onto those of their patients.

The SLHW was mooted first in December 1911. 'It had then long been recognised', stated the hospital's prospectus, that 'the demand among women for medical and surgical treatment by members of their own sex was growing, and growing rapidly'.[168] Additionally, the NHW was unable to cope with the overwhelming need for its services; an equivalent was required south of the river.[169] The outpatient department opened in April 1913, while its in-patient equivalent, built anew, was declared open in July 1916.[170] Temporary in-patient accommodation had been

---

Social Intervention in Britain's Mortality Decline c.1850–1914: a Re-Interpretation of the Role of Public Health', *SHM*, 1.1 (April 1988), 1–38. For wartime health, see J.M. Winter, *The Great War and the British People*, second edition (Basingstoke: Palgrave Macmillan, 2003).

[167] Millicent Garrett Fawcett, 'Women's Work in War Time', *Contemporary Review*, CVI (December 1914), 775–782; 779, in *LSMWRFHPC, Vol. V.*

[168] 'A Brief Account of its Origin and Progress', *The South London Hospital for Women* (n.d.; c.1917–1918), p. 5, H24/SLW/A/44/002, LMA.

[169] H. Franklin, 'A New Hospital for Women', *Daily News and Leader*, 12 October 1912, in *SLHWPC.*

[170] 'Women as Hospital Doctors. South London Enterprise', *St James's Gazette*, 3 April 1913; 'The Queen at Clapham. Her Majesty Opens the Women's Hospital, (unidentified, but definitely local newspaper; July 1916), ibid.

provided from 1914 at a nursing home called Warrington Lodge.[171] Support for the hospital was impressive; the majority of funding was provided by anonymous benefactors, keen to support women treating their own sex.[172] The initial Committee which established the institution was composed of Maud Chadburn, surgeon at the NHW, and Eleanor Davies-Colley, the first female FRCS, along with a number of other medical women.[173] Patients would not require a subscriber's letter, in similar fashion to the RFH, and they would be treated gratuitously, excepting a contribution of 3d. a week for the cost of medicine. To prevent the dreaded abuse of hospital benevolence, so feared by late nineteenth- and early twentieth-century institutions, an almoner would ensure that only suitable cases would receive free treatment.[174] From the outset, however, it was also proposed that the hospital should have special consultation hours for patients who would be sent by their own general practitioners and who could not afford to see a consultant. Furthermore, paying wards would enable those with a small income, although not affluent enough to pay nursing-home fees, to receive hospital and, specifically, surgical, treatment, in addition to their own private or small, shared rooms. As we saw in chapter 2, not all patients were typically working class in early twentieth-century hospitals, but the majority would have been. This still popular perception that institutions were for charity cases only meant both that the middle class avoided them or, alternately, that they took advantage of beds in general hospitals which should have been for the exclusive use of the poorest in society.[175] As Prochaska has remarked, middle-class women 'were known to dress down to avoid payment'.[176] The SLHW decided to cater for potential variations in 'small' income by

---

171 'The South London Hospital for Women. Munificent Gift to Building Fund', *Clapham Observer*, Friday, 5 March 1915, ibid; SLHW Advisory Medical Council Minutes: April 1913–May 1934, 11 May 1914; 9 June 1914, H24/SLW/A/19/001.

172 The anonymous donors were never identified, even in any of the hospital's many committee meetings, and appeared only as 'some friends of medical women'. For their initial contribution, see SLHW Board of Management Minutes, Volume I (July 1912–September 1915), Saturday, 30 November 1912, H24/SLW/A/04/001. For details of donations, see SLHW Trustee Minutes: 1913–1924, H24/SLW/A03. By 1916, they had donated £71,000. See a vote of thanks on Wednesday, 9 February 1916, in Board of Management Minutes, Volume II (October 1915–December 1918), H24/SLW/A/04/002.

173 Promotion Committee Minutes of the SLHW, 8 December 1911, H24/SLW/A1/1.

174 See Keir Waddington, *Charity and the London Hospitals, 1850–1898* (Woodbridge: Boydell Press, 2000) and 'Unsuitable Cases'. For the almoner system, see Cullen, 'The First Lady Almoner.

175 The latter point is implied by Elizabeth Sloan Chesser when she states that such women 'should not be occupying the free wards intended for the very poor in ordinary hospitals'. See 'A New Women's Hospital', *Standard*, 3 August 1912, in *SLHWPC*.

176 Prochaska, *Philanthropy*, p. 74.

offering a rising scale of cost for private beds. This was initially from £3 3s. 0d. weekly for a single room, £2 2s. 0d. for a bed in a ward containing two beds, and £1 1s. 0d. weekly for a stay in the eight-bed cubicle ward.[177] By providing this 'special feature',[178] the hospital was assigning 14 of its projected 80 beds to private patients. This was publicised as a 'much-needed innovation'.[179] The SLHW was therefore filling a considerable gap for those who needed an operation, but could not usually be considered necessitous.

Whereas the LSMW had been castigated for solely promoting their own cause, the SLHW was more careful in its publicity. The 'Aims and Objects' of the institution were listed in the second *Annual Report* for 1913:

1. To meet the great and growing demand on the part of women for medical treatment by members of their own sex.
2. To provide, in addition to ordinary hospital accommodation, private wards for women of limited means at an inclusive charge of from one to three guineas a week.
3. To afford further scope for post graduate training for medical women.[180]

Here, patients were listed first and second, while benefits for medical women came last. The focus of the founding committee on the opportunities for postgraduate clinical experience also differed from the LSMW's plea for future medical women, rather than those already qualified. During the war, evidently conscious of the pressure of conditions, as well as the way in which appeals from the LSMW had been received, the Press Committee of the hospital decided in November 1915 that it was inadvisable to proceed with articles on the present disabilities of medical women.[181] Interestingly, it was the SLHW's Medical Council which had vetoed this suggestion.[182] Instead, press coverage considered more appropriate was that concerning the work of the hospital, rather than its personnel. That the hospital instigated the wonderfully named Drawing-Room Meeting Propaganda Sub-Committee implied how seriously they

---

[177] This information is announced in many different articles advertising the hospital. See, for example, Lady Chance, 'A New Hospital for Women. South London Scheme', *Standard*, 14 October 1912, *SLHWPC.*; *SLHW Fourth Annual Report for the Year 1915* (London: Printed by The Women's Printing Society, Limited, 1916), p. 26.

[178] *Second Annual Report for the Year 1913* (1914), p. 11.

[179] 'A New Hospital for Women', *Observer*, 15 December 1912, in *SLHWPC.*

[180] *Second Annual Report*, p. 6.

[181] Press Committee of the SLHW, 24 November 1915, H24/SLW/A10/1.

[182] There is no record, however, of this being brought up in the AMC's minutes, but as the suggestion was made initially at the meeting of the Press Committee on 17 July 1914, it may have been discussed privately.

took the business of advertising their services. Unlike the grand society occasions most hospitals utilised to squeeze more support out of the aristocracy, the SLHW used the titled on their board to write to the newspapers, as well as organise more intimate drawing-room meetings. Lists of who should write to which paper were found in the meetings of the Press Committee, showing how carefully the institution matched its patrons to different press outlets. For example, the Press Sub-Committee reported in April 1913 that the following would be asked to write in support of the hospital:

Lady Robert Cecil to The Times; Lady Castlereagh to Morning Post; Lady Hulse to Daily Telegraph; Mr Franklin to Daily News; Mr Courtney to Pall Mall, and Observer; Lady Dupplin to The Queen; Lady Emmott or Mrs Talbot to The Westminster; Lady Willoughby de Broke to The Standard; Mrs J.P. Boyd-Carpenter to The Guardian; Miss Emily Davis [sic] to Manchester Guardian; Lady Thrift to Surrey Comet; Lady Busk or Lady Brassey to Daily Chronicle; Lady Chance to Sunday Times.

Also letters to the suffrage and Anti-Suffrage papers, and Mrs P. Lawrence to be asked to write an article in Votes for Women.[183]

The latter sentence was telling; even opponents in the suffrage question had women's interests at heart, so why not appeal to both? Politics could be put aside when the health of the nation was at stake. Actresses were contacted, who would be able to offer sketches or speak at meetings. Their attendance was encouraged both because of their rhetorical flair, but also in the hope that they would be impressed by the provision of paying wards and form a league to support the use of a private bed.[184] During the war the management of a variety of theatres contributed collecting boxes to the hospital, including the Alhambra, Empire, Wyndham's and Gaiety. Debenham and Freebody's, the department store, also donated to the cause in the same year.[185] Garden-parties were proposed, not just for the upper classes, but also for local businessmen.[186] Early-closing day was also taken into account when recommending dates for fundraising events.[187]

Indeed, the importance of propinquity was recognised from the start, especially in the form of printed advertisements; after all, local people would form the core patient base of the hospital, at least in the outpatient department. Newspapers from 1912 to 1917, held in the hospital's

---

[183] Press Committee Minutes, Wednesday, 9 April 1913, H24/SLW/A10/1.
[184] Drawing-Room Meeting Propaganda Sub-Committee Minutes: November 1912–June 1914, 1 October 1913, H24/SLW/A10/2.
[185] 'Collecting Boxes', Fifth Annual Report for the Year 1916 (1917), p. 51.
[186] Drawing-Room Meeting Sub-Committee, 7 May 1913.
[187] Ibid., 23 April 1913.

press scrapbook, include cuttings from the *South London Press*, *Clapham Observer*, *Wandsworth Boro' News*, *Camberwell and Peckham Times*, *Sydenham Boro' Gazette*, *Sydenham Boro' News*, and *Balham News-Letter*. Minutes from the Propaganda Sub-Committee made clear the aim of stimulating interest locally. Speakers at meetings to drum up funding were to appeal 'very strongly to the neighbourhood'.[188] In May 1914, it was suggested that a special South London Committee be formed to work in the area on increasing local residents' commitment to the institution.[189] Specific areas were identified and targeted. For example, 'Richmond Propaganda' formed an item on the minutes of a meeting in the spring of 1914.[190] Meetings were held in schools, as well as drawing rooms; Blackheath High School was the venue for an 'at home' intended to support the SLHW in May 1913.[191] Such locations were deliberate, as the hospital wanted to stress its private wards to professional women, including teachers, and to encourage them to set up leagues to support beds for their members. This was a successful manoeuvre, as the Teachers' League and Professional and Business Women's League established connections with the hospital and endowed beds in the private wards.[192] As the RFH's gynaecological patient base revealed in chapter 2, women requiring surgical treatment did not always consult their own sex before entering hospital; however, an exception can be made for professionals, who, as statistics proved, were more likely to visit female doctors. Or, as the *Daily News and Leader* put it in October 1912, '[w]orking women and the thinking Society women almost invariably consult a woman doctor in preference to a man'.[193] Publicity for the hospital repeatedly stressed the ways in which 'gentlewomen' had been overlooked in medical and surgical provision.[194] As a consequence, appeals were directed towards women of this class, locally and further afield, to support themselves should they need hospital treatment.

At the SLHW's Annual Meeting in 1915, Maud Chadburn defended the institution against contemporary expectations that war had brought male and female medical professionals closer together. In opposition to the belief that barriers were breaking down, she re-erected them, precisely for the sake of her patients. Chadburn responded to the claim that 'almost

[188] Ibid., 7 May 1913.   [189] Ibid., 29 May 1914.   [190] Ibid.

[191] *Blackheath Local Guide and Advertiser*, 10 May 1913, in *SLHWPC*.

[192] 'The Teachers' League and Professional and Business Women's League', *Second Annual Report*, p. 11.

[193] 'Ministering Angels. Striking Scheme for Establishing a new Hospital for Women', *Daily News and Leader*, 22 October 1912, in *SLHWPC*.

[194] 'The South London Hospital for Women'. By a Medical Woman, *Queen*, 9 November 1912, ibid.

everyone agreed that men and women should work together and that it was the best and healthiest so to be' with a riposte:

It was simply the result of a demand, the overwhelming demand on the part of women workers – the class of women who as patients entered the general and private wards of hospitals – for more accommodation under women doctors (Applause). These patients had plenty of hospitals staffed by men doctors and they did not ask for education in ideals as giving them a mixed staff would be, but they asked for hospital accommodation where they could be under women doctors, and so the South London Hospital for Women appeared and has been a wonderful success (Applause). [. . .]

The times were not yet ripe for men and women working together on equal terms. One very rarely found the terms equal and anything less than equal terms was bad for men and women.[195]

In amongst all the excitement of wartime opportunities, Chadburn presented an oddly dated, yet compellingly realistic argument in favour of a hospital for women run by women as a 'product of the times'. Her stance was analogous to those supporting the inward-looking fortress of the LSMW, who said 'No, thanks very much' to co-education. By turning around the contemporary fascination with women's opportunities on the home front, she claimed that it was 'unreasonable and impossible to expect medical men to vacate their valuable posts on London hospital staffs in order to give medical women a chance of development'. Women, she argued vehemently, 'must find opportunities for themselves'.[196] Their male colleagues were 'perhaps even secretly thankful that women were making new posts for themselves rather than trying to acquire some of the men's positions (Applause)'. Although ideal, it was unlikely that appointments would be thrown open to men and women equally for some years to come. If the present staff of the hospital waited for this to occur, 'they would live and die without their opportunity'; so, too, would several other generations of their successors.[197] Women could not abandon their roles as professionals for their own sex because it was neither productive for them, nor fair to their patients. And, with hospital beds being given over to wounded soldiers and sailors, it was only right that there should be increased accommodation for their wives, sisters, mothers, and daughters. 'The health of the women of the country became increasingly important as this war continued with its terrible toll of their best men', continued Chadburn. It was contingent upon those left behind to see

[195] 'The South London Hospital for Women. Clapham's Great Female Institution', *Clapham Observer*, 4 June 1915, ibid.
[196] 'The South London Hospital for Women', *Common Cause*, 11 June 1915, ibid.
[197] *Clapham Observer*, 4 June 1915.

that the families of these men were neither neglected nor their menfolk troubled or distracted from their important fight on the Continent. Neither was it simply the working classes who were affected. The 'financial position of the professional classes and of the people of small means', concluded Chadburn, would make the demand for the private wards – of which this hospital was to have a large number – greater than ever (Applause)'.[198] The SLHW, argued its founder, was both necessary and vital to the preservation of the health of men, women and children, today and in the future.

During the war years, the demand for the hospital was indeed high. Established by 'women surgeons of repute', it is hardly surprising that publicity focused specifically upon the need for female surgical assistance in cases where the 'dread' of examination by men led to neglect, unnecessary suffering and the advancement of conditions which would become inoperable because of the delay.[199] In addition to the 'modest and refined' nature of the middle classes, however, cost could also be factored into the awful prospect of physical and mental discomfort.[200] Surgical treatment, skilled nursing and the luxuries of a nursing home could not be afforded by women of small means.[201] '[H]undreds of brave women workers to whom at present illness means unnecessary tragedy' would receive an 'inestimable blessing' from the privacy of paying wards.[202] Unsurprisingly, surgical procedures grew enormously at the SLHW during the Great War. The institution 'desired to point out', in its *Annual Report* for 1915, that the 'heavy toll levied by the war upon the manhood of the country makes the health of the women and children a matter of national importance'.[203]

From a mere 40 in 1914, when surgery was being carried out in Warrington Lodge, the hospital was carrying out 770 operations by 1918 on its own new premises; 440, or just over 57 per cent of which were major procedures (Figure 5.4).[204] Most importantly, given the hospital's remit to care specifically for those suffering from ailments peculiar to the female sex, at least 198, or 45 per cent, of those major operations

---

198 Ibid.
199 Miss A.E.A. Baker, 'What is Wanted. South London Hospital for Women', *Kentish Independent*, 30 November 1912, ibid.
200 'Drawing Room Meeting', *Kentish Independent*, 29 November 1913, ibid.
201 'A New Women's Hospital. Consultations and Paying Wards for Ladies of Small Means', *Evening Standard*, 22 October 1912, ibid.
202 Olga Hartley, 'A New South London Hospital for Women', *Gentlewoman*, 3 May 1913, p. 30, ibid.
203 *Fourth Annual Report for the Year 1915* (1916), p. 13.
204 *Seventh Annual Report*, p. 34.

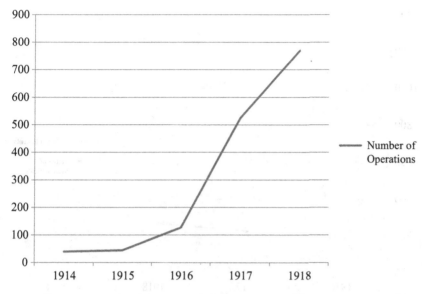

Figure 5.4 Number of Operations: SLHW, 1914–1918.[205]

in 1918 were for the diseases of women.[206] The figures for private patients were interesting to compare with the overall numbers of in-patients (Figure 5.5). For the two years where figures are available, the private patients form 23.2 per cent of all seen in 1917 and 23.3 per cent in 1918. Given there were only 14 beds assigned to private patients, 20.9 per cent of 67 in 1917, and 17.5 per cent of the whole 80 available by 1918, demand was clearly high. In the 1917 *Annual Report*, indeed, the hospital remarked specifically on the numbers in private wards. The comments revealed a distinction in wartime between the working-class rise in standards, wages and access to treatment and middle-class financial burdens. As the 'Almoner's Report' made clear in 1915, the great desire both for skilled and unskilled labour because of the economic and industrial situation caused by the war was coupled with an increase in the cost of living. However, for workers, this was counterbalanced by the increase in wages.[207] For those members of the middle classes on

---

[205] Calculated from Third to Seventh *Annual Reports* for the years 1914 to 1918, published between 1915 and 1919.

[206] The figure could be higher. There were also 44 laparotomies, which are not further explained.

[207] 'Almoner's Report', *Fourth Annual Report*, pp. 29–30; p. 29.

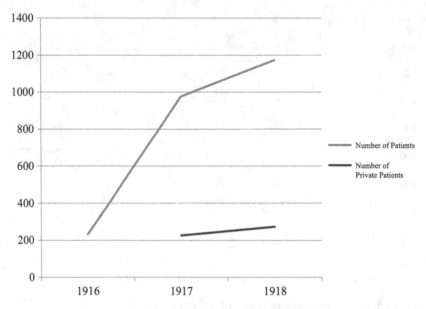

Figure 5.5 Patients: SLHW, July 1916–December 1918.[208]

'limited means', there was no such boom. As the 1917 *Annual Report* claimed, the sliding-scale of the cost of the private wards was 'proving an especial boost to those whose incomes have been reduced as a result of the War'.[209] With the prolongation of the conflict more and more women came under that category and the SLHW was there to support them if they were in ill-health or required surgery.

Conclusion

As this chapter has considered, there was a range of opportunities open to those women who chose to stay in Britain and assist in the care of the civilian population. For some, this meant treating men surgically for the first time; for others the health of women and children needed to be protected while the country was at war. It was undoubtedly one of the worst times to keep hospitals running, let alone securely establish them, as the SLHW showed. Although it tried to attract female staff, sometimes the desire to try something more than their usual patient base meant it

[208] Calculated from Fifth to Seventh *Annual Reports* for the years 1916 to 1918, published between 1917 and 1919.
[209] *Sixth Annual Report*, p. 7.

was extremely difficult to recruit suitable women to look after their own. As Emily Hill wrote in the *National Weekly*, in 1917, this desertion of potential medical and surgical staff, which affected all British hospitals, was coupled with

the enormous price of food, fuel and drugs, the irresistible claims of the wounded and sick from the battlefield, the consequent scarcity of nurses, together with the insistent calls of the Government to give every shilling that we can spare, and even the shillings we cannot spare, to help the country, have all imposed a heavy strain on the management and on the staff.[210]

It is no wonder that the writer of 'A Lament', whose poem opened this chapter, envied the lives of her surgical counterparts abroad. In contrast to the penny-pinching at home, at Royaumount Elizabeth Courtauld indulged in condensed milk on bread, and army rations which contained 'many things civilians can't [have] now-a-days'.[211] Ruth Verney's recollections of Salonika were that they had '[l]ots of tinned food and so on. Oh we did very well for food really'.[212] A lack of material goods, though, was not compounded by restrictions in salary on the home front, as women profited from the need for their services. Those who did not forget that they were 'locum tenens for wartime' must have accepted their lot when the war ended. And those, like Maud Chadburn, who insisted that the time was still not right for the mingling of men and women professionally, must have felt vindicated with the success of the SLHW in 'safeguarding the new generation of citizens' through protecting 'suffering women' and ensuring a 'far-reaching effect in the future'. The 'preservation, the conservation of life'[213] was not far from any of the women's minds whose experiences were considered in this chapter, whoever they decided to treat. That they had multiple possibilities in the first place was contingent upon the exceptional wartime conditions. If the shine on their halo has not resonated as brightly as their frontline colleagues, this should not devalue the importance of their work. How each chose to operate during the Great War years revealed that 'Adoctoring' on the home front was neither as dull nor as unchallenging as the anonymous poet implied.

---

[210] Emily Hill, 'The South London Hospital for Women and Children, Clapham Common', *National Weekly*, 16 June 1917, 635–6; 636, in *SLHWPC*.
[211] Courtauld to Ruth, Royaumont, 28 August 1918, in WWI/WO/023, LC.
[212] Verney, Tape 477.
[213] Elizabeth Sloan Chesser, 'Women's Work for Women. The Needs of the Hospitals' [unknown publication], 1915, in *SLHWPC*.

Conclusion

In April 2014, Clare Marx became the first female president of the Royal College of Surgeons in its 214-year history. In an interview following her election, Marx observed that she had never thought of herself as a 'female surgeon'. 'No-one said to me', she continued, 'this is not a world you can enter. I had no negative feedback, just what I regarded as teasing.'[1] Marx considers herself 'lucky' and is aware that other women of her generation have been less fortunate. Nonetheless, that any woman could enjoy such an experience was the product of a remarkable revolution in surgical attitudes and practices. Now more than half of applicants to medical school are women, 29.5 per cent of surgical trainees were female in 2014, and women are represented across all surgical specialties, yet the perceived macho culture of surgery and intergenerational tensions dampen enthusiasm for potential recruits.[2]

This book has told the first chapter in the story of this transformation, but has also indicated historical reasons why there are still challenges for those 'less fortunate' women in surgery, including divisions over the ways in which to practise. Unlike Marx, women in the mid-nineteenth century were told that they could not and would not dare to enter the operating theatre and they received critical and derogatory comments about their capabilities when confronted with the stresses and strains of practice. I have considered the ways in which the first women to enter the medical profession picked up scraps of surgical learning piecemeal, awed by their own stamina in the face of operations which they were told they would not withstand. Unable initially to practise in general hospitals, women set up their own, which became specialist surgical centres. The surgery performed there was a process of trial and error, where skills were, eventually, learnt through experience. This book has

---

[1] Luisa Dillner, 'Interview: Clare Marx: "No one said to me this is a world you cannot enter"', *BMJ* 2015;350:h462 [accessed 16 May 2016].

[2] http://surgicalcareers.rcseng.ac.uk/wins/statistics [accessed 16 May 2016]; Mary Ann Elston, *Women and Medicine: The Future* (London: Royal College of Physicians, 2009). For the American context, see More, *Restoring the Balance*.

also, through a study of patient records, explored the experiences of those who came under the female surgical knife, as a counterpoint to the histories of those who wielded it. As well as providing an insight into the patient reaction to hospitalisation, such an investigation contributes to the understanding of, as Risse and Harley Warner put it, 'the broader conditions of social life'.[3] Case notes can give the historian an unusually detailed picture of the everyday lives and struggles of the poorest in society. That the women patients who entered the Royal Free Hospital had very little contact with women medical practitioners beforehand made the encounter between them and their female surgeons particularly fascinating. What those patients were willing to undergo when they were suffering from agonisingly painful malignancies and the corresponding way in which their surgeons sought to treat them provided a key refutation to the argument that women moved away from surgical procedures in the 1910s. In line with the experimental bent of surgery in the late nineteenth and early twentieth centuries, female surgeons adopted, adapted and honed their operative skills.[4] They were anxious to buy time, as they saw it, for their patients, choosing risky surgery over less invasive radium or X-ray applications, which were offered only to the dying and later were in cruelly short supply even for terminal cases due to the Great War. This book's final sections returned to the scenario conjured up by those who, more than half-a-century earlier, had described a room of Semiramis-like figures amputating limbs. The changing attitudes towards women surgical practitioners were revealed when necessity required their expertise both near the Great War battlefields and on the home front.

That *British Women Surgeons* has been in part a whiggish history of progress was inevitable. At the beginning of the period covered by this volume, there were no women surgeons; at the end, female-only surgical teams had operated across Europe for Allied countries more eager to co-opt them than their own. Women had proved by their actions that they could be surgeons.[5] Even in Britain, however, there was an acceptance of women's valuable contribution to the war effort. By 1918, very few thought it unwomanly or unseemly to be a doctor. Not everyone supported their cause, but women had sufficient confidence in their abilities to laugh at misplaced prejudice. In 1915, 'As Others See Us' was published by A.F. in the *Magazine* of the LSMW. It responded to an article

---

[3] Risse and Harley Warner, 'Reconstructing Clinical Activities', 194.

[4] See the excellent recent issue of *Medical History*, edited by Nicholas Whitfield and Thomas Schlich, which considered *Skill in the History of Medicine and Science*, 59.3 (July 2015).

[5] Olga Hartley, 'Women's Work. I. The New Hospital for Women', *Conservative and Unionist Women's Franchise Review*, [n.d. noted – 1912], 244, in *SLHWPC*.

by a male medical student which claimed that women practitioners aped their male counterparts.[6] A.F. joked:

> For me there is no earthly hope,
> For I have used a stethoscope,
> And heard through it the very sounds
> A man would hear.
>
> I see the error of my ways.
> I'll try to find some symbol
> That may express my heart-felt grief.
> I'll choose these methods, when I can,
> That shall the least appeal to Man:
> And when I sew my muscles up,
> I swear I'll use a thimble.

Women did not need to 'ape' men. Neatly twisting the original, A.F. implied the opposite: the 'sewing' of surgery meant it was already feminised. Female participation in the Great War was seen by the suffrage periodical *Votes for Women* as one of the 'few inspiring incidents of this terrible period', but even less politically-orientated publications had supported the cause of the locum tenens for wartime. The belief, by the end of the conflict, was that the woman surgeon would now never be able to look back, whatever happened in the future.[7] A *Lancet* article entitled 'Surgery in 1918' could as easily be applied to 'The Woman Surgeon in 1918'. If the future was uncertain and unsolved, this was due only to forward movement: 'if it may be said that on many points surgery is in a state of flux, this is only a sign of progress'.[8] Between 1860 and 1918, women surgeons learnt to negotiate and to work around the slamming shut of briefly-opened professional doors. That more would close upon them in the next decade should not detract from their achievements over the nearly 60-year span of this book. There would be more tantalising opportunities just beyond those swinging doors and further battles to fight; the trick was, as it always had been, to operate skilfully through the openings. And, of course, they would not forget to wear a thimble while sewing.

---

[6] A.F. 'As Others See Us', *L(RFH)SMWM*, X.62 (November 1915), 127–8; 128. The poem responded to an article by J.A. in the 'G___'s Hospital Gazette'.

[7] 'Women Doctors and the War', *Votes for Women*, 26 February 1915, in *LSMWRFHPC Volume IV*.

[8] 'Surgery in 1918', *Lancet*, 191.4923 (5 January 1918), 28–9; 28.

Bibliography

PRIMARY SOURCES

ARCHIVES

Autograph Letter Collection, Women's Library, London School of Economics.

Records of Birmingham and Midland Hospital for Women, Birmingham City Archives, Library of Birmingham.

Bruntsfield Hospital and Elsie Inglis Memorial Maternity Hospital Archives, Lothian Health Services Archive, Edinburgh University Library.

Records of Elizabeth Garrett Anderson Hospital (formerly New Hospital for Women), London Metropolitan Archives.

Elizabeth Garrett Anderson Letters and Papers, Ipswich Record Office, Suffolk.

Records of Hampstead General Hospital, Royal Free London, NHS Foundation Trust, London Metropolitan Archives.

Liddle Collection, Brotherton Library, Leeds.

Records of London (Royal Free Hospital) School of Medicine for Women, London Metropolitan Archives.

Records of Royal Free Hospital, Royal Free London, NHS Foundation Trust, London Metropolitan Archives.

Scottish Women's Hospitals Collection, Glasgow City Archives, Mitchell Library, Glasgow.

Records of South London Hospital for Women and Children, London Metropolitan Archives.

PERIODICALS

Archives of the Roentgen Ray
Blackwood's Magazine
British Journal of Radiology
British Journal of Surgery (BJS)
British Medical Journal (BMJ)
Common Cause
Journal of the American Medical Association (JAMA)
Journal of Obstetrics and Gynaecology of the British Empire (JOGBE)
Lancet
London (Royal Free Hospital) School of Medicine for Women Magazine (L(RFH) SMWM)
Medical Record: A Weekly Journal of Medicine and Surgery

Medico-Chirurgical Transactions
Proceedings of the Royal Society of Medicine (PRSM)
Punch

BOOKS AND ARTICLES

Ball, Sir Charles B., *The Rectum: Its Diseases and Developmental Defects* (London: Hodder and Stoughton/Oxford University Press, 1908).

Berry, James, *A Manual of Surgical Diagnosis* (London: J. and A. Churchill, 1904).

Between the Lines: Letters and Diaries from Elsie Inglis' Russian Unit, ed. Audrey Fawcett Cahill (Bishop Auckland: The Pentland Press, 1999).

Black, Clementina, *Sweated Industry and the Minimum Wage* (London: Duckworth & Co., 1907).

Blackwell, Elizabeth, *Essays in Medical Sociology* (London: Bell, 1902).
  Pioneer Work in Opening the Medical Profession to Women. Autobiographical Sketches (London and New York: Longmans, Green and Co., 1895).

Bland-Sutton, John, *Tumours Innocent and Malignant*, second edition (London: Cassell and Company, Ltd, 1901).

Cripps, Harrison, *On Diseases of the Rectum and Anus*, fourth edition (New York and London: Macmillan, 1914).

Erichsen, John Eric, *The Science and Art of Surgery*, fourth edition (London: Walton and Maberley, 1864).

Gardener, H. Bellamy, *Surgical Anaesthesia* (New York: William Wood and Co., 1909).

Garrett Anderson, Louisa, *Elizabeth Garrett Anderson 1836–1917* (London: Faber and Faber, 1939).

Henry, Lydia Manley, 'The Treatment of War Wounds by Serum Therapy', PhD thesis, University of Sheffield, 1920.

Hutchins, B.L., *Women in Modern Industry* (London: G. Bell and Sons Ltd., 1915; republished Wakefield: E.P. Publishing Limited, 1978).

Hutton, Isabel, *Memories of a Doctor in War and Peace* (London: Heinemann, 1960).

Keetley, Charles Bell, *The Student's Guide to the Medical Profession* (London: Macmillan, 1878).

Keith, Skene, *Textbook of Abdominal Surgery* (Edinburgh and London: Young J. Pentland, 1894).

Kelly, Howard A., *Medical Gynecology* (New York and London: D. Appleton and Company, 1908).
  Operative Gynecology. Volume I, second edition (New York and London: D. Appleton and Company, 1906).

Lazarus-Barlow, W.S., '"Cancer Ages": A Statistical Study Based on the Cancer Records of the Middlesex Hospital', in *Archives of the Middlesex Hospital V: Fourth Report from the Cancer Research Laboratories* (London: Macmillan and Co, Ltd, 1905), pp. 26–46.

Legg, J. Wickham, *A Treatise on Haemophilia* (London: H.K. Lewis, 1872).

McLaren, Barbara, *Women of the War* (London: Hodder and Stoughton, 1917).

Maternity. Letters from Working Women (London: G. Bell & Sons Ltd, 1915), ed. Gloden Dallas (London: Virago, 1978).

Mummery, P. Lockhart, *Diseases of the Colon and their Surgical Treatment* (Bristol: John Wright and Sons; London: Simpkin, Marshall, Hamilton, Kent and Co., 1910).

Murray, Flora, *Women as Army Surgeons* (London: Hodder and Stoughton, n.d. [1920]).

Murrell, Christine M., 'The Medical Profession Including Dentistry', in Edith J. Morley, ed., *Women Workers in Seven Professions: A Survey of their Economic Conditions and Prospects* (London: George Routledge & Sons, 1914), pp. 137–67.

Octavia Wilberforce: The Autobiography of a Pioneer Woman Doctor, ed. Pat Jalland (London: Cassell, 1989).

Parkes, Charles T., *Clinical Lectures in Abdominal Surgery and Other Subjects* (Chicago: Chicago Medical Book Co., 1899).

Riddell, Lord, *Dame Louisa Aldrich-Blake* (London: Hodder and Stoughton, 1926).

Scharlieb, Mary, *Seven Lamps of Medicine* (Oxford: Horace Hart, 1888).

Reminiscences (London: Williams and Norgate, 1924).

Weinberg, M. et P. Séguin, *La Gangrène gazeuse: Bactériologie, Reproduction expérimentale, Sérotherapie* (Paris: Masson et Cie, 1918).

SECONDARY SOURCES

Abel-Smith, Brian *The Hospitals 1800–1948: A Study in Social Administration in England and Wales* (London: Heinemann, 1964).

Alexander, Wendy, *First Ladies of Medicine: the Origins, Education and Destination of Early Women Medical Graduates of Glasgow University* (Glasgow: University of Glasgow Wellcome Unit for the History of Medicine, 1987).

Amidon, Lynne A., *An Illustrated History of the Royal Free Hospital* (London: The Special Trustees for the Royal Free Hospital, 1996).

Bittel, Carla, *Mary Putnam Jacobi and the Politics of Medicine in Nineteenth-Century America* (Chapel Hill, NC: University of North Carolina Press, 2009).

Blocker, Jack S. Jnr., David M. Fahey, and Ian R. Tyrell, eds., *Alcohol and Temperance in Modern History: A Global Encyclopaedia. Volume I* (Santa Barbara, CA: ABC-CLIO, 2003).

Brock, Claire, 'Risk, Responsibility and Surgery in the 1890s and early 1900s', *Medical History*, 57.3 (July 2013), 317–37.

Bryder, Linda, *Below the Magic Mountain: A Social History of Tuberculosis in Twentieth-Century Britain* (Oxford: Clarendon Press, 1988).

Bourke, Joanna, *The Story of Pain: From Prayer to Painkillers* (Oxford: Oxford University Press, 2014).

Burney, Ian, *Bodies of Evidence: Medicine and the Politics of the English Inquest, 1830–1926* (Baltimore, MD: Johns Hopkins University Press, 2000).

Cantor, David, 'Cancer Control and Prevention in the Twentieth Century', *Bulletin of the History of Medicine*, 81.1 (Spring 2007), 1–38.

Carden-Coyne, Ana, *The Politics of Wounds: Military Patients and Medical Power in the First World War* (Oxford: Oxford University Press, 2014).

Chamberland, Celeste, 'Partners and Practitioners: Women and the Management of Surgical Households in London, 1570–1640', *Social History of Medicine*, 24.3 (December 2011), 554–69.

Clark-Kennedy, A.E., *London Pride: The Story of a Voluntary Hospital* (London: Hutchinson Benham, 1979).

Cocroft, Wayne D., 'First World War Explosives Manufacture: The British Experience', in Roy MacLeod and Jeffrey A. Johnson, eds., *Frontline and Factory: Comparative Perspectives on the Chemical Industry at War, 1914–1924* (Dordrecht: Springer, 2006), pp. 31–46.

Coleman, Julie, *A History of Cant and Slang Dictionaries. Volume III: 1859–1936* (Oxford: Oxford University Press, 2008).

Cooter, Roger, *Surgery and Society in Peace and War: Orthopaedics and the Organisation of Modern Medicine, 1880–1948* (Basingstoke: Macmillan, 1993).

Crofton, Eileen, *The Women of Royaumont: A Scottish Women's Hospital on the Western Front* (East Linton: Tuckwell Press, 1996).

Crowther, M. Anne and Marguerite Dupree, *Medical Lives in the Age of Surgical Revolution* (Cambridge: Cambridge University Press, 2007).

Cullen, Lynsey T., 'The First Lady Almoner: The Appointment, Position, and Findings of Miss Mary Stewart at the Royal Free Hospital, 1895–1899', *Journal of the History of Medicine and the Allied Sciences*, 68.4 (October 2013), 551–82.

Cullen, Lynsey T., 'Patient Records of the Royal Free Hospital, 1902–1912', PhD thesis, Oxford Brookes University, 2011.

Dally, Ann, *Women Under the Knife: A History of Surgery* (London: Hutchinson Radius, 1991).

Davin, Anna, 'Imperialism and Motherhood', *History Workshop Journal*, 5 (1978), 9–65.

Digby, Anne, *The Evolution of British General Practice 1850–1948* (Oxford: Oxford University Press, 1999).

Making a Medical Living: Doctors and Patients in the English Market for Medicine, 1720–1911 (Oxford: Oxford University Press, 1994).

Durbach, Nadia, *Bodily Matters: The Anti-Vaccination Movement in England, 1853–1907* (Durham, NC and London: Duke University Press, 2005).

Dyhouse, Carol, 'Driving Ambitions: Women in Pursuit of a Medical Education, 1890–1939', *Women's History Review*, 7.3 (1998), 321–43.

Ellis, Harold, *The Cambridge Illustrated History of Surgery* (Cambridge: Cambridge University Press, 2009).

Elston, Mary Ann, '"Run by Women, (mainly) for Women": Medical Women's Hospitals in Britain, 1866–1948', in Anne Hardy and Lawrence Conrad, eds., *Women and Modern Medicine* (Amsterdam: Rodopi, 2001), pp. 73–107.

'Women and Anti-Vivisection in Victorian England, 1870–1900', in Nicolaas A. Rupke, ed., *Vivisection in Historical Perspective* (London and New York: Croom Helm, 1987), pp. 259–94.

Women and Medicine: The Future (London: Royal College of Physicians, 2009).

Elston, Mary Ann C., 'Women Doctors in the British Health Services: A Sociological Study of their Careers and Opportunities, PhD thesis, University of Leeds, 1986.

Fishman, William, *East End 1888* (Nottingham: Five Leaves, 1988/2005).

Fox, Daniel M. and Christopher Lawrence, *Photographing Medicine: Images and Power in Britain and America since 1840* (New York and London: Greenwood Press, 1988).

Gardner, James Stewart, 'The Great Experiment: The Admission of Women Students to St Mary's Hospital Medical School, 1916–1925', *Medical History*, 42.1 (January 1998), 68–88.

Geddes, Jennian, The Doctors' Dilemma: Medical Women and the British Suffrage Movement', *Women's History Review*, 18.2 (April 2009), 203–18.

'Deeds *and* Words in the Suffrage Military Hospital in Endell Street', *Medical History*, 51.1 (January 2007), 79–98.

'The Women's Hospital Corps: Forgotten Surgeons of the First World War', *Journal of Medical Biography*, 14.2 (May 2006), 109–17.

Gillis, Jonathan, 'The History of the Patient History Since 1850', *Bulletin of the History of Medicine*, 80.3 (Fall 2006), 490–512.

Goldberg, Daniel S., 'Suffering and Death among Early American Roentgenologists: The Power of Remotely Anatomizing the Living Body in Fin de Siècle America', *Bulletin of the History of Medicine*, 85.1 (Spring 2011), 1–28.

Granshaw, Lindsay, *St Mark's Hospital: A Social History of a Specialist Hospital* (London: King Edward's Hospital Fund for London, 1985).

Guy, Jean M., 'Edith (1869–1938) and Florence (1870–1932) Stoney, Two Irish Sisters and Their Contribution to Radiology during World War I', *Journal of Medical Biography*, 21.2 (May 2013), 100–7.

Harrison, Mark, *The Medical War: British Military Medicine in the First World War* (Oxford: Oxford University Press, 2010).

Heaman, E.A., *St Mary's: The History of a London Teaching Hospital* (Liverpool and Montreal: Liverpool University Press / McGill-Queen's University Press, 2003).

Howell, Joel D., *Technology in the Hospital: Transforming Patient Care in the Early Twentieth Century* (Baltimore, MD and London: Johns Hopkins University Press, 1995).

'"Soldier's Heart": The Redefinition of Heart Disease and Specialty Formation in Early Twentieth-Century Great Britain', *Medical History: Supplement S5: The Emergence of Modern Cardiology*, 29 (January 1985), 34–52.

Jacyna, Steven, 'The Laboratory and the Clinic: The Impact of Pathology on Surgical Diagnosis in the Glasgow Western Infirmary, 1875–1910', *Bulletin of the History of Medicine*, 62.3 (Fall, 1988), 384–406.

Jordanova, Ludmilla, *Sexual Visions: Images of Gender in Science and Medicine between the Eighteenth and Twentieth Centuries* (Madison, WI: University of Wisconsin Press, 1989).

Kelly, Laura, *Irish Women in Medicine, c.1880s–1920s: Origins, Education and Careers* (Manchester: Manchester University Press, 2013).

Knight, Pamela, 'Women and Abortion in Victorian and Edwardian England', *History Workshop Journal*, 4 (Autumn 1977), 57–69.

Lawrence, Christopher, ed., *Medical Theory, Surgical Practice: Studies in the History of Surgery* (London and New York: Routledge, 1992).

Lawrence, Margot, *Shadow of Swords: A Biography of Elsie Inglis* (London: Michael Joseph, 1971).

Leneman, Leah, 'Medical Women at War, 1914–1918', *Medical History*, 38.2 (April 1994), 160–77.

Lockhart, Judith, 'Women, Health and Hospitals in Birmingham: The Birmingham and Midland Hospital for Women', PhD thesis, University of Warwick, 2008.

Lomax, Scott C., *The Home Front: Sheffield in the First World War* (Barnsley: Pen and Sword Military, 2014).

Löwy, Ilana, *A Woman's Disease: The History of Cervical Cancer* (Oxford: Oxford University Press, 2011).

'"Because of their Praiseworthy Modesty, They Consult Too Late": Regime of Hope and Cancer of the Womb, 1800–1910', *Bulletin of the History of Medicine*, 85.3 (Fall, 2011), 356–83.

Preventive Strikes: Women, Precancer and Prophylactic Surgery (Baltimore, MA: Johns Hopkins University Press, 2010).

'Breast Cancer and the "Materiality of Risk": The Rise of Morphological Prediction', *Bulletin of the History of Medicine*, 81.1 (Spring, 2007), 241–66.

McKeown, Thomas, *The Modern Rise of Population* (London: Edward Arnold, 1976).

Manton, Jo, *Elizabeth Garrett Anderson* (London: Methuen, 1965).

Monger, David, 'Nothing Special? Propaganda and Women's Roles in Late First World War Britain', *Women's History Review*, 23.4 (2014), 518–42.

Morantz-Sanchez, Regina, 'Negotiating Power at the Bedside: Historical Perspectives on Nineteenth-Century Patients and their Gynaecologists', *Feminist Studies*, 26.2 (2000), 287–309.

Conduct Unbecoming a Woman: Medicine on Trial in Turn-of-the-Century Brooklyn (New York: Oxford University Press, 1999).

More, Ellen S., *Restoring the Balance: Women Physicians and the Profession of Medicine, 1850–1995* (Cambridge, MA and London: Harvard University Press, 1999).

Moscucci, Ornella, 'The British Fight against Cancer: Publicity and Education, 1900–1948', *Social History of Medicine*, 23.2 (August 2010), 356–73.

'The "Ineffable Freemasonry of Sex": Feminist Surgeons and the Establishment of Radiotherapy in Early Twentieth-Century Britain', *Bulletin of the History of Medicine*, 81.1 (Spring 2007), 139–63.

'Gender and Cancer in Britain, 1860–1910: The Emergence of Cancer as a Public Health Concern', *American Journal of Public Health*, 95.8 (August 2005), 1312–21.

The Science of Woman: Gynaecology and Gender in England, 1800–1929 (Cambridge: Cambridge University Press, 1990).

Murphy, Caroline, 'A History of Radiotherapy to 1950: Cancer and Radiotherapy in Britain, 1850–1950', PhD Thesis, University of Manchester, 1986.

Nolte, Karen, 'Carcinoma Uteri and "Sexual Debauchery" – Morality, Cancer and Gender in the Nineteenth Century', *Social History of Medicine*, 21.1 (April 2008), 31–46.

Perkin, Harold, *The Rise of Professional Society: England Since 1880*, second edition (London and New York: Routledge, 2002).

Pickstone, John V., 'Contested Cumulations: Configurations of Cancer Treatments through the Twentieth Century', *Bulletin of the History of Medicine*, 81.1 (Spring 2007), 164–96.

Poovey, Mary, '"Scenes of an Indelicate Character": The Medical "Treatment" of Victorian Women', *Representations*, 14 (Spring 1986), 137–78.

Prochaska, F.K., *Philanthropy and the Hospitals of London: The King's Fund, 1897–1990* (Oxford: Clarendon Press, 1992).

Riha, Ortrun, 'Surgical Case Records as an Historical Source: Limits and Perspectives', *Social History of Medicine*, 8.2 (August 1995), 271–83.

Risse, Guenter B. and John Harley Warner, 'Reconstructing Clinical Activities: Patient Records in Medical History', *Social History of Medicine*, 5.2 (August 1992), 183–205.

Risse, Guenter B., 'Hospital History: New Sources and Methods', in *Problems and Methods in the History of Medicine*, eds. Roy Porter and Andrew Wear (London: Routledge, 1987), pp. 175–204.

Schlich, Thomas, 'Negotiating Technologies in Surgery: The Controversy about Surgical Gloves in the 1890s', *Bulletin of the History of Medicine*, 87.2 (Summer 2013), 170–97.

The Origins of Organ Transplantation: Surgery and Laboratory Science, 1880–1930 (Rochester, NY: University of Rochester Press, 2010).

'Surgery, Science and Modernity: Operating Rooms and Laboratories as Spaces of Control', *History of Science*, 45.3 (September 2007), 231–56.

and Ulrich Tröhler, eds., *The Risks of Medical Innovation: Risk Perception and Assessment in Historical Context* (Abingdon and New York: Routledge, 2006).

Scotland, Thomas and Steven Heys, eds., *War Surgery 1914–1918* (Solihull: Helion and Company, 2013).

Skill in the History of Medicine and Science, Special Issue of *Medical History*, eds. Nicholas Whitfield and Thomas Schlich, 59.3 (July 2015).

Snow, Stephanie, *Operations Without Pain: The Practice and Science of Anaesthesia in Victorian Britain* (Basingstoke: Palgrave Macmillan, 2006).

Stanley, Peter, *For Fear of Pain: British Surgery, 1790–1850* (Amsterdam: Rodopi, 2003).

Szreter, Simon, 'The Importance of Social Intervention in Britain's Mortality Decline c.1850–1914: a Re-Interpretation of the Role of Public Health', *Social History of Medicine*, 1.1 (April 1988), 1–38.

Thomas, Adrian K. and Arpan K. Banerjee, *The History of Radiology* (Oxford: Oxford University Press, 2013).

Thomas, Onfel, *Frances Elizabeth Hoggan* (Newport: n.p., 1971).

Thomson, Elaine, 'Women in Medicine in Late Nineteenth and Early Twentieth-Century Edinburgh: A Case Study', PhD thesis, University of Edinburgh, 1998.

Timmermann, Carsten and Elizabeth Toon, eds., *Cancer Patients, Cancer Pathways: Historical and Sociological Perspectives* (Basingstoke: Palgrave Macmillan, 2012).

Waddington, Keir, *Charity and the London Hospitals, 1850–1898* (Woodbridge: Boydell Press, 2000).

'Unsuitable Cases: The Debate over Outpatient Admissions, the Medical Profession and late-Victorian London Hospitals', *Medical History*, 42.1 (January 1998), 26–46.

Wangensteen, Owen H. and Sarah D. Wangensteen, *The Rise of Surgery: From Empiric Craft to Scientific Discipline* (Folkestone: Dawson, 1978).

Weisz, George, *Divide and Conquer: A Comparative History of Medical Specialization* (New York: Oxford University Press, 2006).

Whitehead, Ian R., *Doctors in the Great War* (Barnsley: Pen and Sword Military, 1999/2013).

Wilde, Sally, *The History of Surgery: Trust, Patient Autonomy, Medical Dominance and Australian Surgery, 1890–1940*: www.thehistoryofsurgery.com.

'Truth, Trust, and Confidence in Surgery, 1890–1910: Patient Autonomy, Communication, and Consent', *Bulletin of the History of Medicine*, 83.2 (Summer 2009), 302–30.

and Geoffrey Hurst, 'Learning from Mistakes: Early Twentieth-Century Surgical Practice', *Journal of the History of Medicine and Allied Sciences*, 64.1 (January 2009), 38–77.

'The Elephants in the Doctor–Patient Relationship: Patients' Clinical Interactions and the Changing Surgical Landscape of the 1890s', *Health and History*, 9.1 (2007), 2–27.

'See One, Do One, Modify One, Prostate Surgery in the 1930s', *Medical History*, 48 (2004), 351–66.

Winter, J.M., *The Great War and the British People*, second edition (Basingstoke: Palgrave Macmillan, 2003).

Witz, Anne, *Professions and Patriarchy* (London and New York: Routledge, 1992).

Woollacott, Angela, *On Her Their Lives Depend: Munition Workers in the Great War* (Berkeley and Los Angeles, CA and London: University of California Press, 1994).

Worboys, Michael, *Spreading Germs: Disease Theories and Medical Practice in Britain, 1865–1900* (Cambridge: Cambridge University Press, 2000).

Wyman, A.L., 'The Surgeoness: The Female Practitioner of Surgery 1400–1800', *Medical History*, 28.1 (January 1984), 22–41.

Index

abdominal surgery, 5, 31–2, 38, 42–4,
  48–52 *and passim*
  in Great War, 193
  patient reactions to, 64–6
Abel Smith, Brian, 275
Aldrich-Blake, Louisa
  'Aldrich-Blake Method' for excision of
    rectum, 145–7
  and Croix de Guerre, 231
  and first MS, 18n53
  and Great War service, 182, 258–60
  and rectal surgery, 145–51, 179
  and surgical patients (male and female)
    at RFH, 259–70, 271, 274–5
  and surgical precautions, 153
  at the NHW, 47n70, 134, 153
Alexander, Wendy, 3n6
Amidon, Lynne A., 67n121, 258n90
anaesthesia, 3, 4, 5, 15–16
  and death from, 114
  and goitre, 53–5
  and haemophilia, 115–16
  and heart problems, 116–17
  and patient perception of advances in
    surgery, 91
  and patient resistance to, 110–11,
    173
  and patient resistance under, 114
  and physical injuries from, 115
  and pregnancy, 111
  and respiratory problems, 117–18
  and respiratory problems with
    Wertheim's, 169–70
  and sickness from, 115
  and virginity, 112–13
  as a cure, 113–14
  at the NHW, 32–4, 52–7
Anderson, Agnes, at Royaumont, 187,
  189
  on patient behaviour, 227n201
Anderson, Annie, 53–4
Anderson, Elizabeth Garrett

and accusations of over-zealous surgical
  practices by Elizabeth Blackwell, 50–2
and female medical student's aptitude
  for dissection and surgery, 9–10
and lack of inclination towards surgery,
  27–8
and 'manual control' of NHW, 47
and replacement of outsiders with
  female surgeons at NHW, 58n105
and resignation from NHW, 46, 47, 57
and St Mary's Dispensary, 20, 26
and surgical problems at NHW, 28–45,
  54, 57
and women's suitability for surgery,
  16–17
as a medical student, 8–9
Anderson, Florence, 199
Anderson, Louisa Garrett
  and CBE, 231
  and Elizabeth Garrett Anderson's
    dislike of surgery, 28
  and value of pathology in cancer
    diagnosis at NHW, 151–3
  and wartime encouragement of LSMW
    students, 237, 242
  and WHC, 2, 183–4, 256, 275
  and WHC B.I.P.P. trials, 72, 196
  and WHC press coverage, 197
  and Women's Hospital for Children,
    191–2
  on Ethel Vaughan-Sawyer, 69n2
  on Mary Scharlieb's surgical skills, 16
antisepsis, 5, 11, 39n43, 134
asepsis, 2, 3, 4, 5, 39n43, 70, 134
  and patient confidence, 88
  difficulties achieving during Great War,
    211
Association of Registered Medical Women,
  97
Atkins, Louisa
  at the BMHW, 17–18
  at the NHW, 36–42, 44

297

Printed in the United States
By Bookmasters